Polypharmacy in Psychiatry Practice
Volume II

Michael S. Ritsner
Editor

Polypharmacy in Psychiatry Practice
Volume II

Use of Polypharmacy in the "Real World"

Springer

Editor
Michael S. Ritsner
Technion - Israel
Institute of Technology
Sha'ar Menashe Mental Health Center
Hadera, Haifa, Israel

ISBN 978-94-007-5798-1 ISBN 978-94-007-5799-8 (eBook)
DOI 10.1007/978-94-007-5799-8
Springer Dordrecht Heidelberg New York London

Library of Congress Control Number: 2013932219

Printed on acid-free paper

Springer is part of Springer Science+Business Media (www.springer.com)

I dedicate this book to my dear grandchildren Ron, Miriam, Diana and Daniel Ritsner who are funny, smart, obstinate, and sometimes downright willful

About the Editor

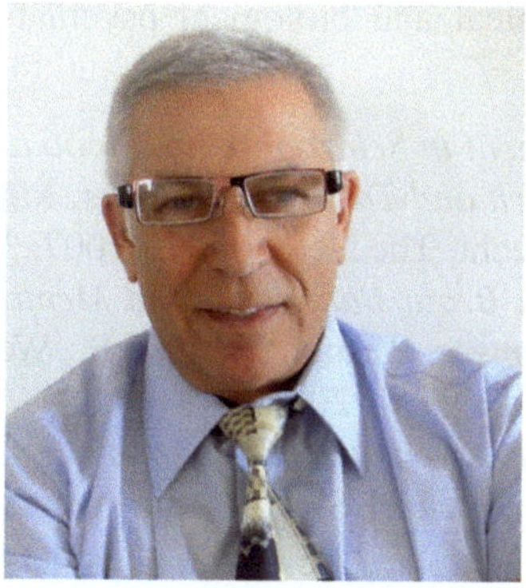

Michael S. Ritsner, M.D., Ph.D.

Dr. Ritsner, MD, PhD is a physician and scientist who spent his career of over 35 years caring for patients and studying the nature and treatment of mental illness. Dr. Ritsner is a Professor of Psychiatry at the Rappaport Faculty of Medicine, Technion – Israel Institute of Technology (Haifa), Israel.

Dr. Ritsner graduated from the Khabarovsk State Medical University, and received his PhD in Psychiatry from the Siberian State Medical University in 1975 (Tomsk, Russia). After gaining clinical practice as a neurologist and clinical psychiatrist he joined the Siberian State Research Center at the Russian Academy of Medical Sciences (Tomsk) as a Head of the Psychiatric Genetics Department in 1981. In 1990 he emigrated to Israel where he chaired a Psychiatry Department and the Research Unit at Talbieh Mental Health Center (Jerusalem). Since 1998 Dr. Ritsner directs the Acute Department of the Sha'ar Menashe Mental Health Center, and Cognitive & Psychobiology Research Laboratory affiliated to the Rappaport Faculty of Medicine, Technion.

Particular areas of interest include schizophrenia spectrum disorders, genetic epidemiology, neuropsychiatric biomarkers, the role of neurosteroids in schizophrenia, novel neuroprotective treatments, and cognitive and quality of life impairments. Dr. Ritsner's research has been supported by grants from the Stanley Foundation. He also currently serves as Principal Investigator of a multi-site research team searching and testing novel agents with neuroprotective properties for treatment of the debilitating effects of schizophrenia and related psychotic disorders.

Dr. Ritsner is the co-author of two books on neuropsychiatry and editor of three books and two handbooks, and has published more than 140 peer-reviewed journal articles, reviews, and more than 20 book chapters. He has given more than 200 presentations including as invited speaker at scientific conferences and medical education events.

This monograph is yet another milestone toward achieving his goals of providing a comprehensive up-to-date state-of-the-art overview of the literature that addresses the challenges facing clinical and biological psychiatry. This series follows 12 volumes:

1. *Quality of Life Impairment in Schizophrenia, Mood and Anxiety Disorders. New Perspectives on Research and Treatment*. Ritsner, Michael S.; Awad, A. George (Eds.), Springer, Dordrecht. The Netherlands, 2007, 388 p.
2. *Neuroactive Steroids in Brain Functions, and Mental Health. Novel Strategies for Research and Treatment*. Ritsner, Michael S.; Weizman A. (Eds.), Springer Science + Business Media, B.V., 2008. 559 p.
3. *The Handbook of Neuropsychiatric Biomarkers, Endophenotypes, and Genes*. Volumes I–IV. Ritsner, Michael S. (Ed.), Springer Science + Business Media, B.V., 2009.

   - Volume I: *Neuropsychological Endophenotypes and Biomarkers*. 231 pp.
   - Volume II: *Neuroanatomical and Neuroimaging Endophenotypes and Biomarkers*. 244 pp.
   - Volume III: *Metabolic and Peripheral Biomarkers*. 231 pp.
   - Volume IV: *Molecular Genetic and Genomic Markers*. 232 pp.

4. *Brain Protection in Schizophrenia, Mood and Cognitive Disorders*. Ritsner, Michael S. (Ed.), Springer Science + Business Media, B.V. 2010. 663 p.
5. *Handbook of Schizophrenia Spectrum Disorders*. Volumes I–III. Ritsner, Michael S. (Ed.), Springer Science + Business Media, B.V. 2011.

   - Volume I: *Conceptual Issues and Neurobiological Advances*. 494 pp.
   - Volume II: *Phenotypic and Endophenotypic Presentations*. 526 pp.
   - Volume III: *Therapeutic Approaches, Comorbidity, and Outcomes*. 461 pp.

6. *Polypharmacy in Psychiatric Practice*. Volumes I–II. Ritsner, Michael S. (Ed.), Springer Science + Business Media, B.V. 2013.

Dr. Ritsner served as Associate Editor, *Quality of Life Research* (an international journal of quality of life aspects of treatment, care and rehabilitation, Amsterdam, The Netherlands); Board Member, *American Journal of Neuroprotection and*

Neuroregeneration (USA); *CNS & Neurological Disorders-Drug Targets* (Italy); and member of the Scientific Committee, International Society for the Study of Neuroprotection and Neuroplasticity (Romania). Referee activity: *CNS Drugs, Quality of Life Research, Psychiatry Research, Clinical Drug Investigation, Social Psychiatry and Psychiatric Epidemiology, Biological Psychiatry*, etc.

Web: http://md.technion.ac.il/lecturers/lecturer_desc.asp?lecturerID=393

Preface

To the best of my knowledge, this might be the first comprehensive, clinically oriented two-volume collection on the polypharmacy (co-administration of more than one medication) or the use of multiple preparations to treat psychotic, cognitive, mood and anxiety disorders. Despite the large number of psychotropic medications currently available, effective management of mental disorders continues to be a challenging task. Although monotherapy may be desirable, most patients require combinations of two or more psychotropic drugs. Polypharmacy aims to address different aspects of treatment resistance, especially insufficient response of positive and negative symptoms, cognitive disturbances, affective comorbidity, obsessive-compulsive syndromes and side-effects of antipsychotic agents. At the same time, evidence based guidelines in support of polypharmacy and augmentative strategies are scant.

This monograph is divided into four parts. Volume I contains two parts including chapters that serve as an introduction and overview of conceptual issues. Key topics include: a rational polypharmacy, receptor binding targets, drug interactions, preclinical and clinical investigation in this field, dosing regimens, multiple medication use in forensic psychiatry, a naturalistic trial, adjunctive strategies, and multiple medication use for the treatment of somatic symptom disorders.

Volume II contains two parts including chapters that focus on antipsychotic polypharmacy for schizophrenia; clinical practice in USA, Czech Republik, Ukraine, and Italy; polypharmacy and associated phenomena; clozapine combinations; and metabolic syndrome. The authors discuss combination therapy for bipolar disorder, major depressive disorder, obsessive-compulsive syndromes in schizophrenia, and potentially inappropriate medication use among elderly patients with dementia. Finally, each volume includes an Appendix that contains 'Annotated Bibliography on Polypharmacy' and 'List of Psychotropic Medications'.

Since many of the contributors to this collection are internationally known experts, they not only provide up-to-date state-of-the-art overviews, but also clarify some of the ongoing controversies and future challenges and propose new insights for future research. The contents of these volumes have been carefully planned, organized, and edited. Of course, despite the assistance provided by the contributors, I alone remain responsible for the content of this monograph including any errors or omissions.

Editing this book has been an exciting journey that brought several incredible people into my life. First and foremost, I am grateful and thankful to all contributors for their excellent cooperation. I wish to thank the entire staff, heads of departments, and the medical director of the Shaar-Menashe Mental Health Center, Dr. Alexander Grinshpoon, M.D, MHA, Ph.D, for their commitment, and support. Thanks to Peter Butler and Dr. Martijn Roelandse, publishing editors, who did their utmost to promote this project. And of course, I would like to thank my lovely wife Stella for her tolerance of me having my head stuck in my computer. Without her love, patience and support I would not have completed this project.

I sincerely hope that this book will extend the knowledge in the complex field of treatment of psychiatric disorders and will be of interest to a broad spectrum of readers including psychiatrists, neurologists, neuroscientists, endocrinologists, pharmacologists, general practitioners, geriatricians, graduate students, and health care providers in the field of mental health.

Haifa
September, 2012

Michael S. Ritsner

Contents

Contributors

Peter F. Buckley M.D. Department of Psychiatry and Health Behavior, Medical College of Georgia, Georgia Health Sciences University, Augusta, GA, USA

André F. Carvalho, M.D., Ph.D. Department of Clinical Medicine and Psychiatry Research Group, Faculty of Medicine, Federal University of Ceará, Fortaleza, CE, Brazil

Tricia L. da Silva, M.A. Mood and Anxiety Disorders Program, Centre for Addiction and Mental Health, Toronto, ON, Canada

Luigi Ferrannini, M.D. Department of Mental Health, ASL3 Genovese, Genoa, Italy

Konstantinos N. Fountoulakis, M.D., Ph.D. 3rd Department of Psychiatry, Division of Neurosciences, School of Medicine, Aristotle University of Thessaloniki, Thessaloniki, Greece

Lucio Ghio, M.D. Department of Neuroscience, Ophthalmology and Genetic, Psychiatry Section, University of Genoa, Genoa, Italy

Xenia Gonda Department of Clinical and Theoretical Mental Health, Faculty of Medicine, Semmelweis University, Budapest, Hungary

Simona Gotelli, M.D. Department of Neuroscience, Ophthalmology and Genetic, Psychiatry Section, University of Genoa, Genoa, Italy

Heinz Grunze Institute of Neuroscience, Academic Psychiatry, Campus of Aging and Vitality, Wolfson Research Centre, Newcastle University, Newcastle, UK

Thomas N. Hyphantis, M.D., Ph.D. Department of Psychiatry, Medical School, University of Ioaninna, Ioaninna, Greece

Apostolos Iacovides 3rd Department of Psychiatry School of Medicine, Aristotle University of Thessaloniki, Thessaloniki, Greece

Hiroto Ito Department of Social Psychiatry, National Institute of Mental Health, Tokyo, Japan

Rena Kurs, B.A. Medical Library, Sha'ar Menashe Mental Health Center, Hadera, Israel

Vladimir Lerner, M.D., Ph.D. Ministry of Health, Faculty of Health Sciences, Ben Gurion University of the Negev and Be'er Sheva Mental Health Center, Be'er Sheva, Israel

Jan Luzny, M.D. Mental Hospital Kromeriz and Palacky University Olomouc, Praha, Czech Republic

Danielle S. Macêdo, Ph.D. Department of Physiology and Pharmacology, Faculty of Medicine, Federal University of Ceará, Fortaleza, CE, Brazil

Stamatia Magiria 3rd Department of Psychiatry, School of Medicine, Aristotle University of Thessaloniki, Thessaloniki, Greece

Roger S. McIntyre, M.D., FRCPC Department of Psychiatry, University of Toronto, Toronto, ON, Canada

Mood Disorders Psychopharmacology Unit, University Health Network, Toronto, ON, Canada

Yong K. H. Michael, M.D., M.Med (Psychiatry) Department of Psychological Medicine, Jurong Health Alexandra Hospital, Singapore, Singapore

Masaru Mimura, M.D., Ph.D. Department of Neuropsychiatry, Keio University School of Medicine, Tokyo, Japan

Chanoch Miodownik, M.D. Ministry of Health, Faculty of Health Sciences, Ben Gurion University of the Negev and Be'er Sheva Mental Health Center, Be'er Sheva, Israel

Fuminari Misawa Yamanashi Prefectural KITA Hospital, Yamanashi, Japan

Werner Natta, M.D. Department of Neuroscience, Ophthalmology and Genetic, Psychiatry Section, University of Genoa, Genoa, Italy

Yasuyuki Okumura Department of Social Psychiatry, National Institute of Mental Health, Tokyo, Japan

Anand K. Pandurangi, MBBS, M.D. Division of Inpatient Psychiatry, Department of Psychiatry, Virginia Commonwealth University, Richmond, VA, USA

Schizophrenia Program and Brain Stimulation Therapies Program, Virginia Commonwealth University, Richmond, VA, USA

Arun V. Ravindran, MBBS, M.Sc., Ph.D., FRCPC, FRCPsych. Departments of Psychiatry, Psychology and Institute of Medical Sciences, University of Toronto, Toronto, ON, Canada

Mood and Anxiety Disorders Program, Centre for Addiction and Mental Health, Toronto, ON, Canada

Oksana E. Samokhvalova, M.D., Ph.D. Department of Psychiatry, Central Military Hospital – Military University Hospital Prague, Prague, Czech Republic

Viktor P. Samokhvalov, M.D., Ph.D., D.Sc. Deutsch-Russische Gesellschaft für Psychiatrie, Psychotherapie und psychosoziale Gesundheit, Nürnberg, Germany

Norman Sartorius, M.D., Ph.D. Association for the Improvement of Mental Health Programmes, Geneva, Switzerland

Frederike Schirmbeck, Dipl.-Psych Department of Psychiatry and Psychotherapy, Medical Faculty Mannheim, Central Institute of Mental Health, University of Heidelberg, Mannheim, Germany

Melina Siamouli 3rd Department of Psychiatry, School of Medicine, Aristotle University of Thessaloniki, Thessaloniki, Greece

Kang Sim, MBBS (Melb), M.Med (Psychiatry), PG Dip Psychotherapy (Distinction) Institute of Mental Health (IMH), Singapore, Singapore

Yong Loo Lin School of Medicine, National University of Singapore, Singapore, Singapore

Takefumi Suzuki, M.D., Ph.D. Department of Neuropsychiatry, Keio University School of Medicine, Tokyo, Japan

Inokashira Hospital, Tokyo, Japan

Hiroyuki Uchida, M.D., Ph.D. Department of Neuropsychiatry, Keio University School of Medicine, Tokyo, Japan

Georgij N. Verbenko, M.D. Department of Psychiatry, Crimean Medical University, Simferopol, Crimea, Ukraine

Viktoria A. Verbenko, M.D., Ph.D. Department of Psychiatry, Crimean Medical University, Simferopol, Crimea, Ukraine

John T. Vernon, M.D. Department of Psychiatry, Virginia Commonwealth University, Richmond, VA, USA

Koichiro Watanabe, M.D., Ph.D. Department of Neuropsychiatry, Kyorin University School of Medicine, Tokyo, Japan

Fujii Yasuo Yamanashi Prefectural KITA Hospital, Yamanashi, Japan

Mathias Zink, M.D. Department of Psychiatry and Psychotherapy, Medical Faculty Mannheim, Central Institute of Mental Health, University of Heidelberg, Mannheim, Germany

Part I
Antipsychotic Polypharmacy

Chapter 1
Antipsychotic Polypharmacy in Schizophrenia: 'Secret Sauce or Wild Abandon?'

Peter F. Buckley

Abstract The treatment of schizophrenia has paradoxically become increasingly complex with the greater availability and choice among antipsychotic medications. At the same time, there is still substantial unmet need, as confirmed by recent large pragmatic trials in schizophrenia, which provides the therapeutic context for antipsychotic polypharmacy. For patients and clinicians, then, the question of "why and when do I combine medications?" is now very challenging. All available evidence suggests that antipsychotic polypharmacy is common in clinical practice. Additionally, it is a topic of enduring interest among clinicians who are always eager to understand the information contributing to key therapeutic strategies. This chapter will provide a current appraisal of the extant evidence-base that informs the daily decision making process that is the clinician's dilemma: how should I use antipsychotic polypharmacy to its best advantage in my practice? The chapter will also critically evaluate the extent to which polypharmacy truly impacts tolerability considerations in treating schizophrenia.

Abbreviations

AP	Antipsychotic polypharmacy
CATIE	Clinical Antipsychotic Trials of Intervention Effectiveness
EPS	Extrapyramidal side effects
FGA	First generation antipsychotic
NT	Neurotransmitters
PRN	Pro re nata
SGA	Second general antipsychotic

P.F. Buckley, M.D. (✉)
Department of Psychiatry and Health Behavior, Medical College of Georgia, Georgia Health Sciences University, Augusta, GA, USA
e-mail: pbuckley@georgiahealth.edu

M.S. Ritsner (ed.), *Polypharmacy in Psychiatry Practice, Volume II: Use of Polypharmacy in the "Real World"*, DOI 10.1007/978-94-007-5799-8_1,

1.1 Introduction

Few aspects, if any, of the psychopharmacology of schizophrenia draw more skepticism and negative attention than the practice of antipsychotic polypharmacy (AP). This is certainly not surprising, although perhaps the extent of clamor is disproportionate given the prevalence of AP – in the sense that most of us practice polypharmacy in some of our patients and yet we still decry the practice publically [1–3].

Although always a topic of intense interest, this is particularly so now as services curtail expenses on medications and also see to implement quality improvement process – AP has been a target in both circumstances [4–6]. Notwithstanding these considerations, the prevalence and extent of AP over time [7], in tandem with the 'one-off' accounts of great patient successes that we regularly hear from our astute clinician colleagues (vide infra), suggest that there is some merit – sometime, somehow, some circumstances – to this practice. While the latter argument may appear contrarian, more recent evidence is supportive of this commonplace practice. An influential meta-analysis [8] panning some 20 years of psychopharmacology reports a modest beneficial effect of AP. A more recent 6-month randomized trial with a comparable naturalistic follow-up period showed similar symptomatic outcomes between AP and antipsychotic monotherapy [9]. An accompanying editorial asks the question of the day *"When is polypharmacy an advantage?"* [2].

This chapter, appearing as one of many among a compendium solely dedicated to this vexing issue, will succinctly review the rationale(s) for AP. Since the topic of AP is given such comprehensive coverage in this book, an attempt is made in this chapter to minimize overlap with other contributions. To that end, aspects of prevalence and clinical impact of AP are well-covered in other chapters.

1.2 Why Do We Practice Antipsychotic Polypharmacy?

There are many and varied reasons why a clinician may resort to AP [10]. These are highlighted in Table 1.1 and are discussed further below. As described in other chapters, foremost among the reasons for AP is the failure of all our current antipsychotics to achieve the kind of superior therapeutic responses that our patients and we, as clinicians, expect. Lieberman and Stroup [11] provide a sobering account of the U.S. federal study CATIE (Clinical Antipsychotic Trials of Intervention Effectiveness) which, inter alia, showed overall comparability in outcomes across a broad range of drugs. Moreover, many patients discontinued medications altogether or moved on to the next phase of the study, thus displaying a high degree of customer dissatisfaction with current medications. It might be considered that the advent of second generation antipsychotics (SGAs) in long-acting injectable formulations might provide an added therapeutic advantage, thus lessening the need to resort to AP for either failed monotherapy and/or medication non-adherence. This does not appear to be the case and there is some data toward the opposite [12]. Thus, a sustained need exists and this continues to propel AP as a reasonable therapeutic

Table 1.1 Rationale for antipsychotic polypharmacy in schizophrenia

Pharmacodynamics	Targeting different receptors
	Boosting receptor blockade
	Use of different formulations in combination
	Prolong metabolism of primary agent
	Selective receptor target fine tuning agonist – antagonist effects
Efficacy-related	Boost overall response
	Target residual symptoms
	Target different symptoms
	Prevent relapse
	"Don't rock the boat"
	Sustained-suspended AP due to aborted switching ("Psychopharmacologic purgatory", P. Weiden, M.D.)
Tolerability-related	Permit dose reduction of primary antipsychotic
	Less side-effect burden
Administrative	'Forensic'
	Practice service patterns
	Pharmaceutical marketing

strategy. Moreover, it is plausible that the 'raising of the bar' by setting superior treatment expectations of recovery might engender continued AP.

1.2.1 Pharmacodynamic Considerations

Clozapine, arguably one of the most effective antipsychotics available, has multiple effects on neuroreceptors. Although how it works is still not known, this pleiomorphic receptor profile is given strong consideration as a proposed mechanism of action. Bernardo and colleagues [12] report a low extent of AP in patients on clozapine. To the extent displayed by the receptor binding of the two (or sometimes three) antipsychotic drugs that a clinician might choose for AP, this approach could 'pharmacodynamically mimic' the profile of clozapine … and perhaps thereupon approximate toward its superior efficacy. It is perhaps noteworthy – in reverse argument – that when AP is studied by drug class, there is a trend for less AP among patients who are being treated with olanzapine [5, 13]. However, the converse argument that AP is disproportionately highest among the most neuroreceptor selective of antipsychotics does not appear to hold true [12]. Yet, there is still some rationale for use of AP to either target receptors that are relatively unaffected by the primary antipsychotic and/or to boost a small effect on important target receptor. For example, combining a first generation antipsychotic (FGA) with clozapine theoretically augments the low dopamine (D2) binding that characterizes clozapine [14]. This might be advantageous – or it might disrupt clozapine's 'secret sauce'. Similarly, adding aripiprazole with its partial agonism could prove to be beneficial in providing 'soft touches' of additional D2 antagonism to other antipsychotics of differing D2 antagonism [15]. The same applies to a whole host of other combinations, be they FGA and SGA, SGA and FGA, or SGA and SGA, that might relate to dopamine as well as other receptors. This approach opens up various permutations. Along those lines, a glutamatergic antagonists without affinity for D2 receptors are being developed [16]. It is plausible that this approach might also be tried in AP.

There is also the instance of AP in relation to different formulations of antipsychotic medications. It is not uncommon in clinical practice to on a long-acting antipsychotic as well as an oral agent [12]. The oral agent may be the 'preferred' drug, with the long-acting drug also given to ensure medication adherence.

1.3 Efficacy-Related Reasons for Antipsychotic Polypharmacy

The rationale for pursuing AP to enhance overall efficacy has already been stated. This is also the reason given by experienced clinicians, as exemplified below:

> I have been in practice decades. I treat many schizophrenic patients. I think I try to correct their neurotransmitters (NTs) when not functioning properly. I use one med. It works for a while. Some symptoms return. This means the correction by one med has faded because of tolerance or because of NTs dysfunction occurring elsewhere and not being impacted by the one med (which has a limited number of NTs corrected). So I ADD ANOTHER med which will impact NTs other than the first med. The patient gets better and stays better. (That is a brief sample of my paradigm.) Of course it is more complicated than that but my experience is LOW DOSE COMBOS ARE BETTER THAN HIGH DOSE MONOS…and to stop meds because they fade effectiveness and relapse is to lose the benefit when you are half-way there when targeting the new or refractory symptoms by treating other NTs with a new med ADD-ON makes more sense and is more effective. I have reviewed all the combo studies and am unimpressed especially from my experience – in fact, I think they hint to what I have found. I think the resistance to "polypharmacy" is because the researchers cannot end up with statistically significant findings. Thus monotherapy is a Procrustean Bed!!! But the findings have welcome statistics – hooray! But my patients do not give a damn about that. If the meds are doing what they want and need, they will take them and get and stay better....such is the foxhole practice on the front lines – and it is LOW DOSE COMBOS ARE BETTER THAN HIGH DOSE MONOS. To think the involved NTs (how many are there?) can be corrected by one med is naive and unreasonable. (Sam Nigro, M.D., September 30, 2011)

Correll and colleagues [17] recently sampled the perceptions of doctors involved in AP. While those who preferred AP shared similar attitudes toward AP of those who used this strategy sparingly, they were likely to be of longer duration in clinical practice and to have a specific AP preference. This latter point is important because each clinician has his/her 'favorite' augmentation polypharmacy strategy and this differs between clinicians. Additionally, the present evidence-base for augmentation with AP does not preferentially endorse any individual agent and/or particular combination, thus until recently, AP strategies have not been scientifically unsubstantiated to any adequate extent [1]. This was in part due to the limited inferences from

Table 1.2 The (predominant) use of naturalistic trials to study antipsychotic polypharmacy in schizophrenia

Pros	Cons
Permits individualized treatments	Subject to multiple potential confounds
Results drive by clinician/patient choices	Lacks sufficient scientific rigor
Broad and representative patient populations	Difficult to interpret
Mirrors most closely clinical practice	Response often inadequately measured
Flexibility	Sample may have unappreciated local/site or physician biases
Does not attempt to control for other factors	Often small sample size (retrospective) studies
Can support large observational studies	Variable medication practices
Easier, less expensive, and quicker to conduct quantitative research	Cannot address rationale for AP
Resonates with clinician experiences	Multiple AP combinations exhaust methodological rigor to test each

naturalistic studies – the predominant research methodology in studying AP (Table 1.2). However, Correll and colleagues [8] have synthesized all available literature in a comprehensive meta-analysis of 19 studies that were of superior methodology. In total, 1,229 patients were included in this meta-analysis. While the results were markedly heterogeneous, overall they reported a superior effect – number needed to treat of seven – favoring AP over antipsychotic monotherapy. They also found their result: clozapine AP, short trial duration, polypharmacy occurring simultaneously (hard to disentangle from switching medications), and SGA-FGA combinations. The study is of interest and, given the heterogeneity of included studies, its findings are surprisingly robust. However, the long duration of observation, as well as the inherent drawbacks of the meta-analytic strategy, should temper interpretations thereupon.

Essock and colleagues [9] report on a 6-month randomized trial of AP versus antipsychotic monotherapy. The trial was complicated by high rates of discontinuation early on in the switching phase. Nevertheless, during the 6-month follow-up the symptomatic outcomes were similar. The authors interpreted the clinical significance of their findings as supporting the rationale for transition from AP to monotherapy. That rationale was further buttressed by their finding of almost double the amount of weight gain among patients treated with AP.

The notion that AP can achieve selective benefits in discrete symptom domains is intuitive but still likely implausible [1, 10, 18]. For example, it has been observed that several SGAs have benefits in cognitive functioning and these appear to be different between agents. However, these individual effects on cognitive performance are so marginal that it seems implausible that combining two antipsychotics would result in any clinically meaningful improvement in cognition [19]. Similarly, the response of individual SGAs in treating negative symptoms of schizophrenia has been underwhelming [20]. It is unlikely here, too, that two is better than one. The evidence is not present.

On balance, then, the clinical rationale for AP results on improving symptoms overall and the evidence for this – aside from Correll meta-analysis – is (at best) inconclusive. The dilemma is, however, that group differences, or lack thereof, might obscure clinically meaningful individual differences. This is one of the lessons learned from CATIE [11]. It is also the rationale behind the decision making of astute clinicians (see above comments by Dr. Nigro).

1.4 Tolerability Considerations for Antipsychotic Polypharmacy

If anything, the rationale of adding two antipsychotics in an effort to reduce side-effects seems at first glance counter-intuitive. However, an elegant study by Fleishhacker and colleagues [21] is illustrative of the principle. This group sought to determine the merit of adding aripiprazole to clozapine. Clozapine is the most weight-inducing among all antipsychotics, while aripiprazole is characterized by a relatively low weight gain liability. In this study, adding aripiprazole allowed lower dose of clozapine with a concomitant reduction in weight in the group receiving both drugs. Henderson and colleagues [22] reported a similar effect when aripiprazole is added to olanzapine. Conversely, adding olanzapine to clozapine would seem injudicious as it could be 'doubling up' on the weight gain liabilities of both drugs. Similarly, adding haloperidol to risperidone risks greater extrapyramidal side effects (EPS) liability. On the other hand, adding haloperidol to quetiapine could potentially 'redistribute' the antipsychotic side effect burden between EPS and obesity rather than risk greater obesity at higher doses of quetiapine by monotherapy. Similar potential advantages exist for other SGA-SGA and SGA-FGA permutations, though FGA-FGA combinations appear sterile in this regard. Of course, such approaches are really predicated on the individual patient liabilities to each drug's side effects [3] and these are still highly variable for any given patient. The risk of these combinations is important to evaluate in each patient, especially since weight gain and metabolic liabilities might be cumulative and they would contribute more to long term morbidity and premature mortality [23]. In this regard, it is of interest to note that a recent pharmacovigilance study of all forms of polypharmacy found that the greatest long term risk of death was associated with concomitant use of benzodiazepines [24].

1.5 Administrative Considerations in Antipsychotic Polypharmacy

In the United States, at least, the service delivery model favors a 'don't rock the boat' treatment modality. Patients are seen monthly – or less frequently – for brief (15 min on average) medication checks. This practice pattern could predispose to AP, in that clinicians sensing that a patient is not doing well enough might resort to adding 'a little something else' in favor of the more administratively demanding strategy of changing to a new antipsychotic. Additionally, there is substantial turnover of psychiatrists in the U.S. public mental health system, such that AP might be another preferred strategy which – once started – is sustained across successive treating psychiatrists.

There is also substantial PRN use of antipsychotics in U.S. inpatient units. Whether justified or not, antipsychotics are used as first-line treatments for aggressive behavior [25]. This is another practice pattern that is likely to facilitate AP.

It is also plausible that pharmaceutical marketing practices might contribute to AP. Indeed, antipsychotics have been used for a variety of non FDA-approved circumstances and this – combined with aggressive marketing strategies – could potentiate AP. While there is concern that U.S. psychiatrists are disproportionately vulnerable to conflicts of interest with pharmaceutical companies [26], there is no direct evidence that this has influenced AP in either direction.

1.6 Concluding Remarks

AP is difficult to study and thereupon difficult to draw conclusions about. Accordingly, this book should provide a very useful compendium of disparate information for clinicians. It remains a 'one patient at a time' event whose origins are poorly understood. In a revealing issue of *The American Journal of Psychiatry* that was largely dedicated to polypharmacy, an editorial [2] and accompanying commentary [3] both extol the need for selective research to clarify the rationale for AP and to determine whether AP is indeed some 'secret sauce' or 'wild abandon'.

References

1. Stahl SM (2012) Antipsychotic polypharmacy: never say never, but never say always. Acta Psychiatr Scand 125(5):349–351
2. Tamminga CA (2011) When is polypharmacy an advantage? Am J Psychiatry 168(7):663
3. Goff DC, Dixon L (2011) Antipsychotic polypharmacy: are two ever better than one? Am J Psychiatry 168(7):667–669
4. Stahl SM, Grady MM (2006) High-cost use of second-generation antipsychotics under California's Medicaid program. Psychiatr Serv 57(1):127–129
5. Constantine RJ, Andel R, Tandon R (2010) Trends in adult antipsychotic polypharmacy: progress and challenges in Florida's Medicaid program. Community Ment Health J 46(6):523–530
6. Baandrup L, Allerup P, Lublin H, Nordentoft M, Peacock L, Glenthoj B (2010) Evaluation of a multifaceted intervention to limit excessive antipsychotic co-prescribing in schizophrenia outpatients. Acta Psychiatr Scand 122(5):367–374
7. Dussias P, Kalali AH, Citrome L (2010) Polypharmacy of schizophrenia. Psychiatry (Edgemont) 7(8):17–19
8. Correll CU, Rummel-Kluge C, Corves C, Kane JM, Leucht S (2009) Antipsychotic combinations vs monotherapy in schizophrenia: a meta-analysis of randomized clinical trials. Schizophr Bull 35(2):443–457

9. Essock SM, Schooler NR, Stroup TS, McEvoy JP, Rojas I, Jackson C, Covell NH (2011) Effectiveness of switching from antipsychotic polypharmacy to monotherapy. Am J Psychiatry 168:702–708
10. Zink M, Englisch S, Meyer-Lindenberg A (2010) Polypharmacy in schizophrenia. Curr Opin Psychiatry 23(2):103–111
11. Lieberman JA, Stroup TS (2011) The NIMH-CATIE schizophrenia study: what did we learn? Am J Psychiatry 168(8):770–775
12. Bernardo M, Coma A, Ibañez C, Zara C, Bari JM, Serrano-Blanco A (2012) Antipsychotic polypharmacy in a regional health service: a population-based study. BMC Psychiatry 12(1):42
13. Procyshyn RM, Honer WG, Wu TK, Ko RW, McIsaac SA, Young AH, Johnson JL, Barr AM (2010) Persistent antipsychotic polypharmacy and excessive dosing in the community psychiatric treatment setting: a review of medication profiles in 435 Canadian outpatients. J Clin Psychiatry 71(5):566–573
14. Friedman JI, Lindenmayer JP, Alcantara F, Bowler S, Parak M, White L, Iskander A, Parrella M, Adler DN, Tsopelas ND, Tsai WY, Novakovic V, Harvey PD, Davis KL, Kaushik S (2011) Pimozide augmentation of clozapine inpatients with schizophrenia and schizoaffective disorder unresponsive to clozapine monotherapy. Neuropsychopharmacology 36(6):1289–1295
15. Kane JM, Correll CU, Goff DC, Kirkpatrick B, Marder SR, Vester-Blokland E, Sun W, Carson WH, Pikalov A, Assuncáo-Talbott S (2009) A multicenter, randomized, double-blind, placebo-controlled, 16-week study of adjunctive aripiprazole for schizophrenia or schizoaffective disorder inadequately treated with quetiapine or risperidone monotherapy. J Clin Psychiatry 70:1348–1357
16. Kantrowitz J, Javitt DC (2012) Glutamatergic transmission in schizophrenia: from basic research to clinical practice. Curr Opin Psychiatry 25(2):96–102
17. Correll CU, Shaikh L, Gallego JA, Nachbar J, Olshansky V, Kishimoto T, Kane JM (2011) Antipsychotic polypharmacy: a survey study of prescriber attitudes, knowledge and behavior. Schizophr Res 131(1–3):58–62
18. Shiloh R, Zemishlany Z, Aizenberg D, Radwan M, Schwartz B, Dorfman-Etrog P, Modai I, Khaikin M, Weizman A (1997) Sulpride augmentation in people with schizophrenia partially responsive to clozapine: a double-blind, placebo-controlled study. Br J Psychiatry 171:569–573
19. Goldberg TE, Keefe RS, Goldman RS, Robinson DG, Harvey PD (2010) Circumstances under which practice does not make perfect: a review of the practice effect literature in schizophrenia and its relevance to clinical treatment studies. Neuropsychopharmacology 35(5):1053–1062
20. Buckley PF, Stahl SM (2007) Pharmacological treatment of negative symptoms of schizophrenia: therapeutic opportunity or cul-de-sac? Acta Psychiatr Scand 115(2):93–100
21. Fleischhacker WW, Heikkinen ME, Olié JP, Landsberg W, Dewaele P, McQuade RD, Loze JY, Hennicken D, Kerselaers W (2010) Effects of adjunctive treatment with aripiprazole on body weight and clinical efficacy in schizophrenia patients treated with clozapine: a randomized, double-blind, placebo-controlled trial. Int J Neuropsychopharmacol 13(8):1115–1125
22. Henderson DC, Fan X, Copeland PM, Sharma B, Borba CP, Boxill R, Freudenreich O, Cather C, Evins AE, Goff DC (2009) Aripiprazole added to overweight and obese olanzapine-treated schizophrenia patients. J Clin Psychopharmacol 29:165–169
23. Baandrup L, Gasse C, Jensen VD, Glenthoj BY, Nordentoft M, Lublin H, Fink-Jensen A, Lindhardt A, Mortensen PB (2010) Antipsychotic polypharmacy and risk of death from natural causes in patients with schizophrenia: a population-based nested case–control study. J Clin Psychiatry 71:103–108
24. Tiihonen J, Suokas JT, Suvisaari JM, Haukka J, Korhonen P (2012) Polypharmacy with antipsychotics, antidepressants, or benzodiazepines and mortality in schizophrenia. Arch Gen Psychiatry 69(5):476–483
25. Buckley PF, Miller BJ, Lehrer DS, Castle DJ (2009) Psychiatric comorbidities and schizophrenia. Schizophr Bull 35(2):393–402
26. Insel TR (2010) Psychiatrists' relationships with pharmaceutical companies: part of the problem or part of the solution? JAMA 303(12):1192–1193

Chapter 2
Antipsychotic Polypharmacy in USA

Anand K. Pandurangi and John T. Vernon

Abstract Fifty-six million prescriptions were dispensed for antipsychotics in the USA in 2010, at an estimated cost of $16.1 billion, and 90% of these were for atypical antipsychotics (IMS Institute for Healthcare Informatics: The use of medicines in the United States: review of 2010). Co-prescription of two (or more) antipsychotics or so-called polypharmacy is estimated from 2 to >50% depending on the population surveyed. Antipsychotic polypharmacy is of considerable importance from multiple perspectives such as its sheer volume, quality and safety of care, and cost. There is much variability in this practice based on age group, primary and co-morbid diagnoses, practice setting, health insurance status, etc. A thorough understanding of the associated factors is necessary to know what drives and maintains polypharmacy practice

Psychiatric, pharmacological and systems-of-care factors separately or together influence physician co-prescribing of two or more antipsychotics. Psychiatric factors include partial response to monotherapy, co-morbid psychiatric syndromes including behavioral challenges, and adverse effects or intolerance of high dose monotherapy, including but not limited to extra-pyramidal symptoms, metabolic effects and sedation. Pharmacological factors include variable receptor effects and pharmacokinetics. The third set of factors that sustains polypharmacy include the need to produce rapid clinical response, pressures of managed care, patient preferences and family concerns about specific symptoms and behaviors, the cross-titration trap, and the need to obtain treatment adherence.

A.K. Pandurangi, M.B.B.S., M.D. (✉)
Department of Psychiatry, Virginia Commonwealth University, P.O. Box 980710, Richmond, VA 23298, USA

Schizophrenia Program and Brain Stimulation Therapies Program, Richmond, VA, USA
e-mail: apandurangi@mcvh-vcu.edu

J.T. Vernon, M.D.
Department of Psychiatry, Virginia Commonwealth University, P.O. Box 980710, Richmond, VA 23298, USA

M.S. Ritsner (ed.), *Polypharmacy in Psychiatry Practice, Volume II: Use of Polypharmacy in the "Real World"*, DOI 10.1007/978-94-007-5799-8_2,

This chapter describes the scope of antipsychotic polypharmacy in the USA in different clinical settings, and why clinicians find it necessary to prescribe multiple antipsychotics. We review the clinical and research evidence for and against antipsychotic polypharmacy and its practice in USA, and discuss the challenges confronting the patient, clinician, healthcare managers and policy makers. Cost of polypharmacy and interventional studies to change or reduce the practice of polypharmacy are also reviewed.

Antipsychotic polypharmacy will likely persist due to clinical necessity. Rather than pursue prescriptive, prohibitive, and/or regulatory approaches to complex patient management, it may be pragmatic to develop rational and cost-effective polypharmacy guidelines, and encourage translational research that will assist clinicians in cost-effective, evidence-based practices while meeting the unique needs of their patients.

Abbreviations

AAP	Atypical Antipsychotic
AP	Antipsychotic
APM	Antipsychotic Monotherapy
APP	Antipsychotic Polypharmacy

2.1 Introduction

Antipsychotic polypharmacy (APP) is a common practice around the world. In the USA such polypharmacy rates have been found to be around 2–7% in general medical practices, around 15% in outpatient psychiatric settings, between 20 and 30% in schizophrenia patients, and >50% in the long term course of treatment for patients with schizophrenia [2–7]. There is much variability in these rates. Whereas data captured by cross sectional studies in large populations of patients counting co-prescriptions at any one point in time reveal APP in the 10–25% range, studies that examine how patients fare over a longitudinal course of treatment such as 1- or 2-years, indicate that 30–50% of patients receive APP at some point in this course. APP is by no means a novel phenomenon. In 1974, Sheppard and Beyel [8] surveyed psychiatrists in New York, Pennsylvania, California, and Texas and found APP was prevalent, and sometimes combinations of up to six neuroleptics were used! Chlorpromazine-trifluperazine was the most common combination.

The practice of APP has sustained despite the fact that various guidelines for the treatment of Schizophrenia, and literature reviews of the evidence for and against APP generally suggest that it should be a practice of last resort [9, 10]. The most significant factor sustaining APP appears to be the fact that antipsychotic monotherapy (APM) for schizophrenia has significant limitations [3, 11]. Treatment non-response with monotherapies is estimated at up to 30%. American Psychiatric Association (APA) practice guidelines from 2004 acknowledge that an additional 30% of patients have only partial response to APM [10]. In this context, APP is by no means universally dismissed in the available literature. Polypharmacy is an accepted practice in the treatment of chronic, complex and multifactorial disorders such as hypertension, diabetes, epilepsy, etc [12]. Nor does APP inherently lead to increased adverse effect burden. The latter is determined by the specific drugs and doses [13]. The idea of rational APP has been put forward. Preskorn and Lacey [14] describe criteria for so-called rational co-pharmacy to include the following: evidence for benefit from combination therapy, evidence for improved efficacy over monotherapy, equal or improved safety/tolerability compared to monotherapy, pharmacokinetic/dynamic simplicity and minimal interactions, and combination of drugs that do not antagonize each other or have completely overlapping mechanisms of action. Used in an informed pharmacologic/pharmacokinetic fashion, there may very well be benefits [4, 15]. However as Stahl [16] has observed such benefits are not established in well controlled trials, and unlike polypharmacy in other medical disorders, it is not necessarily proved that the different receptor-binding profiles of antipsychotic medications represent sufficiently distinct mechanisms of action. Finally, in judging the appropriateness of APP, one has to keep in mind not just the diagnostic indication or similarity in efficacy of the drugs being used, as the determining factors but also quality of daily life.

Thus any review of APP and the state-of-the-art needs to consider the limitations of APM, potential benefits and side effects, evidence for and against APP, realities of clinical practice, and cost – benefit of APP in a comprehensive and balanced manner.

2.2 Prevalence of APP in the USA

There are numerous estimates of the practice of APP throughout the world. In the United States, APP for patients with Schizophrenia is around 17% with a range between 10 and 30% in most studies. In comparison, APP was estimated at somewhat higher rates in other countries, 30% in the United Kingdom, 46–90% in East Asian countries, 25% in Spanish community practice and 45% in Spain's hospitals [17]. However, prevalence rates of APP in the USA vary from a low of 3% to as much as 55% and this range is too wide to be of much use. Understandably APP rates in general medical ambulatory practices are low and range between 0.04% to about 3.7% [18, 19], while in psychiatry settings, the rates range from 7% in closely monitored systems such as the Veterans Administration, between 20 and 30% in community hospitals and practices, and >50% in long term facilities [2–7, 20, 21] (Table 2.1).

Table 2.1 Review of select APP studies in USA

Author/Year	Setting, design, year (s)	Sample size	APP rate	Comments
Williams (1999) [22]	General hospital and clinics of Indianapolis; Retrospective, 1995	316	19.2% received AAP over 1 year	
Covell (2002) [23]	Outpatient Mental Health & Addiction Clinics in Connecticut, Crosssectional & Longitudinal, 1999	400	Cross sectional = 11% Longitudinal rate = 35%	APP down by 40% (1 month) and 90% (2-years) with intervention
Weissman (2002) [19]	Veteran Outpatients with schizo phrenia, 1998–2001	~2,900	SGA+SGA 15–17% SGA = SGA = 78% SGA + FGA = 20%	More APP in younger patients
Botts et al. (2003) [24]	National Ambulatory Medical Care Survey 1993–2000. Random 1-week samples	232,439 General physician office visits	0.04% APP. Prevalence increased over study period	2 FGAs up to 1997; 1 FGA + 1 SGA after 1997
Faries (2005) [2]	University, community, and Veterans hospital settings. Random sample in 6 states in USA. Naturalistic study. 1997–2003	2,327 Schizophrenia Care and Assessment Program	APP = 64% (two or more AP, >60-days)	Olanzapine had lower rates of APP
Morrato (2007) [4]	Medicaid data 5- western USA states (89% from California), Schizophrenia 1998–2003	55,481 on APP	APP = 6.4% Two or more AP, > 60 days	Highest rates in younger males, Asian or Black Lowest rates in >65 years

Eissen (2008) [18]	Public Mental Health Cross sectional study 1-month in 2002	6,666	APP=15% FGA + SGA=474, 7.1% SGA + SGA=527, 7.9%	
Yu and Ben-Hamadi (2009) [25]	Medicaid claims in Pennsylvania, Schizophrenia, on olanzapine or quetiapine, matched on age, sex, race and comorbidity.	2,321 in each group	16.7% Olanzapine 18.6% Quetiapine	Olanzapine had lower APP
Lee and Walker (2010) [26]	California Medicaid program. All Claims		3.7%	
Boaz and Constantine (2011) [27]	Florida Medicaid patients on Risperdal Consta injections, 2003–2007	3,364 patients 4,546 injections	APP=43% =>2 AP, > 21 days)	
Aggarwal and Sernyak (2012) [28]	Connecticut Mental Health Center. Patients on long acting injections. 2009–2010	124	AP=46%	Highest incidence in Hispanics, and alcohol dependence
Citrome (2012) [29]	IMS PharMetrics Data 2003–2009. Patients with commercial insurance.	4,446	APP=25–40% and included at least one SGA	
Dolder (2011) [5]	Retrospective, inpatients, >55 years; Schizophrenia, Bipolar, and/or Dementia 2006–2010, North Carolina		APP=12.5% SGA + SGA=54% Schiz/ Bipolar=21% Dementia=8%	Quetiapine most common SGA in APP

2.3 APP Rates in the Treatment of Children and Adolescents

Data is very sparse on how much APP is prevalent in children and adolescents and if the reasons for APP are the same as in adults. Available studies are mostly restricted to Medicaid populations – in USA Medicaid is a form of public health insurance for the poor, and show APP rates of 7–8%. Diagnosis of any psychoses including schizophrenia, co-pharmacy with a mood stabilizer or antidepressant, and Foster care placement for more than 30 days are most associated with APP [30, 31].

2.4 Current Practice Guidelines and Adherence

The Texas Medication Algorithm project was initiated in 1995 to develop an algorithm for using a standardized systematic approach to psychopharmacology for treatment of Schizophrenia, Bipolar I Disorder and Major Depressive Disorder based on expert consensus. The TMAP update from April 2008 [9] advises that three antipsychotic monotherapy trials (including clozapine) should be completed before attempting APP, namely augmenting clozapine with another antipsychotic. If polypharmacy with clozapine is not successful, TMAP recommends returning to antipsychotic monotherapy before resorting to atypical APP or combination of atypical and typical APP. The American Psychiatric Association Guidelines from 2004 [10] conclude that there is no significant evidence for improved outcomes with APP, with the possible exception of augmentation of clozapine. However trial of APP was still mentioned as a treatment option for some patients with treatment resistant illness.

Whereas guidelines are developed with much thought and effort, they are of limited value unless they address ground realities, and practitioners are trained in their use, and embrace them. Adherence to guidelines is variable. For example, many deviations are noted from PORT [32] and APA Guidelines [10] for management of schizophrenia, such as infrequent use of depot antipsychotic medications, underutilization of clozapine, underdosing or overdosing of SGA, and 16% APP prior to exhausting other recommended options [33]. The Joint Commission for Accreditation of Healthcare Organizations (TJC) is concerned about such deviations and now includes the use of APP in its core psychiatric measure for assessment of quality of care [34].

All guidelines recommend the use of clozapine as "third line" treatment in schizophrenia, however it is estimated only 25% of eligible patients receive a trial of clozapine. The APA estimates only 7% of schizophrenia patients receive clozapine and the national rate within the Veterans Administration was only 2.7%. Further, as more atypicals have become available there may be a gradual decline in clozapine utilization [19]. Likewise, all the guidelines allow for polypharmacy to augment clozapine. However, despite the evidence favoring this, numerous authors have found clozapine to be used minimally in polypharmacy [5]. Thus, ironically, one of the few APP interventions with evidence appears to be underutilized, again pointing to a need for training practitioners in the use of guidelines.

Adherence to guidelines tends to be mediocre for various reasons. For one, numerous guidelines exist and they are not fully consistent with each other. None take into consideration the real world challenges and constraints physicians face [35]. Guidelines derive from studies that exclude typical patients seen in practices (floridly psychotic, co-morbid psychiatric and medical disorders, suicidal, aggressive, etc.). While a systematic algorithmic approach to pharmacotherapy may maximize the possibility of eventually matching a patient with an effective medication, this process can be excruciating for patients, families, and physicians. Establishing treatment failure with adequate monotherapy could take as long as 16 weeks.

2.5 Factors Associated with APP

A variety of factors are associated with APP. Individual-specific factors include diagnosis of schizophrenia, alcohol and substance abuse, and more severe illness. Biancosino [36] found that history of prior APP is a reliable predictor of future APP. Group factors may include younger age especially 18–34 years, ethnic groups such as Black, Hispanic and Asians, facility/institutional placement, free-standing psychiatry hospitals, and presence of multiple psychiatric co-morbidities [4, 5, 16, 28, 37]. Some medications such as quetiapine are somewhat more associated with being part of the APP than others such as olanzapine [2, 25]. There is also geographic variation with California having higher rates and states such as Wyoming with lower rates [4, 5]. Most frequent combinations used in APP are (i) aripiprazole and quetiapine, followed by (ii) risperidone and quetiapine, (iii) aripiprazole and risperidone, (iv) risperidone and olanzapine, and (v) quetiapine and olanzapine.

Newer agents: There is as yet no literature on APP involving the newer agents such as paliperidone, iloperidone, asenapine, and lurasidone. Since their pharmacologic profiles are mostly similar to existing atypicals, no major new benefit is to be expected from using them in APP. One can however expect APP involving these agents will gradually increase as their usage increases.

Interestingly, reasons documented for discontinuation of APP are the same as those for APM, namely lack of improvement, intolerable side effects, and non-adherence, and thus APP tends to become less prevalent by the time of discharge from long term care. Despite this, in nearly half the patients APP is in-fact continued, resulting in the high rates of 50–60% noted in longitudinal studies.

2.6 Factors Associated with Less APP

It is worth looking at what factors discourage polypharmacy or are not associated with it as much. Lower rates of APP are found in areas with increased awareness of national/local guidelines, more participation in local educational activities and research among doctors, and lower perception of an overwhelming work load and time pressures among nurses. It has also been found that patients begun on typical antipsychotics and/or receiving smaller doses of an antipsychotic seem less vulnerable to APP [38, 39]. However, it is not known if this is due to socio-economic factors, patient preferences or lesser severity of illness. Such patients also become more non-compliant during the course of treatment, again for reasons not known but could include improvement, discomfort with being on medications for too long, side effects, etc. Lower rates are also seen in certain geographic locations and institutions such as correctional facilities. Again the reasons for this are not known. We can speculate less availability of medications, less promotion by Pharma, limited resources and, providers who may not be comfortable practicing more aggressive pharmacotherapy, such as general physicians and nurse providers may be relevant.

2.7 Patterns of Polypharmacy

Various practicing patterns may be recognized with APP: (i) patient is typically started on monotherapy and quickly acquires a second medication, often due to lack of rapid response, occurrence of a side effect, and/or pressures of the Managed Care system, (ii) another avenue to APP is the common practice of starting the second AP with the intent of transitioning from one AP to another AP. However, rather than being a transitional phenomenon, APP continues as a maintenance strategy. This is referred to as the cross-titration trap, (iii) another common source of APP is the practice of using "as needed" (PRN) medication often used in hospitals and group facilities [40], (iv) Another form of APP occurs in the course of longitudinal care, when a physician targets non-psychotic symptom clusters with a second antipsychotic. For example, for symptoms such as insomnia, agitation, irritability/aggression, anxiety or depression, once the physician believes the optimum or maximum benefit from the first medication has been obtained, or that any further increase in dose will likely increase in side effects, he/she adds the second antipsychotic with the hope/belief that the second antipsychotic is more suitable than the primary antipsychotic for such symptoms and more rational than a symptomatic agent such as sedative-hypnotic or antidepressant, (v) APP of an oral AP and a long acting injection of an AP is yet another pattern. In this, the physician is either unsure of compliance with the oral AP and uses the LAI as an adjunct and more reliable formulation, or wishes to obtain sustained antipsychotic effects with the LAI, and more immediate daily effects from the oral formulation. While these goals could be achieved with oral and LAI formulation of the same AP, such as haloperidol, fluphenazine, risperidone, olanzapine and paliperidone, with other AP medications LAI formulations are not available.

Despite the pattern described in item 4 above, polypharmacy in treatment of schizophrenia is not limited to antipsychotics. Using data from SDI Physician Drug and Diagnosis Audit database, May 2009 through April 2010, consisting of a survey of 3,200 practitioners from various specialties, Dussias and Citrome [7] found one medication was used in 53% of visits, two medications were used in 29% of visits, and three or more medications were used in 18% of visits. Of medication regimens that involved antipsychotic treatments (97%), APM was used in 56%. Antipsychotic medications were augmented by an antidepressant medication in 20% of the regimens. Lithium and antiepileptic augmentation occurred in 15% of regimens, anti-anxiety medications (unspecified classes) were used to augment antipsychotics in 7% of regimens and anticholinergic augmenting agents were used in 6% of regimens. It should be noted here that not only is evidence for APP limited, evidence from RCTs is minimal for augmentation of antipsychotic agents with lithium and anticonvulsants such as valproate and lamotrigine.

2.8 Reasons for APP

Choice of antipsychotic polypharmacy is generally thought to be informed by a complex interplay among psychopharmacologic theory, physician prescribing attitudes, and socio-cultural context including issues surrounding systems of care. This is no exception in the United States. The better known reasons for APP were mentioned above in outlining the practice patterns that lead to APP, including APM failure, cross titration trap, attempt to reduce or avoid adverse effects from high dose APM, and consequently improving adherence [3]. Physician interviews confirm the biggest reason for APP is the need to further reduce positive symptoms. For example, in a study conducted in 1999–2000 at two Veterans Administration Medical Centers, reported by Sernyak [41] 61% of the responders mentioned this as a reason. Other reasons included improving negative symptoms (20%), need to decrease dose/amount of primary antipsychotic (9%), and need to reduce extrapyramidal symptoms (5%). Failure of APM was cited in 65% of patients and cross-titration was cited in 39% of patients. Only 46% of the cross-titration patients actually completed switch back to APM within a year. In another survey of psychiatric medical providers conducted at Zucker Hillside Hospital in New York between 2006 and 2007, justifications for APP were generally appropriate, and involved cross titration, failure of clozapine trial, evidence from positive controlled trials, and patient inability to tolerate clozapine [38].

We discuss below both the well recognized reasons as well as others to provide a more comprehensive list for APP.

1. Lack of response or partial response [3]: As noted earlier most studies document 30% non-response to antipsychotic monotherapy, and another 30% have partial response. The clinician may appropriately attempt to enhance the response of his/her patient through APP. To achieve the improved efficacy:

   To achieve the enhanced efficacy, the physician may combine medications that have different receptor-binding profiles to take advantage of potential for multiple mechanisms for treating psychosis and widen the scope of benefits. Surveys of antipsychotic polypharmacy in the United States would seem to reflect practitioner consensus that there must be at least some non-overlapping antipsychotic effects/mechanisms of different antipsychotic medications. Clozapine and quetiapine with their lower affinity for D2 receptor blockade are theorized to benefit by combining with an agent with higher D2 affinity [3, 42–44]. The literature provides some support to this approach, mostly to augmenting clozapine and there are fewer studies to support quetiapine although there are case series and case reports. There are also negative trials [44]. The limited evidence in support of APP from randomized controlled trials favors combination of clozapine with risperidone or amisulpride/sulpride. However, in the United States, as we have observed earlier, clozapine tends to be underused despite the best-practice guidelines for its use as both monotherapy and combination therapy in patients with treatment resistant schizophrenia. Given the low rates of clozapine use and the lack of availability of amisulpiride/sulpiride in the United States, it seems that much APP in the United States is based on a rationale that does not have the current backing of controlled trials. Interestingly, despite the low rate of clozapine use in clinical practice in the USA, research into APP has centered on augmentation of clozapine. This is reflected in the preponderance of studies from USA examining addition of risperidone to clozapine in APP.

A meta-analysis by Goodwin et al. [44] showed small positive effect of antipsychotic combination but the effect limited to studies that began with combination dosing, involved clozapine, and involved treatment longer than 10 weeks. Randomized clinical trials in which risperidone or amisulpiride/sulpiride were used to augment clozapine have produced mixed results [3, 6, 7, 18]. Beyond controlled trials, there is an extensive case report literature for both clozapine and non-clozapine APP but not surprisingly suffers from numerous limitations, particularly the absence of the ABA design [3, 45]. This leaves doubt as to whether any improvement noted in these reports is due to the combination or the new drug. Also, if APP is introduced too soon in the treatment such as acute inpatient care, the improvement on two drugs could simply be due to longer trial duration of the first drug. Further even the benefits noted in the case reports are variable from case to case, and do not allow for any generalization.

APP not only does not guarantee increased efficacy, in a few instances may actually make the psychosis worse. There are several case series reporting worsening of psychosis, especially with aripiprazole in the combination [45, 46].

2. **Differences in safety and tolerability profiles**: Certain combinations of antipsychotics are believed to be safer, such as causing less EPS with use of SGA, less prolactin with aripirazole, less weight gain and metabolic effects with ziprasidone, etc. Thus the physician is understandably attempting to hold on to the efficacy of the first drug while minimizing its adverse effects with the choice of a second agent.

   The most consistent benefits appear to be reduction in adverse effects, such as weight gain, metabolic effects (with ziprasidone and ariprazole), and prolactinemia (with aripiprazole). Weight loss and improvement in fasting total cholesterol and triglyceride levels have been noted with clozapine augmentation with aripiprazole, and with quetiapine, and olanzapine augmentation with aripiprazole [44, 45, 47–50].

Interestingly, physicians respond to more visible side effects such as tardive dyskinesia and weight gain and not to less visible metabolic effects. In the 2005–2007 National Ambulatory Medical Care Survey with 1898 office visits for patients receiving antipsychotics, it was observed that obese patients were less likely to receive antipsychotics with higher potential to cause metabolic side effects; however, patients with metabolic conditions did not have a lower likelihood of receiving the same antisychotics [51].

There is no controlled trial literature on reducing EPS through APP, although there are sporadic case reports of improvement in tardive dyskinesia by augmenting with a lower D2 potency agent.

Risks of Increased Adverse Effects: APP could also lead to increased adverse effects. Unlike efficacy where a double blind placebo controlled RCT is the gold standard, for adverse effects case reports serve as a good source of information. There are many case reports highlighting the increased burden of adverse effects with APP. For example, oculogyric crisis and elevated clozapine levels in a patient undergoing cross taper from clozapine to risperidone, increased prolactin levels in patients treated with both clozapine and risperidone compared to clozapine monotherapy, agranulocytosis upon addition of risperidone, and emergence or worsening of compulsive behaviors [45]. APP may create greater risk of adverse effects and longer hospital stays [3].

There may also be increased metabolic side effects including diabetes and cardiac risks in APP [44], and this may correlate with the increased number of antipsychotics and increased duration of APP [3]. Other adverse effects in this situation include increased confusion, hypotension, EPS, falls (in the geriatric population), presumably from higher blood levels of the offending agent.

More seriously there is a concern [52] about the increased risk of pharmacokinetic-pharmacodynamic interactions and possible increase in mortality from APP. However some reassurance may be derived from the fact that a case control study in Denmark with 193 matched patients with schizophrenia/psychosis diagnosis did not show any association [53] and concluded that APP was not associated with increased mortality from "natural causes" (excluding suicide, homicides, accidents, and unexplained death). It has been felt that the results of early studies suggesting increased mortality with APP in schizophrenia have not been replicated in recent studies [12], with exception of higher doses of antipsychotics, which may be associated with increased cardiac mortality.

3. Cross-taper treatment plans also provide an understandable context for APP. Again the evidence indicates that this quickly becomes maintenance therapy in more than 50% of patients. Physicians are appropriately concerned that removing one agent from an APP treatment plan may cause relapse/worsening of psychosis. This scenario is an extension of the cross-titration trap. It has been noted that

75% of cases of APP were inherited with prescriber hesitance to switch to monotherapy in 40% of cases but successful switch in 28% [38]. Successful cross titration is possible was demonstrated in an unblinded randomized trial [13] in which 66% of patients could be switched without problems, and there was no difference in symptom control or hospitalizations between those switched to APM versus those continuing on APP. In this study, physicians with more than 10% APP were more likely attending physicians who had practiced 10 years longer than colleagues, saw relatively more patients, continued APP upon the recommendation of the previous prescriber, and had overall fewer concerns about AP. Quetiapine and clozapine were most likely to be involved in AP.

4. Improved compliance: As result of improved efficacy and/or reduced adverse effects, APP is supposed to promote improved adherence to treatment, which is a major challenge in the treatment of schizophrenia. However the notion of needing lower doses of the two agents during APP is not always borne out by data. For example, De Torre et al. [3] observed that APP patients had higher rather than lower doses of antipsychotics compared to monotherapy. This results in higher costs and could also decrease compliance [3].
5. Multiple simultaneous diagnoses: Since the DSM-III, multiple diagnoses are allowed and encouraged when criteria are met. Physicians tailor the medications to symptom clusters of each diagnosis, resulting in APP. Thus quetiapine and aripiprazole may be used to treat depression and mood symptoms, while haloperidol, risperidone or olanzapine may be prescribed for positive psychosis, in the same patient. Similarly, one antipsychotic such as quetiapine may be prescribed to target manic symptoms of excitement, irritability and hyperactivity while another such as haloperidol or risperidone may be prescribed to target psychosis.
6. Substance abuse: As noted earlier, amongst individual factors associated with APP, the presence of substance abuse is often a marker of multiple psychopathologies, immediate gratification, medication seeking and poor compliance. Each of these factors may lend the patient and/or physician to APP.
7. Third part payers including care managers (health insurance companies) pressure physicians to increase drug doses and/or add medications, as justification for approving days in the hospital, to expedite discharges and to reduce total hospital length of stays [4].
8. Increased availability of antipsychotics: Within 10-years, from 1992 to 2002, five different SGAs became available to the physician. Since then four-more atypical antipsychotics (iloperidone, paliperidone, asenapine and lurasidone, and three long acting preparations (risperidone long acting, paliperidone long acting and olanzapine long acting) have become available in the USA, and one long acting formulation (aripprazole long acting) is slated to become available soon. It is tempting to the physician to make use of one or more of these agents/formulations to the benefit the refractory and/or non-compliant patient. Unlike

conservative methods of practice, where typically the public and private general psychiatrist waited for academic psychiatrists to prescribe new agents and share their experience, there is now greater physician comfort with trying new antipsychotics as soon as they become available.

9. Marketing practices: In the same period mentioned above, marketing and promotional practices by Pharma became more competitive and creative, luring physicians to use more medications. Whereas no single Pharma promotes APP, the net effect of increased marketing including direct to patient marketing takes a patient more rather than less towards APP.
10. Uncoordinated systems of care – it is intent of the inpatient physician to transition from one antipsychotic to another but the outpatient physician is unaware of the treatment plan. The outpatient physician feels compelled to keep the two agents as maintenance, rather than risk the (perceived) liability from relapse. This is a different type of cross titration trap and is more due to the fragmented system of mental health care, rather than patient or illness-driven factors.
11. Patient/Family concerns: Often patients desire/demand specific effects from medications, such as improved sleep, reduced anxiety, improved mood etc. The targets chosen by the physician may be different (for example, reducing hallucinations and delusions). Family members also have specific expectations and suggest/demand physicians target symptoms such as aggression, sleep etc. These factors combine to create the need for APP.

Thus illness, treatment and patient driven factors cause APP. Systems of care, (modest) evidence from trials and case reports, availability of different agents promote it. Presumed reduction in risk of relapse and side effects, co-morbid psychiatric disorders with diverse constellation of symptoms, and the law of inertia perpetuate it.

2.9 Interventional Studies to Reduce APP

Research programs designed to reduce APP by psychiatrists in the United States have shown some success. These appear to focus mostly on combining dissemination of best-practice information with feedback involving audit and instruction from institution leadership. However, these studies do not indicate whether or not there are differences in patient outcomes after reducing APP. We mention a few programs to give the reader a sense of the methodology and outcomes.

The Psychiatric Services and Clinical Knowledge Enhancement System (PSYCKES) [54] was initiated in three phases in New York State between 2005 and 2010, with a network of 18 psychiatric hospitals with purpose of reducing APP defined as use of more than two antipsychotics for more than 60 days. In phase I, physicians were provided access to clinical practice guidelines, quality indicator reports, and individual patient treatment histories combined with requirement for clinical directors and chief medical officer to approve addition of a third antipsychotic for any patient in the hospital. In phase II, patient specific feedback to providers, hospital leadership and state level oversight were implemented, and in phase III, state-level oversight and feedback were removed and the remainder of the program was continued. APP decreased from 16.9/1,000 to 9.7/1,000 inpatients during phase 1, then to 3.9/1,000 inpatients in phase 2, maintained at 3.9/1,000 in phase 3, but returned to 9.6/1,000 inpatients after 36 months from initiation in 2004. Limitations of the study include lack of information about the effect of the reduction in APP on specific patient outcomes.

Patrick et al. [37] report on a program designed to reduce APP at a Northeastern state hospital by providing feedback from the chief of psychiatry to 14 psychiatrists in 2001–2002. Individual interviews were conducted to include data comparing prescribing practices with anonymous peers. The psychiatrists were directed to reduce APP by 10%. Decline in APP from 42% (197 patients) to 31% (127 patients) was achieved, and 8/14 psychiatrists achieved at least 10% reduction in APP. In case of patients receiving depot medications, there was no significant reduction in APP.

Goren and Beck (2008) [55] tested the use of education and monthly audit feedback to physicians and nursing staff and meetings with the chief of service, on reducing APP in acute inpatient settings, in academic and community hospitals in the Cambridge Health Alliance between 2007 and 2008. They were 389 patients with ~34% APP at baseline which declined to 21.8% after 1-year and 12.2% by 2-years. Interestingly and consistent with our previous discussion, use of clozapine in APP was below 1% throughout the study.

Constantine [56] reviewed APP from 2003 to 2006 in the Florida Medicaid program (fee-for-service claims only) to determine the effect of a quality improvement program started in 2005, setting guidelines on the treatment of Schizophrenia in Florida, sending reminders to physicians writing for 2 or more AP within 60 days, and selecting nonresponsive physicians for peer-to-peer consultation on physician prescribing practices. Of 51,756 patients receiving antipsychotics, 21% experienced APP with a preponderance of white male patients with diagnosis of schizophrenia or schizoaffective disorder. APP prevalence rates declined from 18.8 to 16.5% temporally correlating with the onset of the quality improvement program, although causation could not be established.

It is thus clear that a combination of education, consultation, prescription, feedback and proscription can reduce the rates of APP. The critical elements missing in these interventional studies are data on patient outcomes. More importantly, whether the specific reasons for which APP was initiated in the first place were overcome by a return to APM is not known.

2.10 Antipsychotic Polypharmacy and Cost (USA)

APP in the United States involves SGA medications more than 90% of the times, which proves to be quite burdensome in terms of cost. SGA medications accounted for a large proportion of increased spending on mental health drugs in 1996–2001.

In 2010, the total cost of antipsychotic medications dispensed in the USA was estimated at $16.1 billion. SGA polypharmacy is estimated to cost three times more per patient compared to APM for patients [4, 17, 57].

Aparasu and Bhatara [58] using the 2003 Medical Expenditure Panel Survey data estimated 1-month of an FGA cost ~$40 in comparison to ~$164 for an SGA. By this dataset, APP with two SGAs would cost 4-times the cost of APP with two FGAs. Valuck et al. [59] conducted a retrospective cohort study using Medicaid claims data from California, Nebraska, Oregon, Utah, and Wyoming (55,383 patients) to examine APP expenditures (drug and non-drug) from 1998 to 2002. Average annual prevalence of APP was 6% with 70–80% of total healthcare dollars going to prescriptions. APP related drug and non-drug costs were an additional $2,079 for 1 year over APM related drug and non-drug costs. Of note, in this study clozapine prescription led to a decline in total costs even compared to FGA monotherapy.

Thus, the burden is on the practitioners of APP to demonstrate that the cost-benefit ratio of their practice is acceptable.

2.11 Conclusions and Future Research Needs

APP is widespread and here to stay. Between 1 and 7% of all psychiatric patients in the USA, and 10–30% of patients with schizophrenia appear to receive APP at one time or another. Twenty-five to fifty percent of patients with schizophrenia receive APP during some time in their treatment life. Clinical settings and available resources dictate the extent of APP. APP combination most often is an SGA + SGA or FGA + SGA.

APP has modest supportive evidence in a few specific circumstances, namely (i) augmenting clozapine effects to obtain more D2 antagonism, (ii) improving tolerability by reducing side effects of the primary effective drug by addition of drugs such as aripiprazole or ziprasidone, and (iii) augmentation of an oral medication with a long acting injection. In these three scenarios APP could provide additional benefit over APM. Continuation of APP out of a fear of relapse, using APP to beat the system (using two drugs of similar action to stay under prohibited dose limits), use of two similar drugs in the hopes of additive efficacy seem to be without any evidence and reflect poor practice.

APP is however practiced beyond these situations primarily because of limitations of available medications in both efficacy and tolerability, and the real challenges of refractory symptom clusters in psychotic disorders, especially schizophrenia. In the USA, it is exacerbated and sustained by the demands of a fast-moving and (unfortunately) fragmented care delivery system that may have conflicting goals, and to a smaller extent availability of many antipsychotics, promotion by Pharma, and possibly by physicians believing 'more is better'. However, it is not simply a result of bad or irresponsible clinical practice, and clinicians have justifiable and logical reasons for APP. APP does not 'go away' simply by developing treatment manuals if they are disconnected with the real world challenges, or by interventions to force a change in physician behavior. Such methods are temporary fixes and APP returns. Proscriptive methods will become unnecessary when more effective and safer treatments become available.

The costs of atypical polypharmacy are considerable and sooner than later will bring more external regulation unless physicians become more cost-sensitive. The burden is on the psychiatric profession and specifically practitioners of APP to demonstrate that the cost-benefit ratio of their practice is acceptable and does not warrant external regulation.

Research into the causes and pathophysiology of psychotic disorders, and development of therapies with new mechanisms of action, are the true answers to APP. In the mean time, (i) understanding the diversity of patients and their unique needs including the specific challenges of schizophrenia such as paranoia, aggressive behaviors, poor insight, and family burden, (ii) translational research on the most effective drug regimens and dosing, and (iii) promoting the use of interventions such as long acting injections and clozapine are likely to yield more rational practice and greater patient benefits.

References

1. IMS Institute for Healthcare Informatics (2010) The use of medicines in the United States: review of 2010, Parsippany, New Jersey
2. Faries D, Ascher-Svanum H, Zhu B, Correll C, Kane J (2005) Antipsychotic monotherapy and polypharmacy in the naturalistic treatment of schizophrenia with atypical antipsychotics. BMC Psychiatry 5:26
3. López de Torre A, Lertxundi U, Hernández R, Medrano J (2012) Antipsychotic polypharmacy: a needle in a haystack? Gen Hosp Psychiatry 34(4):423–432, Epub 2012 Mar 27. PMID: 22460003
4. Morrato EH, Dodd S, Oderda G, Haxby DG, Allen R, Valuck RJ (2007) Prevalence, utilization patterns, and predictors of antipsychotic polypharmacy: experience in a multistate Medicaid population, 1998–2003. Clin Ther 29(1):183–195
5. Dolder CR, McKinsey J (2011) Antipsychotic polypharmacy among patients admitted to a geriatric psychiatry unit. J Psychiatr Pract 17(5):368–374
6. Correll CU, Rummel-Kluge C, Corves C, Kane JM, Leucht S (2009) Antipsychotic combinations vs monotherapy in schizophrenia: a meta-analysis of randomized controlled trials. Schizophr Bull 35(2):443–457
7. Dussias P, Kalali AH, Citrome L (2010) Polypharmacy of schizophrenia. Psychiatry (Edgmont) 7(8):17–19
8. Sheppard C, Beyel V, Fracchia J, Merlis S (1974) Polypharmacy in psychiatry: a multi-state comparison of psychotropic drug combinations. Dis Nerv Syst 35(4):183–189
9. Moore TA, Buchanan RW, Buckley PF, Chiles JA, Conley RR, Crismon ML, Essock SM, Finnerty M, Marder SR, Miller DD, McEvoy JP, Robinson DG, Schooler NR, Shon SP, Stroup TS, Miller AL (2007) The Texas Medication Algorithm Project antipsychotic algorithm for schizophrenia: 2006 update. J Clin Psychiatry 68(11):1751–1762
10. American Psychiatric Association (2004) Practice guidelines for the treatment of patients with schizophrenia. American Psychiatric Press, Arlington
11. Gibson A, Patel NC, Lauriello J, Buckley P (2008) Anti-psychotic combinations: blind step or logical? Curr Psychiatry 7:41–48

12. Goff DC, Dixon L (2011) Antipsychotic polypharmacy: are two ever better than one? Am J Psychiatry 168(7):667–669
13. Essock SM, Schooler NR, Stroup TS, McEvoy JP, Rojas I, Jackson C, Covell NH (2011) Schizophrenia Trials Network. Effectiveness of switching from antipsychotic polypharmacy to monotherapy. Am J Psychiatry 168(7):702–708, Epub 2011 May 2. PMID:21536693
14. Preskorn SH, Lacey RL (2007) Polypharmacy: when is it rational? J Psychiatr Pract 13(2):97–105
15. Ereshefsky L (1999) Pharmacologic and pharmacokinetic considerations in choosing an antipsychotic. J Clin Psychiatry 60(Suppl 10):20–30, PMID:10340684
16. Stahl SM, Grady MM (2006) High-cost use of second-generation antipsychotics under California's Medicaid program. Psychiatr Serv 57(1):127–129
17. Gallego JA, Bonetti J, Zhang J, Kane JM, Correll CU (2012) Prevalence and correlates of antipsychotic polypharmacy: a systematic review and meta-regression of global and regional trends from the 1970s to 2009. Schizophr Res 138(1):18–28, Epub 2012 Apr 24
18. Eisen C, Shaner R, Unützer J, Fink A, Wells KB (2008) Datapoints: second-generation antipsychotic medication combinations for schizophrenia. Psychiatr Serv 59(3):235
19. Weissman EM (2002) Antipsychotic prescribing practices in the Veterans Healthcare Administration–New York metropolitan region. Schizophr Bull 28(1):31–42
20. Leslie DL, Rosenheck RA (2001) Use of pharmacy data to assess quality of pharmacotherapy for schizophrenia in a national health care system: individual and facility predictors. Med Care 39(9):923–933
21. Ganguly R, Kotzan JA, Miller LS, Kennedy K, Martin BC (2004) Prevalence, trends, and factors associated with antipsychotic polypharmacy among Medicaid-eligible schizophrenia patients, 1998–2000. J Clin Psychiatry 65(10):1377–1388
22. Williams CL, Johnstone BM, Kesterson JG, Javor KA, Schmetzer AD (1999) Evaluation of antipsychotic and concomitant medication use patterns in patients with schizophrenia. Med Care 37(4 Suppl Lilly):AS81–AS86, PMID:10217396
23. Covell NH, Jackson CT, Evans AC, Essock SM (2002) Antipsychotic prescribing practices in Connecticut's public mental health system: rates of changing medications and prescribing styles. Schizophr Bull 28(1):17–29
24. Botts S, Hines H, Littrell R (2003) Antipsychotic polypharmacy in the ambulatory care setting, 1993–2000. Psychiatr Serv 54(8):1086
25. Yu AP, Ben-Hamadi R, Birnbaum HG, Atanasov P, Stensland MD, Philips G (2009) Comparing the treatment patterns of patients with schizophrenia treated with olanzapine and quetiapine in the Pennsylvania Medicaid population. Curr Med Res Opin 25(3):755–764
26. Lee B, Walker V (2008) Polypharmacy as the initial second-generation antipsychotic treatment. Psychiatr Serv 59(7):717, PMID:18586985
27. Boaz TL, Constantine RJ, Robst J, Becker MA, Howe AM (2011) Risperidone long-acting therapy prescribing patterns and their impact on early discontinuation of treatment in a large Medicaid population. J Clin Psychiatry 72(8):1079–1085, Epub 2010 Oct 19. PMID: 21034690
28. Aggarwal NK, Sernyak MJ (2012) Prevalence of concomitant oral antipsychotic drug use among patients treated with long-acting, intramuscular, antipsychotic medications. J Clin Psychopharmacol 32(3):323–328
29. Citrome L, Guo Z, Kalsekar I, Forbes RA, Hebden T (2012) Trends in combination antipsychotic use among persons with commercial insurance: a data snapshot. Innov Clin Neurosci 9(3):17–18
30. Dosreis S, Yoon Y, Rubin DM, Riddle MA, Noll E, Rothbard A (2011) Antipsychotic treatment among youth in foster care. Pediatrics 128(6):e1459–e1466
31. Constantine RJ, Boaz T, Tandon R (2010) Antipsychotic polypharmacy in the treatment of children and adolescents in the fee-for-service component of a large state Medicaid program. Clin Ther 32(5):949–959
32. Lehman AF, Kreyenbuhl J, Buchanan RW, Dickerson FB, Dixon LB, Goldberg R, Green-Paden LD, Tenhula WN, Boerescu D, Tek C, Sandson N, Steinwachs DM (2004) The Schizophrenia Patient Outcomes Research Team (PORT): updated treatment recommendations 2003. Schizophr Bull 30(2):193–217

33. West JC, Wilk JE, Olfson M, Rae DS, Marcus S, Narrow WE, Pincus HA, Regier DA (2005) Patterns and quality of treatment for patients with schizophrenia in routine psychiatric practice. Psychiatr Serv 56(3):283–291
34. The Joint Commission (2008) http://www.jointcommission.org/assets/1/18/HBIPS_CM_selection_form_revised082408.pdf. Retrieved 07 July 2012
35. Moore TA (2011) Schizophrenia treatment guidelines in the United States. Clin Schizophr Relat Psychoses 5(1):40–49, Review
36. Biancosino B, Barbui C, Marmai L, Donà S, Grassi L (2005) Determinants of antipsychotic polypharmacy in psychiatric inpatients: a prospective study. Int Clin Psychopharmacol 20(6):305–309
37. Patrick V, Schleifer SJ, Nurenberg JR, Gill KJ (2006) Best practices: an initiative to curtail the use of antipsychotic polypharmacy in a state psychiatric hospital. Psychiatr Serv 57(1):21–23
38. Correll CU, Shaikh L, Gallego JA, Nachbar J, Olshanskiy V, Kishimoto T, Kane JM (2011) Antipsychotic polypharmacy: a survey study of prescriber attitudes, knowledge and behavior. Schizophr Res 131(1–3):58–62, Epub 2011 Mar 21. PMID: 21419603
39. Baandrup L (2011) How dosing might influence the conclusion in an antipsychotic polypharmacy effectiveness trial. Am J Psychiatry 168(10):1117, author reply 1117. No abstract available. PMID: 21969048
40. Barnes TR, Paton C (2011) Antipsychotic polypharmacy in schizophrenia: benefits and risks. CNS Drugs 25(5):383–399. doi:10.2165/11587810-000000000-00000
41. Sernyak MJ, Rosenheck R (2004) Clinicians' reasons for antipsychotic coprescribing. J Clin Psychiatry 65(12):1597–1600
42. Freudenreich O, Goff DC (2002) Antipsychotic combination therapy in schizophrenia. A review of efficacy and risks of current combinations. Acta Psychiatr Scand 106(5):323–330
43. Josiassen RC, Joseph A, Kohegyi E, Stokes S, Dadvand M, Paing WW, Shaughnessy RA (2005) Clozapine augmented with risperidone in the treatment of schizophrenia: a randomized, double-blind, placebo-controlled trial. Am J Psychiatry 162(1):130–136
44. Goodwin G, Fleischhacker W, Arango C et al (2009) Advantages and disadvantages of combination treatment with antipsychotics: ECNP consensus meeting, March 2008, Nice. Eur Neuropsychopharmacol 19(7):520–532
45. Pandurangi AK, Dalkilic A (2008) Polypharmacy with second-generation antipsychotics: a review of evidence. J Psychiatr Pract 14(6):345–367
46. Avari J, Mahgoub N, Alexopoulos GS (2011) Adding aripiprazole to clozapine worsened delusions and hallucinations: a case report. J Clin Psychopharmacol 31(4):528–531
47. Reinstein MJ, Sirotovskaya LA, Jones LA (1999) Effect of clozapine – quetiapine combination on weight and glycaemic control. Preliminary findings. Clin Drug Invest 18:99–104
48. Henderson DC, Fan X, Copeland PM, Sharma B, Borba CP, Boxill R, Freudenreich O, Cather C, Evins AE, Goff DC (2009) Aripiprazole added to overweight and obese olanzapine-treated schizophrenia patients. J Clin Psychopharmacol 29(2):165–169, PMID: 19512978
49. Fleischhacker WW, Heikkinen ME, Olié JP, Landsberg W, Dewaele P, McQuade RD, Loze JY, Hennicken D, Kerselaers W (2010) Effects of adjunctive treatment with aripiprazole on body weight and clinical efficacy in schizophrenia patients treated with clozapine: a randomized, double-blind, placebo-controlled trial. Int J Neuropsychopharmacol 13(8):1115–1125, Epub 2010 May 12. PMID:20459883
50. Shim JC, Shin JG, Kelly DL, Jung DU, Seo YS, Liu KH, Shon JH, Conley RR (2007) Adjunctive treatment with a dopamine partial agonist, aripiprazole, for antipsychotic-induced hyperprolactinemia: a placebo-controlled trial. Am J Psychiatry 164(9):1404–1410
51. Li C, Mittal D, Owen RR (2011) Impact of patients' preexisting metabolic risk factors on the choice of antipsychotics by office-based physicians. Psychiatr Serv 62(12):1477–1484
52. Joukamaa M, Heliövaara M, Knekt P, Aromaa A, Raitasalo R, Lehtinen V (2006) Schizophrenia, neuroleptic medication and mortality. Br J Psychiatry 188:122–127
53. Khan A (2010) Antipsychotic polypharmacy is not associated with increased mortality from natural causes in patients with schizophrenia compared to monotherapy. Evid Based Ment Health 13(3):90, No abstract available. PMID: 20682830

54. Finnerty MT, Kealey E, Leckman-Westin E, Gupta N, White TM, Engel GM, Opler LA (2011) Psychiatric Services and Clinical Knowledge Enhancement System initiated in 3 phases in NYSOMH network of 18 psychiatric hospitals Long-term impact of web-based tools, leadership feedback, and policies on inpatient antipsychotic polypharmacy. Psychiatr Serv 62(10):1124–1126
55. Gören JL, Parks JJ, Ghinassi FA, Milton CG, Oldham JM, Hernandez P, Chan J, Hermann RC (2008) When is antipsychotic polypharmacy supported by research evidence? Implications for QI. Jt Comm J Qual Patient Saf 34(10):571–582, Review. PMID:18947117
56. Constantine RJ, Andel R, Tandon R (2010) Trends in adult antipsychotic polypharmacy: progress and challenges in Florida's Medicaid program. Community Ment Health J 46(6):523–530, Epub 2010 Jan 23. PMID:20099030
57. Zuvekas SH, Rupp AE, Norquist GS (2005) Spillover effects of benefit expansions and carve-outs on psychotropic medication use and costs. Inquiry 42(1):86–97
58. Aparasu RR, Bhatara V (2006) Antipsychotic use and expenditure in the United States. Psychiatr Serv 57(12):1693
59. Valuck RJ, Morrato EH, Dodd S, Oderda G, Haxby DG, Allen R (2007) Medicaid Pharmacotherapy Research Consortium: how expensive is antipsychotic polypharmacy? Experience from five US state Medicaid programs. Curr Med Res Opin 23(10):2567–2576

Chapter 3
Antipsychotic Polypharmacy in Czech Republic and in Ukraine

Viktor P. Samokhvalov, Oksana E. Samokhvalova, Viktoria A. Verbenko, and Georgij N. Verbenko

Abstract In prescription surveys, use of antipsychotic polypharmacy is common, despite scant supporting evidence. This study investigated the use of monotherapy and different types of polypharmacotherapy among inpatients with acute episodes of schizophrenia in the Czech Republic and in the Ukraine. Two hundred participants were enrolled from two sites: Lnare Psychiatric Clinic, Czech Republic (n = 100) and Psychiatric Hospital №1 in Simferopol, Crimea, Ukraine (n = 100). Each inpatient was evaluated twice with the Positive and Negative Symptom Scale (PANSS) at admission (acute stage) and at discharge (a stabilization stage) from hospital. This study revealed that antipsychotic polypharmacy was prescribed considerably more frequently in the Czech sample (43%) than in the Ukrainian group (29%). The use of combinations of first generation antipsychotics (FGAs) and second generation antipsychotics (SGAs) during hospitalization was six times more prevalent in the Czech Republic (31%) than in the Ukraine (5%; $p < 0.001$); 24% of the Ukranian inpatients received a combination of two or more FGAs, in comparison to 12% of the Czech inpatients ($p < 0.05$) at admission, and the rates decreased to 4% and 9%, respectively, at discharge ($p < 0.05$). Augmentation with off-label prescribed antidepressants and mood stabilizers was far more prevalent in the

V.P. Samokhvalov, M.D., Ph.D., D.Sc. (✉)
Deutsch-Russische Gesellschaft für Psychiatrie, Psychotherapie und Psychosoziale Gesundheit, Nürnberg, Germany
e-mail: samokhvalov@email.cz

O.E. Samokhvalova, M.D., Ph.D.
Department of Psychiatry, Central Military Hospital – Military University Hospital, Prague, Czech Republic
e-mail: anaxo@email.cz

V.A. Verbenko, M.D., Ph.D. • G.N. Verbenko, M.D.
Department of Psychiatry, Crimean Medical University, Simferopol, Crimea, Ukraine
e-mail: vverbenko@mail.ru

M.S. Ritsner (ed.), *Polypharmacy in Psychiatry Practice, Volume II: Use of Polypharmacy in the "Real World"*, DOI 10.1007/978-94-007-5799-8_3,

Ukraine (65 and 54%, at admission and discharge, respectively) than in the Czech sample (40 and 29%, at admission and discharge, respectively). Antipsychotic monotherapy for acute psychosis in the Czech Republic (20%; mainly SGAs) was almost three times more common than in the Ukraine (8%; mainly FGAs; $t=4.63$, $p<0.001$);. When the mental health condition stabilized, antipsychotic monotherapy was increased: from 20 to 33% in the Czech Republic and from 8 to 18% in the Ukraine. International multicenter studies are warranted to investigate the reasons for and the impact of the predominant use of polypharmacy.

Abbreviations

FGA	First generation antipsychotics
NASMHPD	National Association of State Mental Health Program Directors report
PANSS	Positive and Negative Symptom Scale of Schizophrenia
SD	Standard deviation
SGA	Second generation antipsychotics
SSRI	Selective serotonin reuptake inhibitor

3.1 Introduction

Sheppard et al. [1] published the first study of polypharmacy in psychiatry in 1969. Since then, numerous novel antipsychotic agents and other psychotropic preparations for the treatment of schizophrenia have been developed. Polypharmacy has been compounded in elderly patients who have concurrent medical conditions that are treated with non-psychiatric drugs that have psychotropic activity [2–4]. Despite evidence that shows an association between polypharmacy and death in schizophrenia patients, especially from haematological and cardiovascular pathologies, polypharmacy has continued to escalate [5]. However, higher death rates were associated with the absence of treatment with anticholinergic drugs [6]. In addition to the potential dangers of polypharmacy, inefficiency and cost are two noteworthy reasons for discouraging its use [7]. According to the National Association of State Mental Health Program Directors report (NASMHPD), polypharmacy increases the risk of side effects, decreases compliance, diminishes the effects of individual medications, requires the prescription of additional medications to treat side effects, creates more expenses and is dangerous, especially in children and older adults. The NASMHPD has differentiated polypharmacy into categories: same-class polypharmacy, multi-class polypharmacy, adjunctive polypharmacy, augmentation, and total polypharmacy [8].

Polypharmacy should be considered a failure in the treatment of schizophrenia, even though it is often a "necessary harm" that cannot be avoided due to the high resistance and polymorphism of the disorder [9, 10]. For treatment-resistant cognitive symptoms, antipsychotic medication should be combined with cognitive remediation, as to date there is no convincing evidence based pharmacological add-on strategy [11]. In general, the clinical data suggest that polypharmacy cannot be considered an effective treatment for resistant schizophrenia [12]. In particular, in resistant schizophrenia, the traditional combination of clozapine and risperidone has no influence on residual positive symptoms [13].

Evidence suggests that second generation antipsychotics (SGAs), even in resistant cases of schizophrenia, should be prescribed with care [14]. The efficacy of adjunctive benzodiazepine therapy for the treatment of anxiety, depression and hostility is not convincing. The same is true of augmentation with a selective serotonin reuptake inhibitor (SSRI). The use of additional therapy has not been proven to influence quality of life [13]. The recovery period of acute psychosis is longer (more than 6 weeks), compliance decreases, the duration of remission is reduced and the quality of remission worsens [15]. Comparing the courses of monotherapy and polypharmacy, the initial doses are similar. However, the final medication doses in patients treated with polypharmacotherapy are approximately 78% higher than the doses of patients treated with monotherapy, and these differences cannot be explained by the resistant clinical features of schizophrenia [16].

Despite this evidence, schizophrenia is still treated with polypharmacy. In some countries, especially Russia, polypharmacy for the treatment of schizophrenia was considered not only useful but also necessary. The primary Russian textbook on psychiatry even calls polypharmacy the "main principle of therapy of schizophrenia" [17]. The treatment of schizophrenia with polypharmacy has been considered "common sense" [18] and even "a creative problem for the doctor" [19]. Rational approaches are based on the psychopharmacology theory that efficient treatment addresses the clinical profile of positive and negative symptoms and balances the dopaminergic and non-dopaminergic systems, including the adrenergic, glutaminergic and serotoninergic receptor systems. Hence, treatment with polypharmacy is quite logical [20]. Some observations have shown that combined therapy is more effective than monotherapy in some cases. The advantages are appreciable when therapy begins immediately at onset or 10 or more weeks after the failure of monotherapy [21]. Small doses of first generation antipsychotic agents (FGA) equivalent to less than 5 mg of haloperidol per day are most preferable in combination with SGAs [22].

The increasing rates of polypharmacy were triggered by the theory regarding the need for the simultaneous prescription of at least two therapeutic agents at the onset of psychosis [23]. In particular, the combination of antipsychotics and SSRIs used to treat negative symptoms synergistically alters the expression of the ionotropic γ-aminobutyric acid receptor A ($GABA_A$) and related genes in the peripheral mononuclear cells (PMC) of schizophrenia patients [24–26]. Nevertheless, arguments for polypharmacy are mainly based on the personal experience of clinical physicians. The essential psychopharmacology textbook by Stahl (2009) affirms the inefficiency of schizophrenia therapy using high doses SGAs. Combinations of average doses of SGAs with divalproex, lamotrigine or antidepressants, are more effective than a combination of conventional antipsychotics and an SGA or a combination of two SGAs. These findings emphasize the possibility of presymptomatic/prodromal schizophrenia treatments using similar methods [27].

Several authors have reviewed and discussed the use of a combination of antipsychotics in the treatment of schizophrenia [9–15]. In a study of seven psychiatric clinics in Germany, the predictors of polypharmacy in patients with schizophrenia included an increased number of hospitalisations, duration of illness of more than 10 years, and the presence of schizoaffective symptoms [9]. For example, psychiatrists working in the men's unit of a psychiatric hospital who have more than 10 years of experience in psychiatry are more likely to practice polypharmacy [15]. In academic British hospitals, polypharmacy is not as widespread as in community hospitals, where 94–95% of patients are treated with multiple drugs. Similar tendencies exist in the USA [28].

Lack of response to monotherapy does not necessarily indicate polypharmacy [29]. Zink [11] presented advantageous and disadvantageous drug combinations and came to the conclusion that advantageous combinations include combinations of anticholinergic and antipsychotic drugs for the prevention of acute motor dystonias, benzodiazepines and antipsychotics for the treatment of anxiety and agitation, antidepressants and antipsychotics for the treatment of concurrent depression and negative symptoms, lamotrigine and clozapine or SGA and clozapine for the treatment of resistant psychosis, and aripiprazole and clozapine for weight reduction and normalization of metabolism. Disadvantageous combinations include combinations of carbamazepine and clozapine owing to their adverse haematological effects, topiramate and antipsychotics because of their impairment of cognitive function, SGA and FGA due to their low efficacy, and combinations of tricyclic antidepressants and clozapine due to drug-drug interactions. Cross-cultural psychopharmacology studies have shown that polypharmacy is distinctly related to subculture and cultural factors [30–32]. Considering the perfectionistic characteristics of Japanese culture, more than 90% of the incidents of polypharmacy in schizophrenia in Japan cannot be explained solely by economic reasons [33]. Polypharmacy is influenced by cultural factors and patient-family relationships in Europe, especially in Italy [34]. Combinations of medicines are considered appropriate for the treatment of persistent aggression in Australia, Belgium, Canada, Finland, France, Germany, Israel, Italy, Japan, the Netherlands, Great Britain, the USA, countries in East Asia, Russia, Ukraine, and Nigeria. In these countries, it is agreed that polypharmacy should be applied to achieve fast therapeutic effects and to provide treatment if other therapeutic methods have failed [18, 19, 35, 36]. However, the rates of polypharmacy vary from 90% in Japan [33] to 13% in Australia [37] to 30% in England [5]. In the beginning of this century the application of three or more medications for schizophrenia fluctuated from 15 to 35% in Europe [7, 9–11, 38–41]. Doses differ according to the chronicity of disease. For example, patients with chronic psychosis in Hong Kong receive higher doses of antipsychotics and are more likely to receive anticholinergic medications than patients with acute-onset psychosis. This principle is not typical of European countries [42]. The rates of polypharmacy in East Asian countries vary from 13 to 90%, depending on cultural factors, clinical and social distinctions, public health systems, and economic factors, especially the cost of medications, the local traditions of drug prescription and patient choice [43]. However, pharmacogenetic factors are closely connected with ethnicity and culture. For example, the rates of polypharmacy and the average doses of medication are quite different between African-American, Hispanic, Asian and Caucasian patients [44]. In particular, African American patients were less likely to experience antipsychotic polypharmacy [45].

The same differences have been reported in Crimea in Russian, Ukrainian, and Belarusian Slavs and Crimean Tatars belonging to Turkish groups [46]. There are also regional variations that correlate with nursing requests and physician variables such as knowledge, scepticism toward the prescription of medication and time associated pressures that influence rates of polypharmacy [47]. On one hand, doctors do not even try to avoid polypharmacy. It occurs frequently, but is insufficiently studied. In this sense, the "therapeutic option" remains a "dirty little secret" according to Stahl [48]. A small number of international, multicenter randomised clinical investigations proclaim this fact. In particular, schizophrenia is a multifactorial disease with several therapeutic targets that lend themselves to certain medications [41]. Actually, almost all psychotropic drugs are multifunctional and have dose-dependent effects [27]. The target is not necessarily achieved with the use of a combination of two or more multifunctional medications. The number of potential combinations and dosages is a serious obstacle to the design of clinical trials and to the standardization of pertinent scientific research [49]. As a result, treatment with several psychotropic drugs can be considered an art rather than a science [5], and the development of an evidence-base for the use of multiple medications should be a target of future research [50].

We report here patterns of antipsychotic pharmacotherapy including drug class combinations used in the treatment of schizophrenic patients in the acute and stabilization stages during hospitalization in the Czech Republic and in the Ukraine.

3.2 Method

3.2.1 Study Design

This study is a survey of prescribed medications for patients with schizophrenia who were admitted to hospital with an acute psychotic episode in the Czech Republic and in the Autonomous Republic of Crimea, Ukraine. This research included only ethnic Slavs: Czechs (a group of western Slavs), Russians, Ukrainians and Belarusians (eastern Slavs). Eastern and western Slavic populations have the greatest genetic similarity in comparison with surrounding populations, especially northern and southern Slavs [51]. We used a cross-sectional design with repeated registration of psychotropic prescription patterns among 200 schizophrenia inpatients recruited in two hospitals: Lnare Psychiatric Clinic, Czech Republic (N = 100) and Psychiatric Hospital №1 in Simferopol, Crimea, Ukraine (N = 100). Data collection was from 2009 to 2010. Each inpatient was examined twice at admission (an acute stage) and at discharge from hospital (stabilization stage). All participants provided informed consent prior to recruitment to the study.

3.2.2 Assessments

Data collection was conducted via a face to face interview using a standardized protocol which included demographic (sex, age at examination) and background (age at first onset, number of hospitalizations) characteristics, psychiatric symptoms measured with the Positive and Negative Symptom Scale (PANSS), the WHO International Classification of Diseases (ICD-10); length of stay in hospital (days), and information about medications including types of drugs, dosages and adverse effects. On a daily basis, monotherapy (polypharmacy) was defined as the occurrence of one (more than one) ongoing antipsychotic medication prescriptions. The classes of medications reported here were: antipsychotic drugs (first-generation antipsychotic agents, FGAs, and one second-generation antipsychotic agents, SGAs), mood stabilizers, anti-depressants and their combinations. Since almost all patients received a short course of benzodiazepines, it was considered a sporadic background of any therapy. In addition, neuroleptic correctors (mostly anticholinergic agents), groups of prescribed somatic medications and recommended out-patient treatments were also recorded. Both clinical and treatment variables were obtained during the first week after admission and prior to discharge from the hospital. The study did not assess reasons for medication initiation or discontinuation, thus eliminating the ability to evaluate the reasons for any medication changes.

3.2.3 Statistical Analysis

Mean values with standard deviation (SD) are presented. Continuous variables were compared using the two-tailed *t*-test, or the Wilcoxon signed-rank test (z) for assessing the difference in medians. Differences in the frequency of categorical variables were examined with the χ^2 test. Between-group differences (Czech and Ukraine) were analysed using the Statistical Package for Social Sciences (SPSS). For all analyses, the level of statistical significance was defined as $p<0.05$.

3.3 Results

The *patients' sample* included 200 subjects, mean age 41.8 ± 8.3 years (range: 33–50). Mean (±SD) duration of disorder was 19.2 ± 5.4 years (range: 14–24). In the Czech group 70% of the patients presented with ICD-10 paranoid type of schizophrenia (F 20.0), compared to 79% in the Ukraine group ($p<0.05$). The remaining patients had other types of schizophrenia (F 20.1–20.6) 30% and 21%, respectively.

There were no significant differences between the Czech and Ukraine patient groups in the number of hospitalizations (18.2 ± 6.6 versus 12.2 ± 7.9, respectively; $t=0.83$; $p>0.05$), but were differences between groups in length of last hospitalization (38.9 ± 16.4 days versus 58.9 ± 18.2 days, respectively, $t=5.76$, $p<0.001$). In the

Table 3.1 Severity of clinical presentations of schizophrenia inpatients in the Czech Republic and Ukraine (scores)

		Czech Republic	Ukraine	Significance	
PANSS	Assessment	Mean ± SD	Mean ± SD	t	p
Positive scale	Admission	38.1 ± 4.6	28.3 ± 5.4	2.63	<0.001
	Discharge	22.7 ± 3.3	18.4 ± 2.2	n.s.	
Negative scale	Admission	35.7 ± 4.1	32.5 ± 3.6	n.s.	
	Discharge	28.4 ± 3.4	25.3 ± 2.8	n.s.	
General psychopathology	Admission	73.8 ± 3.6	60.8 ± 4.2	2.78	<0.001
	Discharge	51.1 ± 3.3	43.7 ± 2.5	n.s.	

n.s. non significant

Czech Republic, 76% men and 24% women were enrolled (all patients were Czech). In the Ukraine group 66% men and 34% women were enrolled, and all patients were eastern Slavs (Russians, Ukrainians, or Belarusians).

Table 3.1 compares between-group *severity of symptoms* measured with PANSS. As can be seen, at admission the Czech PANSS positive and general psychopathology scales were consistently higher than in the Ukraine group of patients ($p<0.001$). At discharge no statistically significant between group differences in PANSS scores were found. The correlation coefficient of the total PANSS score at admission and the length of hospital stay was $r=0.14$ in the Czech group and $r=0.23$ in the Ukraine group. There were no correlations between the severity of clinical state and duration of hospitalization.

Antipsychotic monotherapy of acute psychosis in the Czech group (20%; mainly SGAs) was almost three times higher than in the Ukraine group (8%; mainly FGAs; $t=4.63$, $p<0.001$; Table 3.2). When the mental health state was stabilized antipsychotic monotherapy was increased: from 20 to 33% in the Czech group and from 8 to 18% in the Ukraine group (Table 3.3).

Antipsychotic polypharmacy (APP) of acute psychosis in the Czech group was 43%, while in the Ukraine group – 29% ($p<0.05$; 38% versus 29%, respectively, at stabilization; Table 3.3). At the same time use of combinations of FGAs and SGAs was about six times higher in the Czech group (31%) than in the Ukraine group (5%; $t=5.23$, $p<0.001$). However, these between-group differences for combinations of FGAs and SGAs did not reach significant levels at stabilization stages (Table 3.3). Furthermore, during acute psychosis twice as many patients in the Ukraine group (24%) than in the Czech group (12%; $t=2.84$, $p<0.05$) received a combination of two or more FGAs, but only 4 and 9%, respectively, at discharge from hospital ($p<0.05$).

Augmentation with off-label prescribed antidepressants (AD) and mood stabilizers (MS) was far more prevalent in the Ukraine (65 and 54%, at admission and discharge, respectively) than in the Czech sample (40% and 29%, at admission and discharge, respectively).

Table 3.2 Drug therapy in schizophrenia at admission in the Czech Republic and Ukraine

	Czech Republic		Ukraine		Significance
Medicines	Mean	%	Mean	%	p
Antipsychotic monotherapy	20	20.0	8	8.0	<0.001
Antipsychotic polypharmacy (APP)	43	43.0	29	29.0	<0.05
FGA+SGA	31	31.0	5	5.0	<0.001
Two or more FGAs	12	12.0	24	24.0	<0.05
Augmentation	37	37.0	63	63.0	<0.001
Add-on antidepressants (AD)	12	12.0	1	1.0	<0.001
Add-on mood stabiliser (MS)	10	10.0	8	8.0	n.s.
Total polypharmacy (APP+AD+MS)	15	15.0	54	54.0	<0.001
Anticholinergic medications	32	32.0	33	33.0	n.s.

Table 3.3 Drug therapy in schizophrenia at discharge in the Czech Republic and Ukraine

	Czech Republic		Ukraine		Significance
Medicines	Mean	%	Mean	%	p
Antipsychotic monotherapy	33	33.0	18	18.0	<0.001
Antipsychotic polypharmacy (APP)	38	38.0	29	29.0	n.s.
FGA+SGA	29	29.0	24	24.0	n.s.
Two or more FGAs	9	9.0	4	4.0	<0.05
Augmentation	29	29.0	53	53.0	<0.001
Add-on antidepressants (AD)	9	9.0	3	3.0	<0.05
Add-on mood stabiliser (MS)	7	7.0	21	21.0	<0.001
Total polypharmacy (APP+AD+AS)	13	13.0	29	29.0	<0.001
Anticholinergic medications	12	12.0	14	14.0	n.s.

Total polypharmacy (APP+AD+AS) was administered to 69 of 200 admitted inpatients (35%), and to 42 discharged patients (21%). This treatment pattern was much more prevalent in the Ukraine than in the Czech Republic (Tables 3.2 and 3.3). Usually one FGA, either haloperidol or zuclopenthixol (Clopixol), was combined with one or two SGAs, such as clozapine, risperidone, paliperidone, olanzapine or aripiprazole, and a mood stabiliser.

There were no between group differences in the number of patients that received *anticholinergic drugs* both at admission (32–33%) and at discharge (12–14%).

No significant between-group differences were found in PANSS scores for patients who received monotherapy and patients who received polypharmacy.

Somatic Therapy: Even though the patients in the Ukraine group were younger, they had higher rates of ischemic heart disease and hypertension and used more hypotensive and cardiovascular medications ($t=3.23$, $p<0.001$ and $t=6.42$, $p<0.001$). These differences may be due to stress from the social environment, and it is impossible to conclude that they received more intensive treatment with FGAs during the course of illness. Moreover, almost every patient received vitamins. In the Czech

Table 3.4 Categories of somatic medications prescribed in schizophrenia inpatients in the Czech Republic and Ukraine

	Czech Republic		Ukraine		Significance
Drugs	Mean	%	Mean	%	p
Hypotensive	10	10.0	25	25.0	<0.001
Cardiovascular	4	4.0	41	41.0	<0.001
Antihistaminic	4	4.0	1	1.0	n.s.
Analgesic	18	18.0	2	2.0	<0.001
Anti-diabetic	4	4.0	2	2.0	n.s.
Antibiotic	15	15.0	5	5.0	<0.001
Gastroenterological	44	44.0	48	48.0	n.s.
Vitamins	15	15.0	70	70.0	<0.001
Thyroid medication	19	19.0	1	1.0	<0.001

group, patients were more likely ($t=5.23$, $p<0.001$) to receive thyroid hormones, and this is possibly explained by the routine screening of thyroid function during hospitalisation (Table 3.4).

3.4 Conclusions and Future Directions for Research

The study of the polypharmacy phenomenon in psychiatry is inherently complex. This study revealed that antipsychotic polypharmacy is prescribed considerably more frequently in the Ukraine than in the Czech Republic:

- *Antipsychotic monotherapy* for acute psychosis in the Czech Republic (20%; mainly SGAs) was almost three times more common than in the Ukraine (8%; mainly FGAs; $t=4.63$, $p<0.001$); when the mental health state was stabilized antipsychotic monotherapy was increased: from 20 to 33% in the Czech Republic and from 8 to 18% in the Ukraine;
- *Antipsychotic polypharmacy* was more prevalent in the Czech sample (43%) than in the Ukraine group (29%); the use of combinations of FGAs and SGAs for acute psychosis was six times more common in the Czech Republic (31%) than in the Ukraine (5%; $p<0.001$); a combination of two or more FGAs, was more frequently received by patients in the Ukraine group (24%) than in the Czech group (12%; $p<0.05$) at admission, but decreased to 4 and 9%, respectively, at discharge ($p<0.05$);
- More than two drug classes were used in 37% of patients. Polypharmacy was far more prevalent in the Ukraine than in the Czech sample.

Various patterns of pharmacotherapy including drug class combinations used in the treatment of schizophrenia were reported. The rates of polypharmacy range from 13% in Australia [37] to 30% in England [5] and to 90% in Japan [33]. The results obtained in our study regarding prescription of psychotropic medications are in accord with those obtained in previous pharmacoepidemiological studies in the same area about psychotropic use [5, 33, 37]. For instance, Pickar et al. [52] reported that 70% of 200 community based schizophrenic patients received an antipsychotic together with medication from another drug class: the most common drug class combinations were antipsychotics and mood stabilizers. A total of 42.5% of patients received more than one antipsychotic drug. Cascade et al. [38] found that 43% of patients received one additional class to supplement their antipsychotic medication, and 10% of patients were prescribed two or more classes of drugs in addition to an antipsychotic agent. The most common classes used to supplement antipsychotic medications in the management of schizophrenia include antidepressants (28%), mood stabilizers (18%), sleep aids (5%), and agents to treat extrapyramidal symptoms (7%), according to Dussias et al. [41] – 20, 15, 7, and 6%, respectively.

Psychopharmacology studies have shown that polypharmacy is influenced by cultural factors and patient-family relationships in Europe [34]; and correlates with subculture and cultural factors [30–32]. The rates of polypharmacy in East Asian countries are associated with cultural, clinical and social factors, public health systems, and economic factors, especially the cost of medication, and the local traditions of drug use [43]. Cross-country differences cannot be explained by economic concerns [33].

As a result, treatment with several psychotropic drugs is an art rather than a science [5], and the development of an evidence-base for the use of multiple medications should be a target of future research [50].

Thus, polypharmacy with psychotropic drugs is a prevalent prescription practice for patients with mental disorders in the in Czech Republic and in the Ukraine. In this non-randomized naturalistic observational study, the most commonly used patterns of antipsychotics and augmentive agents significantly differed between two hospitals in the Czech Republic and in the Ukraine. International multicenter studies are warranted to investigate the reasons for and the impact of the predominant use of polypharmacy.

Acknowledgements The authors express their gratitude to Dr. Vladimir Muchl, the director of the psychiatric hospital in Lnare (Czech Republic) , and Dr. Irina A. Strojevskaja, chief of the acute department of Crimean Psychiatric Hospital № 1(Simferopol, Crimea, Ukraine).

Authors wish to express gratitude to Ms. Rena Kurs, B.A. (Shaar-Menashe Mental Health Center, Hadera, Israel) for editorial assistance.

References

1. Sheppard C, Collins L, Fiorentino D et al (1969) Polypharmacy in psychiatric treatment. Incidence at a state hospital. Curr Therapy Res 11:765–774
2. Praško J, Herman E, Seiferova D (2007) Konziliární psychiatrie. Medical Tribune, Praha
3. Kolvach Z, Holmerova I (2010) Geriatrická farmakoterapie. In: Marek J (ed) Farmakoterapie vnitřních nemocí. Grada Publication, Praha, pp 687–695
4. Hovstadius B, Hovstadius K, Åstrand B et al (2010) Increasing polypharmacy – an individual-based study of the Swedish population 2005–2008. BMC Clin Pharmacol 10:16
5. Langan J, Shajahan P (2010) Antipsychotic polypharmacy: review of mechanisms, mortality and management. Psychiatrist 34:58–62

6. Waddington JL, Youssef HA, Kinsella A (1998) Mortality in schizophrenia. Antipsychotic polypharmacy and absence of adjunctive anticholinergics over the course of a 10-year prospective study. Br J Psychiatry 173:325–329
7. Boschert S (2008) Practical psychopharmacology: polypharmacy in schizophrenia is often expensive, ineffective. Elsevier Global Medical News, 12 Dec
8. Medical Directors Council (2001) Medical directors technical report on psychiatric polypharmacy. National Association of State Mental Health Programs Directors(NASMHPD) Alexandria, Virginia, 9 Oct
9. Janssen B, Weinmann S, Berger M et al (2004) Validation of polypharmacy process measures in inpatient schizophrenia care. Schizophr Bull 30(4):1023–1033
10. Tapp A, Wood AE, Secrest L et al (2003) Combination antipsychotic therapy in clinical practice. Psychiatr Serv 54(1):55–59
11. Zink M, Englisch S, Meyer-Lindenberg A (2010) Polypharmacy in schizophrenia. Curr Opin Psychiatry 23(2):103–111
12. Kreyenbuhl J, Marcus SC, West JC et al (2007) Adding or switching antipsychotic medication in treatment-refractory schizophrenia. Psychiatr Serv 58:983–990
13. Buchman RW, Kreyenbuhl J, Kelly DL et al (2010) The 2009 schizophrenia PORT psychopharmacological treatment recommendation and summary statements. Schizophr Bull 36(1):71–93
14. Schizophrenia: Core Interventions in the Treatment and Management of Schizophrenia in Adults in Primary and Secondary Care (2010) National collaborating centre for mental health, national clinical guideline number 82. The British Psychological Society/The Royal College of Psychiatrists, London
15. Kapiani B (2007) The results of antipsychotic therapy of schizophrenia with connection correlated factors. Ph.D. dissertation Sankt- Petersburg
16. Centorrino F, Goren JL, Hennen J et al (2004) Multiple versus single antipsychotic agents for hospitalized psychiatric patients: case-control study of risks versus benefits. Am J Psychiatry 161:700–706
17. Tiganov AS (1999) Schizophrenia. In: Tiganov AS (ed) Textbook of psychiatry, vol II. Medicine, Moscow, pp 407–555
18. Maljarov SA, Demchenko VA, Vitebskaja TB (2004) What should guide the physician in appointing of combination antipsychotic therapy? Health of Ukraine 96. http://www.health-ua.org/archives/health/738.html
19. Mosolov SN (2010) Actual theoretical problems of diagnostic, classification, neurobiology and therapy of schizophrenia: a comparison of International and Russian experience. Zh Nevrol Psikhiatr Im S S Korsakova 110(6):4–11
20. Freudenreich O, Goff DC (2002) Antipsychotic combination therapy in schizophrenia. A review of efficacy and risks of current combinations. Acta Psychiatrica Scand 106(5):323–330
21. Christoph U, Correll CU, Rummel-Kluge C et al (2009) Antipsychotic combinations vs monotherapy in schizophrenia: a meta-analysis of randomized controlled trials. Schizophr Bull 35(2):443–457
22. Metzer HY, Kostakoglu E (2000) Combining antipsychotics: is there evidence for efficacy? Psychiatric Times 17(9):25–34
23. Stahl SM (2010) Enhancing outcomes from major depression: using antidepressant combination therapies with multifunctional pharmacologic mechanisms from the initiation of treatment. CNS Spectr 15(20):79–94
24. Silver H (2004) Selective serotonin re-uptake inhibitor augmentation in the treatment of negative symptoms of schizophrenia. Expert Opin Pharmacother 5(10):2053–2058
25. Silver H, Chertkow Y, Weinreb O et al (2009) Multifunctional pharmacotherapy: what can we learn from study of selective serotonin reuptake inhibitor augmentation of antipsychotics in negative-symptom schizophrenia? Neurotherapeutics 6(1):86–93
26. Silver H, Susser E, Danovich L et al (2011) SSRI augmentation of antipsychotic alters expression of GABA(A) receptor and related genes in PMC of schizophrenia patients. Int J Neuropsychopharmacol 14(5):573–584

27. Stahl SM (2009) Stahl's essential psychopharmacology. Neuroscientific basis and practical application, 3rd edn. Cambridge University Press, New York
28. Muijen M, Silverstone T (1987) A comparative hospital survey of psychotropic drug prescribing. Br J Psychiatry 150:501–504
29. Goren JL, Parks JJ, Chinassi FA et al (2008) When is antipsychotic polypharmacy supported by research evidence & implication for QI. Jt Comm J Qual Patient Saf 34(10):571–582
30. Sadock BJ, Sadock VA, Ruiz P (eds) (2009) Kaplan and Sadock's comprehensive textbook of psychiatry, vol II, 9th edn. Lippincott Williams & Wilkins, Philadelphia
31. Ghaemi SA (2002) Conceptual and historical background of polypharmacy in psychiatry. In: Ghaemi SA (ed) Polypharmacy in psychiatry. Marcel Dekker Inc, New York, pp 1–34
32. Ghaemi SA (2003) Concepts of psychiatry. A plyralistic approach to mind and mental illness. The John Hopkins Press, Baltimore
33. Ito C, Kubota Y, Sato MA (1999) A prospective survey on drug choice for prescriptions for admitted patients with schizophrenia. Psychiatry Clin Neurosci 53:35–40
34. Tognoni G (1999) Pharmacoepidemiology of psychotropic drugs in patients with severe mental disorders in Italy. Italian Collaborative Study Group on the outcome of severe mental disorders. Eur J Clin Pharmacol 55(9):685–690
35. Barnes TR, Paton C (2011) Antipsychotic polypharmacy in schizophrenia: benefits and risks. CNS Drugs 25(5):383–399
36. Adeponle AB, Obembe AO, Adeyemi SO (2007) Suleiman polypharmacy in psychiatric outpatient practice in northern Nigeria. Afr J Psychiatry 10:215–218
37. Keks NA, Alston K, Hope J et al (1999) Use of antipsychosis and adjunctive medications by an inner urban community psychiatric service. Aust N Z J Psychiatry 33:896–901
38. Cascade EF, Amir HK, Buckley PF (2008) Current management of schizophrenia: antipsychotic monotherapy versus combination therapy. Psychiatry (Edgemont) 5(5):28–30
39. Miller AL (2005) Polypharmacy in schizophrenia: science, art, and fiction. Curr Psychosis Ther Rep 3(2):61–67
40. Ranceva N, Ashraf W, Odelola D (2010) Antipsychotic polypharmacy in outpatients at Birch Hill Hospital: incidence and adherence to guidelines. J Clin Pharmacol 50(6):699–704
41. Dussias P, Kalali AH, Citrome L (2010) Polypharmacy of schizophrenia. Psychiatry (Edgemont) 7(8):17–19
42. Chiu HF, Shum PS, Lam CW (1991) Psychotropic drug prescribing to chronic schizophrenics in a Hong Kong hospital 37(3):187–191. http://www.ncbi.nlm.nih.gov/pubmed/1743903
43. Sim K, Su A, Fujii S et al (2004) Antipsychotic polypharmacy in patients with schizophrenia: a multicentre comparative study in East Asia. Br J Clin Pharmacol 58(2):178–183
44. Pi EH, Simpson GM (2005) Psychopharmacology: cross-cultural psychopharmacology: a current clinical perspective. Psychiatric Serv 56(1)
45. Kreyenbuhl JA, Valenstein M, McCarthy JF et al (2007) Long-term antipsychotic polypharmacy in the VA health system: patient characteristics and treatment patterns. Psychiatric Serv 58:489–495
46. Verbenko NV (2007) Essays of ethnic psychiatry. In: Samokhvalov VP (ed) Simferopol, Dolja
47. Baandrup L, Allerup P, Nordentoft M et al (2010) Exploring regional variation in antipsychotic coprescribing practice: a Danish questionnaire survey. J Clin Psychiatry 71(11):1457–1464, Epub 2010 Oct 19
48. Stahl SM (1999) Antipsychotic polypharmacy. Part 1: therapeutic option or dirty little secret? J Clin Psychiatry 60(7):425–426
49. Miller AL, Craig CS (2002) Combination antipsychotics: pros, cons, and questions. Schizophr Bull 28(1):105–109
50. Taylor D (2010) Antipsychotic polypharmacy – confusion reigns. Psychiatrist 34:41–43
51. Rebala K, Mikulich A, Tsybovsky J et al (2007) Y-STR variation among Slavs: evidence for the Slavic homeland in the middle Dnieper basin. J Hum Genet 52(5):406–414
52. Pickar D, Vinik J, Bartko JJ (2008) Pharmacotherapy of schizophrenic patients: preponderance of off-label drug use. PLoS One 3(9):e3150

Chapter 4
Antipsychotic Polypharmacy in Residential Facilities in Italy: The Gap Between Recommendations and Real World Practice

Lucio Ghio, Werner Natta, Simona Gotelli, and Luigi Ferrannini

Abstract Recent studies based on psychotropic drug use give rise to growing concern about the trend towards psychotropic and antipsychotic polypharmacy, delineating prescriptive practices contrary to treatment recommendations drawn up in international guidelines. An increase in the number of psychotropic medications, in particular antipsychotics, prescribed over the course of years has been noted in all psychiatric settings.

Most studies on psychotropic polypharmacy and antipsychotics' prescription patterns have been carried out either through the use of administrative databases or onsite in acute psychiatric wards. Data related to prescribing practices for patients living in psychiatric residential facilities which, in Italy, have completely replaced mental hospitals for the care of long-term patients, are instead minimal. In this chapter we report the results of drug utilisation studies carried out in Italian residential facilities. These results demonstrate the frequent and alarming distinction between medication treatment recommendations and real world practice in such environments.

Abbreviations

AD	Antidepressant
AP	Antipsychotic
BDZ	Benzodiazepine

L. Ghio, M.D. (✉) • W. Natta, M.D. • S. Gotelli, M.D.
Department of Neuroscience, Ophtalmology and Genetic, Psychiatry Section,
University of Genoa, Genoa, Italy
e-mail: lu.ghio@libero.it

L. Ferrannini, M.D.
Department of Mental Health, ASL3 Genovese, Genoa, Italy

M.S. Ritsner (ed.), *Polypharmacy in Psychiatry Practice, Volume II: Use of Polypharmacy in the "Real World"*, DOI 10.1007/978-94-007-5799-8_4,

BPRS	Brief Psychiatric Rating Scale
CPZeq	Chlorpromazine equivalent
MD	Mood stabilizers
PRN	Pro re nata

4.1 Introduction

Recent studies based on psychotropic drug use give rise to growing concern about the trend towards psychotropic and antipsychotic polypharmacy, delineating prescriptive practices contrary to treatment recommendations drawn up in international guidelines. An increase in the number of psychotropic medications prescribed over the course of years has been noted in all psychiatric settings: in office-based psychiatric practices [1], in hospitals [2–4] and in residential facilities [5–7].

Evidence of an increase in antipsychotic polypharmacy [8, 9], and of the chlorpromazine equivalent (CPZeq) total daily dose of antipsychotic agents [10–12] persisting despite repeated recommendations to the contrary [13], is particularly disturbing.

The rate of antipsychotic polypharmacy varies from 13% [14] to about 50% [15, 16] depending on studies, and has shown an increasing trend towards such prescription patterns in recent years. This is proven in reports that point out a 20-fold increase in patients subject to prescribed polypharmacy with a corresponding 46% increase in the CPZ equivalent total daily dose of antipsychotics between 1989 and 1998 [8] and a 227% increase in the total annual number of antipsychotics prescriptions between 1996 and 2006 [17].

Prescribed antipsychotic polypharmacy has been associated with higher healthcare costs [17, 18], increased anticholinergic drug prescriptions [19, 20], young patient age [8, 21], longer periods of hospitalisation [11, 22], increased use of depot injection [23], above average body weight [4] and is considered the strongest predictor of high levels of antipsychotic dosage [4, 11, 21].

Most studies on antipsychotics' prescription patterns have been carried out either through the use of administrative databases or onsite in acute psychiatric wards. Data related to prescribing practices for patients living in psychiatric residential facilities which, in Italy, have completely replaced mental hospitals for the care of long-term patients, are instead minimal.

In this chapter we report the results of drug utilisation studies carried out in Italian residential facilities. These results demonstrate the frequent and alarming distinction between medication treatment recommendations and real world practice in such environments.

In order to better understand the Italian context we will first describe the main features of Italian residential facilities and the results of drug utilisation studies in both Italian outpatient and acute inpatient settings, which will serve as a comparison to the aforementioned residential facilities.

4.2 Residential Facilities in Italy

Residential facilities were established in Italy after the Reform of 1978 (Law 180), which saw all psychiatric hospitals closed down. The Law 180 stated that as of 1978 no new admissions to existing mental health hospitals would be allowed and that as of 1981 readmission would also cease to continue. The closure of all Italian mental hospitals had been successfully completed by the end of 1999 [24].

As a result of the Reform a community-based model of mental health care was developed and the first non-hospital residential facilities, following specific principles which had been formulated for therapeutic communities, were implemented. Currently mental health care in Italy is delivered by 211 Mental Health Departments, which include small psychiatric hospital units within general hospitals, semi-residential and residential facilities, and mental health outpatients centres, being the hub of a community-based system. Despite the effort to provide effective biological and psychosocial treatment in an outpatients' setting, the Reform could not prevent a substantial number of severely ill patients being admitted over the years to long-term residential facilities, the likes of which have become increasingly numerous.

A national survey of non-hospital residential facilities in Italy [25] found that on the 31st of May, 2000, there were 1,370 facilities with at least four places (a total of 17,138 beds) with an average of 12.5 beds in each facility. Overall, there were 2.98 residential beds for every 10,000 inhabitants, though these results varied greatly between regions. Patients admitted to a residential facility usually have severe difficulties living in the community due to chronic clinical problems, they also have severe disabilities with regard to their daily living skills and very often lack adequate family support. Residents are typically middle aged, and predominantly single males, who have suffered unremitting schizophrenic symptoms since their early adulthoods. Such patients have often never worked and almost half are not involved in any regular activities within the facility [26].

Usually the length of a patient's stay in the facility is very long and the turnover of residents is low. During 1999, more than a third of the residential facilities (37.7%) had not discharged any patients and 31.5% had discharged only one or two in the same year [26].

The length of a patient's admission represents one of the most critical factors for the treatment of patients within residential structures; the extension of treatment periods correlates with phenomena of chronic symptoms not only in the illness but also in therapeutic treatment.

The multiple modes of therapeutic intervention available within residential structures are characterised by ample variety and sparse measurability, so that in an instance of prolonged treatment psychopharmaceutical intervention becomes a central and widespread solution. The clinically assessed appropriateness of such practices is a strong indicator of the quality of psychiatric intervention in such treatment environments.

4.3 Drug Utilisation Studies in Italian Outpatient and Acute Inpatient Facilities

In Italy some studies have been conducted in both in- and out-patient facilities. Data from these studies are comparatively relevant because they describe Italian prescription patterns and may be used as a reference in relation to the results of studies conducted in long term facilities, which will be described in the following paragraphs.

A high variability of prescription patterns is usually reported in the aforementioned studies. Such variability could be partially related to socio-demographic and clinical aspects, though it is more frequently illustrated to be due to a clinician's personal decision to prescribe different medications in the same clinical circumstances [27]. Many studies highlight a poor relationship between a patient's medical prescription and their diagnosis [27, 28], as well as a high rate of psychotropic polypharmacy [29, 30], and a high rate of off-label prescriptions for mood stabilizers [30] with little consideration for subsequent side effects [30].

Tibaldi et al. [29] reported that 82% of outpatients and 98% of acute inpatients were prescribed at least one psychotropic drug and among these 67% of outpatients and 84% of acute inpatients also received an antipsychotic. Antipsychotic polypharmacy was also common (reported in 28% of outpatients and 45% of acute inpatients), but overall antipsychotic total dosage was low; 64% of outpatients received a CPZ equivalent dosage lower than 200 mg/day and an equal proportion of acute inpatients received a dosage lower than 500 mg/day. Mean dosage was between 166 and 375 mg/day CPZeq. The Tibaldi report [29] also showed that one in four patients received benzodiazepine (BDZ) polypharmacy (two or more drugs) while antidepressant polypharmacy was less common (11%).

Ten years later Tognoni et al. [30], surveying a large sample of outpatients, found similar results concerning antipsychotic polypharmacy (with a more widespread use of second generation antipsychotics). Tognoni's results [30] depicted a relationship between the number of drugs prescribed and their consequent side-effects, as well as between antipsychotic polypharmacy and a patient's poor quality of life and health care. Compared with previous studies Tognoni [30] noted a reassuring result in the lower rate of BDZ and antidepressant polypharmacy.

With regard to an acute inpatient setting, a study performed by Santone et al. [31] in 2010 investigated the characteristics of antipsychotic utilisation within a large sample group of patients admitted to acute inpatient facilities. During a 12-day index period, all patients scheduled to be discharged within a week signed up to the study and were assessed.

Santone's study [31] revealed in a sample of 1,022 patients that the percentages of the prescriptions of antipsychotics and antipsychotic polypharmacy were 67.4% and 32.6%, respectively. The most common patterns of antipsychotic polypharmacy included a first-generation and a second-generation antipsychotic (17.6%) or two first generation antipsychotics (7.8%).

Antipsychotic polypharmacy was prescribed more frequently to patients who were admitted coercively, who had poorer insight into their illness, and who showed less cooperation with staff upon admission, however, there were no associations found between prescribed antipsychotic polypharmacy and a patient's violent behaviour or Brief Psychiatric Rating Scale (BPRS) score at discharge.

Overall, the aforementioned drug utilisation studies highlight that the rate of antipsychotic polypharmacy in an outpatient setting has remained constant, the results showing a low to moderate antipsychotic daily dose, whereas in an acute inpatient setting it is apparent that the rate of antipsychotic polypharmacy has decreased from 45 to 33% over the years, nevertheless, the mean daily antipsychotic drug dose is higher in an acute inpatient setting than that of an outpatient setting [12].

4.4 The First Drug Utilisation Study Performed in Italian Residential Facilities

The first study on the prescription of psychotropic drugs in Italian residential facilities was carried out in 2004 through a sample group of 2,962 patients [5]. The study was aimed at evaluating general prescription patterns including patterns of polypharmacy, the variables associated with polypharmacy, correlations between patient diagnosis and drug prescription, and adverse event rates.

All psychotropic drugs available in Italy at the time of the survey were included: these were conventional antipsychotics and atypical antipsychotics (clozapine, olanzapine, risperidone and quetiapine), benzodiazepines, tricyclic antidepressants, as well as other classes of new generation antidepressants, mood stabilizers and other psychotropic drugs. The majority of patients participating in the study were males (63.2%) with a primary diagnosis of schizophrenia (68.2%). The mean age of these patients was 49.5 years and their mean duration of illness amounted to 26.6 years. The average duration of admission for patients in their current facility (at the time of the 2004 study) was 3.5 years. Almost all patients (95.5%) were being treated with a psychotropic drug and 91.6% had also been prescribed at least one antipsychotic.

Overall, 78 different compounds had been prescribed to the patient sample group. Haloperidol (both in its oral and depot forms) was the most frequently prescribed medication, followed by two benzodiazepines (lorazepam and delorazepam) and risperidone. Nine of the 15 most frequently prescribed medications were antipsychotics. Among these clozapine was prescribed to 14.3% of patients studied. This prescription would suggest the presence of a relatively large proportion of treatment-resistant schizophrenic patients. The 12.1% of patients receiving long-acting antipsychotics were more frequently schizophrenic or patients suffering from personality disorders.

Following the prescription of antipsychotics the most commonly prescribed class of drugs were benzodiazepines (69.5%), followed by antiparkinsonians (27%), mood stabilizers (22.7%), and antidepressants (13.7%).

Anti-parkinsonian drug prescription was revealed to be higher in those patients being treated with conventional antipsychotics and in those receiving antipsychotic polypharmacy. Many patients (7.1%) who were not being prescribed antipsychotics were also receiving antiparkinsonian drugs.

Overall, psychotropic polypharmacy (three or more psychotropic drugs) was applied to 53.4% of patients and antipsychotic polypharmacy (two or more antipsychotics) to 39.3% of the same patients. The average amount of drugs received for each patient under treatment was 2.7. An association of two conventional antipsychotics was the most common pattern of antipsychotic polypharmacy prescribed.

Predictors of psychotropic polypharmacy in schizophrenic patients included a medical history of admission to an acute general hospital psychiatric ward, the presence of positive schizophrenic symptoms and lower social functioning, whereas, in all the others patients, the only predictor was a medical history of admission to an acute general hospital psychiatric ward.

Predictors of antipsychotic polypharmacy included a higher score on the aggressiveness as well as the delusion and hallucination items of the administered scales. Overall, this first study carried out in Italian residential facilities in 2004 highlighted that the prescription of psychotropic polypharmacy and antipsychotic polypharmacy was common in such an environment, and more frequently practiced than in inpatient and outpatient facilities. This study was, however, limited by the fact that there was no data collected in relation to prescribed antipsychotic dosage nor the changes in a patients' antipsychotic prescriptions which may have taken place during a patient's stay within the participating facilities.

4.5 Antipsychotic Utilisation and Polypharmacy in Italian Residential Facilities

In order to document current trends of antipsychotic utilisation and polypharmacy compared to earlier studies in the same environment we investigated the antipsychotic drug use and estimated the frequency of antipsychotic polypharmacy in a sample of Italian residential facilities [7]. Unlike earlier studies we collected data on both the antipsychotic dosage and the variation of antipsychotic patterns over the period of stay within the investigated facilities. In addition we investigated any possible relation between the aforementioned data and prescribed psychotropic drugs, anticholinergics, high antipsychotic dosage as well as patients' characteristics.

In this study 15 residential facilities were included. Data were collected through a chart review during a 1-day census. The census took place on a different day for each facility between May and June 2008. Information relating to all patients staying in the facilities was collected. Psychotropic drug prescribing patterns were collected both upon admission and on the given census day. The drug name, class, formulation and daily dose in relation to antipsychotics was collected. In addition, the drug name was collected for the following classes of psychotropic drugs: antidepressants, benzodiazepines, mood stabilizers and anticholinergics. The prescription of non-psychotropic drugs was also investigated.

Table 4.1 Clinical and socio-demographic characteristics (n=362)

	Mean	S.D.
Age (mean, SD)	47.7	(14.8)
	n	%
Gender		
Male	224	(61.9)
Female	138	(38.1)
Primary diagnosis		
Schizophrenia and other psychotic disorders	252	(69.6)
Major affective disorder	23	(6.4)
Personality disorders	50	(13.8)
Other	37	(10.2)
Time spent in the facility		
<1 year	91	(25.1)
1–3 years	102	(28.2)
4–5 years	44	(12.2)
>6 years	125	(34.5)
N. of admissions to acute inpatient facility in the last year		
None	275	(76.0)
1	53	(14.6)
2–4	21	(5.8)
>4	13	(3.6)

At the time of the survey all typical antipsychotics and the following atypical antipsychotics were available in Italy: aripiprazole, clozapine, olanzapine quetiapine and risperidone.

The antipsychotic daily doses, including depot antipsychotics, were converted to CPZ equivalents (mg/day), using published guidelines [32, 33]. In the case of antipsychotic polypharmacy, the total daily dose was calculated by adding up the different CPZ equivalents so that the antipsychotic with the highest CPZ equivalent was considered the main antipsychotic.

Psychotropic polypharmacy was defined as the prescription of at least three different compounds. Antipsychotic polypharmacy was defined as the prescription of at least two different antipsychotics.

The demographic and clinical characteristics of patients are provided in Table 4.1.

The study includes 362 patients with an average age of 47.7 years, 61.9% of whom were males. The most common diagnosis among the participating patients was schizophrenia (69.6%) followed by personality disorders (13.8%) and major affective disorder (6.4%). Other disorders accounted for 10.2%.

Overall 46.7% had spent at least 4 years in their given facilities and 76.0% had had no admission to an acute inpatient facility in the previous year (see Table 4.1). On the census day almost all patients were treated with a psychotropic drug (98.1%) and 92.8% of patients had been prescribed at least one antipsychotic (see Table 4.2).

Table 4.2 Psychopharmacological treatment and antipsychotic prescription pattern at admission to the residential facility and on the census day (N=362)

	Admission		Census day	
	N	%	N	%
Psychopharmacological treatment				
Any psychotropic drug	347	95.9	355	98.1
Antipsychotic	321	88.7	336	92.8
Benzodiazepine	271	74.9	275	76.0
Mood stabilizer	117	32.3	140	38.7
Antidepressant	91	25.1	109	30.1
Anticholinergic	93	25.7	103	28.5
Antipsychotic depot medication	60	16.6	56	15.5
Medication polypharmacy	250	69.1	281	77.5
Antipsychotic treatment				
No antipsychotic	41	11.3	26	7.2
Antipsychotic monotherapy	137	37.8	129	35.6
Clozapine	28	20.4	34	26.4
Olanzapine	20	14.6	21	16.3
Haloperidol	27	19.7	18	14.0
Risperidone	27	19.7	18	14.0
Quetiapine	6	4.4	8	6.2
Levomepromazine	4	2.9	7	5.4
Promazine	6	4.4	7	5.4
Clotiapine	6	4.4	6	4.7
Other	13	9.5	10	7.8
Antipsychotic polypharmacy	184	50.8	207	57.2
Typical plus typical	93	50.5	47	22.7
Atypical plus atypical	8	4.3	15	7.2
Typical-atypical combination	59	32.1	104	50.2

Antipsychotic dose (mean; SD)	457.7; 490.1		577.9; 550.1	
Antipsychotic high dose[a]	42	11.6	62	17.1
Main antipsychotic (at least 10 prescriptions on the census day)				
Clozapine	49	13.5	66	18.2
Risperidone	58	16.0	55	15.2
Olanzapine	26	7.2	46	12.7
Quetiapine	18	5.0	46	12.7
Haloperidol	68	18.8	42	11.6
Clotiapine	54	14.9	37	10.2
Levomepromazine	8	2.2	11	3.0
Promazine	9	2.5	10	2.8
Other	31	8.6	13	3.6
No antipsychotic	41	11.3	26	7.2
Antipsychotic most common prescription pattern				
2 AP + 1 BDZ	35	9.7	25	6.9
1 AP + 1 BDZ	32	8.8	20	5.5
1 AP	21	5.8	20	5.5
3 AP + 1 BDZ	16	4.4	18	5.0
2 AP	23	6.4	16	4.4
1 AP + 1 BDZ + 1 AD	8	2.2	13	3.6
1 AP + 2 BDZ	15	4.1	12	3.3
1 AP + 1 BDZ + 1 MS	12	3.3	11	3.0
2 AP + 2 BDZ	13	3.6	10	2.8
2 AP + 2 BDZ + 1 MS	13	3.6	10	2.8
No antipsychotic	41	11.3	26	7.2

AP Antipsychotic, *BDZ* Benzodiazepine, *AD* Antidepressant, *MS* Mood stabilizer
[a]>1,000 mg CPZ equivalents

A high proportion of patients (76.0%) received at least one benzodiazepine. The proportion of patients receiving psychotropic polypharmacy was 77.5% with an average number of 3.7 drugs prescribed. Five or more psychotropic drugs were prescribed to 32.8% of all patients. Overall 62 different drugs were prescribed. Moreover a PRN medication was prescribed to 25.0% of patients and at least one drug for medical comorbid conditions to 37.0% of patients.

The study showed that delorazepam, lorazepam and flurazepam were the most commonly prescribed benzodiazepines, valproic acid and carbamazepine the most commonly prescribed mood stabilizers, and sertraline, citalopram and paroxetine the most commonly prescribed antidepressants. The most commonly prescribed PRN medication was delorazepam and, overall, 66.7% of PRN medications were benzodiazepines.

The most common associations between drug classes are indicated in Table 4.2, which illustrates a parcelling out of prescription patterns, all of which are below 7% in frequency. It is remarkable that among the first five most common combinations, three include some form of antipsychotic polypharmacy.

Clozapine, risperidone, olanzapine and quetiapine were the most commonly prescribed antipsychotics. Atypical prescription increased compared to prescription patterns upon admission where haloperidol was the most commonly prescribed antipsychotic. The variations in prescribing patterns are confirmed by the changes to the typical:atypical ratio from admission to the census day (2.02:1 vs 1.35:1).

There were 35.6% of patients taking antipsychotic monotherapy, while the amount of patients receiving antipsychotic polypharmacy was 57.2%. More than three different antipsychotics were prescribed to 22.9% of patients. The most common antipsychotics combinations included one atypical and one (or more) typical drug(s), but no antipsychotics combination appeared to be prevalent.

Antipsychotic total daily dose (in CPZ equivalents) was 577.9 mg/day. Overall 22.9% of patients were receiving a dose lower than 200 mg/day, 31.5% a dose between 201 mg and 500 mg/day, 18.2% a dose between 501 and 800 mg/day and 27.3% a dose higher than 800 mg/day. There were 17.1% (62) of patients receiving a dose higher than the suggested maximum dose (1,000 mg/day). Patients with a diagnosis of schizophrenia or other psychotic disorders were most likely to be prescribed a dose of antipsychotic higher than 800 mg/day ($p<0.001$; OR 3.04). As expected, there was a significant association between the total daily dose and the number of antipsychotics prescribed ($p<0.01$). In contrast with earlier studies, antipsychotic polypharmacy was unrelated to the number of admissions to an acute general hospital psychiatric ward in the previous 12 months and to a patient's age. Of patients taking an antipsychotic 70.1% were also receiving a benzodiazepine, 35.4% of patients a mood stabilizer and 27.0% an antidepressant.

The prescription of anticholinergic medication was related both to the total antipsychotic dose and to the number of prescribed antipsychotics. Patients taking anticholinergic drugs were in fact prescribed 789.7 mg/day of CPZ equivalents while patients not taking anticholinergic drugs were prescribed 504.6 mg/day ($p<0.0001$). Of patients treated with antipsychotic monotherapy 13.2% were also receiving anticholinergic drugs, but this proportion increased to 29.8% when two antipsychotics were administered.

Table 4.3 Changes in antipsychotic and psychopharmacological prescriptions from admission to census day for patients staying less than 1 year (n=91)

	Admission		Census day			
	N	%	N	%	Test	p
Antipsychotic depot medication	13	14.3	18	19.8	–	0.06[b]
Medication polypharmacy	72	79.1	69	75.8	–	0.51[b]
Antipsychotic polypharmacy	42	46.2	44	48.4	–	0.80[b]
Antipsychotic dose (mean; SD)	465.6; 513.5		503.2; 586.2		Z=−1.38	0.17
Antipsychotic high dose[a]	11	12.1	12	13.2	–	1.00[b]

[a] >1,000 mg CPZ equivalents
[b] Binomial distribution used

Overall, psychopharmacological treatment denotes substantial deviations from guideline recommendations. This is particularly demonstrated through the extensive and specific use of benzodiazepines, the prescription of mood stabilizers to a percentage of patients much higher than those patients suffering from a bipolar disorder, and the utilisation of antipsychotics in almost all patients studied, regardless of their diagnosis. However, the most interesting findings of the study were related to the changes in prescribing patterns over a patient's length of stay in the facility. Prescription changes from admission to the census day were analysed. This analysis took into account the amount of time each patient spent in the facility, in order to provide a comparable time frame for all the patients in each of the four control groups. The four groups were identified according to the time spent in the facilities. This comparison focused on antipsychotic and psychotropic polypharmacy, depot medications and antipsychotic dosage.

For the first group of patients (those whose length of stay was less than 1 year; see Table 4.3) no statistically significant changes were noted in the mean antipsychotic dose and in the use of depot medications although there was an increase in the frequency of prescribing antipsychotic polypharmacy. The second group of patients (those whose length of stay was between 1 and 3 years; see Table 4.4) showed a statistically significant increase in the average dose of antipsychotics from 491.9 to 620.2 CPZ equivalents. A similar significant increase (from 521.1 to 622.8 CPZ equivalents) was observed in the third group of patients (those staying between 4 and 5 years; see Table 4.5).

Long-term patients (those staying more than 6 years; see Table 4.6) made up the largest group and showed a statistically significant increase in medication polypharmacy (from 61.6 to 76.8%), in antipsychotic average dose (from 401.7 to 581.9 CPZ equivalents) and in the amount of patients receiving more than 1,000 mg/day of CPZ equivalents (from 8.8 to 17.6%). A slight yet insignificant decrease in depot medications was noted. Overall changes in prescribing patterns seem to be related to time spent in the facility: few changes occurred to short-term patients, while more significant changes occurred to longer-term patients.

Table 4.4 Changes in antipsychotic and psychopharmacological prescriptions from admission to census day for patients staying 1–3 years (n = 102)

	Admission		Census day			
	N	%	N	%	Test	p
Antipsychotic depot medication	19	18.6	16	15.7	–	0.61[b]
Medication polypharmacy	72	70.6	81	79.4	–	0.08[b]
Antipsychotic polypharmacy	53	52.0	58	56.9	–	0.42[b]
Antipsychotic dose (mean; SD)	491.9; 503.0		620.2; 593.8		Z = −2.58	< 0.05
Antipsychotic high dose[a]	13	12.7	18	17.6	–	0.30[b]

[a]>1,000 mg CPZ equivalents
[b]Binomial distribution used

Table 4.5 Changes in antipsychotic and psychopharmacological prescriptions from admission to census day for patients staying 4–5 years (n = 44)

	Admission		Census day			
	N	%	N	%	Test	p
Antipsychotic depot medication	7	15.9	7	15.9	–	1.00[b]
Medication polypharmacy	29	65.9	35	79.5	–	0.15
Antipsychotic polypharmacy	18	40.9	22	50.0	–	0.42
Antipsychotic dose (mean; SD)	521.1; 659.3		622.8; 497.9		Z = −2.12	<0.05
Antipsychotic high dose[a]	7	15.9	10	22.7	–	0.45[b]

[a]>1,000 mg CPZ equivalents
[b]Binomial distribution used

A trend towards an increase of antipsychotic and psychotropic polypharmacy and higher doses of antipsychotics over the period of stay within the facilities was nonetheless present in each group.

The length of stay in facilities was the only variable related to the prescription changes after controlling all other variables.

Analysis conducted on the complete sample confirm the role a patient's length of stay plays in changes to his/her prescription: the switch to a different main antipsychotic (antipsychotic with the highest CPZ equivalent) was related to the duration of stay within the facility ($p < 0.0001$); in particular, patients who had spent at least 3 years had a 2.48 OR (C.I. 1.62–3.79) of being administered a different main antipsychotic.

Table 4.6 Changes in antipsychotic and psychopharmacological prescriptions from admission to census day for patients staying more than 6 years (n = 125)

	Admission		Census day			
	N	%	N	%	Test	p
Antipsychotic depot medication	21	16.8	15	12.0	–	0.21[b]
Medication polypharmacy	77	61.6	96	76.8	$\chi^2=8.31$	<0.01
Antipsychotic polypharmacy	71	56.8	83	66.4	$^2=2.63$	0.11
Antipsychotic dose (mean; SD)	401.7; 381.4		581.9; 502.9		Z = −3.33	<0.01
Antipsychotic high dose[a]	11	8.8	22	17.6	–	<0.05[b]

[a]>1,000 mg CPZ equivalents
[b]Binomial distribution used

Treatment augmentation was also related to the duration of stay within the facility: patients placed in monotherapy at admission who then went on to spend at least 3 years in the facility had an OR = 2.04 (C.I. 1.17–3.58) of receiving antipsychotic polypharmacy.

Compared to earlier studies in the same clinical environment [5, 6] a significant increase in the use of psychotropic polypharmacy and antipsychotic polypharmacy was observed. According to our results, patients receiving antipsychotic polypharmacy were 77.5% versus 53% [5] and those receiving antipsychotic polypharmacy were 57.2% versus 23% [6] and 39.3% [5].

Our sample was similar to those of the aforementioned studies in terms of diagnosis, average patient age and sex. However, differences lie in the patients' length of stay (our sample being composed of double the amount of patients staying more than 6 years in a given facility compared to those who participated in the Tomasi study [5]) and for the level of assistance provided by the facilities included (both earlier studies having also recruited patients from group homes and sheltered housing facilities).

Taking into account our data (which demonstrates that the increase in medication polypharmacy is related to time spent in the facilities and not to different types of facility), we can hypothesise that the variable of time represents a possible explanation for differences compared to earlier studies as well as being a possible risk factor for polypharmacy. The longer the patient's term the higher the risk of prescribed polypharmacy.

Similar results were found in acute inpatient facilities where polypharmacy has been associated with long-term hospitalisation [4, 22]. In a residential setting this finding could be related to the severity of illness and treatment resistance or may be a reaction on the part of the prescribers to the chronicity of the patients' illness.

Our findings denote increased odds for longer-term patients of a switch from antipsychotic monotherapy to polypharmacy and of a switch to a different main antipsychotic. These results could also indicate that chronic treatments may lose their effectiveness over the course of time.

Long term facilities certainly host a significant proportion of seriously ill patients (as the high percentage of clozapine use seems to confirm) which could partially justify the use of polypharmacy, despite the lack of research based evidence demonstrating its superior effectiveness. Nevertheless, some studies did not identify psychopathology as a predictor of polypharmacy [34] and have shown that a switch from antipsychotic polypharmacy to monotherapy has been beneficially linked to the patients' overall clinical status [11, 35]. Furthermore, the increased risk of adverse effects related to polypharmacy should be cautionary to clinicians, especially when treating patients over a period of years [36] as is the case with the majority of patients being hosted in long term facilities.

This is especially true if we take into account our findings depicting a general tendency towards increasing prescriptions of all classes of psychotropic drugs during patient's stay in the facility and an increased use of antipsychotic polypharmacy among more common combination prescriptions.

These findings are consistent with earlier reports that show a growing trend over the last 10 years for the administration of psychotropic polypharmacy in every setting [1, 8, 17].

It is remarkable that in our study this practice is more widespread than that of acute inpatient facilities [12, 37], where, by definition, patients are treated in the more severe phase of their illness.

As we pointed out antipsychotic polypharmacy is the strongest predictor of high dose and prescriptions above the maximum recommended dosage.

Compared to other studies conducted in Italy reporting antipsychotic doses (only done with hospitalised patients or outpatients), our study showed a particularly high frequency of high dose prescriptions [12, 29]. As for polypharmacy the tendency to increase the mean dose of antipsychotic over the patients' length of stay seems to be related to the duration of time spent in the investigated facilities.

The highest doses prescribed were usually a consequence of prescribing medium doses of two or more drugs, rather than that of prescribing high doses of a single drug. A possible explanation for this practice is that the prescriber is not always aware of exceeding, along with polypharmacy, the maximum recommended dose, and maybe through the administration of multiple medium doses the prescriber unconsciously overrode this concern. This hypothesis seems to be consistent with a recent survey denoting clinicians' reasoning behind antipsychotics polypharmacy which stresses, among other motives, the intent to avoid high doses of a single drug [38].

Another hypothesis is that with chronically ill psychotic patients who are typically limited when it comes to receiving benefits from treatment, antipsychotic polypharmacy and high doses might reflect hopes for greater effectiveness of treatment and this prescribing habit could be read as a reaction of the prescribers to the chronicity of the illness. However, this strategy lacks compelling evidence for the superior effectiveness of the aforementioned polypharmacy and high dosage, and may increase the cost of healthcare and the risk of possible side effects. This is confirmed by our findings of a twofold increase in anticholinergic prescriptions when a second antipsychotic is added.

This prescribers factor could therefore influence the prescription patterns regardless of the severity of the illness [39]. The absence in our results of a more frequent and specific antipsychotic combination and the high variability of overall prescriptions is consistent with this hypothesis. This observation should be further investigated, but it is interesting to note that, in our study, patient related factors such as young age and admission to a general hospital's acute psychiatric ward in the previous 12 months were not associated with antipsychotic polypharmacy contrary to the evidence of previous studies [5, 21].

4.6 Conclusions and Future Directions

Drug utilisation studies are necessary in order to provide a clear picture of real-world treatment patterns, further allowing us to identify areas which need change and improvement.

As we previously reported, the two main drug utilisation studies in Italian long-term facilities show a large gap between recommendations and real-world practice. Indeed they show a weak relationship between diagnosis and psychotropic treatment, a high rate of polypharmacy, and a trend towards increasing antipsychotic polypharmacy and dosage.

The rate of psychotropic and antipsychotic polypharmacy as well as antipsychotic high dosage seem to increase either over the years (when comparing our results with those of Tomasi et al. [5]) or (according to our own results) over the length of patient's stay within the facilities.

These data support, on the one hand, the clinicians' cultural tendency towards an increase in psychotropic polypharmacy (as has been proven in studies carried out over the last 10 years), and on the other hand, they show that such prescriptions are common even in long-term facilities where treatment goals should also be reached through non-pharmacological interventions aimed towards rehabilitation. The results instead affirm the contrary; that longer treatment periods lead to an increased risk of polypharmacy.

The evidence that approximately 50% of the patients living in residential facilities have little to no involvement in rehabilitation activities [26] raises more than one question with regard to the function and the purpose of long term psychiatric facilities. What is the relationship between the increase in a patient's psychotropic polypharmacy for the duration of his/her admission, low patient turn-over (45% of patients stay in the same facility for more than 4 years), and minimum involvement in rehabilitation activities?

Even if we can answer that long-term facilities usually host severely ill and chronic patients, it has to be noted that, when long term psychiatric facilities opened in Italy, psychotropic drug treatment was considered an effective, though not substantial, intervention, and had to be used in the lowest possible dosages in order to allow for a patient's participation in rehabilitation activities. Nowadays, psychotropic drug treatment seems to have taken on a determining role and in some cases it is the only delivered treatment.

In this current scenario the studies have outlined, the risk is in adopting the practice of increasing the dosage of psychotropics to deal with the severity of a patient's illness, rather than increasing the patient's available global care. However, as has been highlighted, the severity, chronicity and treatment resistance of certain illnesses usually found in patients of long-term facilities, places clinicians in a predicament in which they may be forced to rely on their clinical experience, and perhaps intuition, to design antipsychotic polypharmacy treatment protocols for real-world practice, especially where they have no specific practice guidelines to rely on for antipsychotic polypharmacy. The consequence being the aforementioned parcelling out of psychotropic combinations, often without a pharmacological rationale. The variability of prescriptive practice seems to suggest, as Klein [40] claimed, that in clinical psychopharmacology the scientifically based knowledge necessary to make prescription rational and informed is not available, since the research is more inclined to focus on the development and registration of new drugs, rather than on the improvement of the use of existing ones.

In order to attain such knowledge, it would be desirable to perform pragmatic, randomised clinical trials in order to replace subjective clinical impression with a more rational approach to antipsychotic polypharmacy, based on a pharmacodynamic and pharmacokinetic understanding of drug action.

Furthermore, we would suggest that more drug utilisation studies be implemented in order to raise awareness regarding the rate of polypharmacy and the appropriateness of its use, although we acknowledge that the mere carrying out of these studies would not be sufficient enough to improve prescribing practice.

As has been demonstrated in our study [7], carried out at a distance of 4 years from Tomasi's original study [5], prescribing patterns in residential facilities have not improved, rather they have worsened. We believe it would be useful to offer specific training courses on the rational implementation of psychotropic drug prescription in the same facilities which have been subjected to our investigations once a drug utilisation study has been completed. Given the large gap between treatment recommendations and real-world practice in residential facilities, more effective strategies for distributing evidence-based knowledge are necessary in order to turn scientific results into everyday practices.

References

1. Mojtabai R, Olfson M (2010) National trends in psychotropic medication polypharmacy in office-based psychiatry. Arch Gen Psychiatry 67:26–36
2. McCue RE, Waheed R, Urcuyo L (2004) Polypharmacy in patients with schizophrenia. J Clin Psychiatry 64:984–989
3. Barbui C, Ciuna A, Nosè M et al (2005) Drug treatment modalities in psychiatric inpatient practice: a 20-year comparison. Eur Arch Psychiatry Clin Neurosci 255(2):136–142
4. Centorrino F, Cincotta SL, Talamo A (2008) Hospital use of antipsychotic drugs: polytherapy. Compr Psychiatry 49(1):65–69
5. Tomasi R, De Girolamo G, Santone G (2006) The prescription of psychotropic drugs in psychiatric residential facilities: a national survey in Italy. Acta Psychiatr Scand 113:212–223

6. Schorr SG, Loonen AJM, Brouwers JRBJ et al (2008) A cross-sectional study of prescribing patterns in chronic psychiatric patients living in sheltered housing facilities. Int J Clin Pharmacol Ther 46:146–150
7. Ghio L, Natta W, Gotelli S et al (2011) Antipsychotic utilisation and polypharmacy in Italian residential facilities: a survey. Epidemiol Psychiatr Sci 20:171–179
8. Centorrino F, Eakin M, Bahk W et al (2002) Inpatient antipsychotic drug use in 1998, 1993 and 1989. Am J Psychiatry 159:11
9. Ganguly R, Kotzan JA, Miller LS et al (2004) Prevalence, trends, and factors associated with antipsychotic polypharmacy among medicaid-eligible schizophrenia patients, 1998–2000. J Clin Psychiatry 65:1377–1388
10. Tempier RP, Pawliuk NH (2003) Conventional, Atypical and combination antipsychotic prescriptions: a 2 year comparison. J Clin Psychiatry 64:673–679
11. Centorrino F, Goren J, Hennen J et al (2004) Multiple versus single antipsychotic agents for hospitalized psychiatric patients: case-control study of risk versus benefits. Am J Psychiatry 161:4
12. Mauri MC, Regispani F, Beraldo S et al (2005) Patterns of clinical use of antipsychotics in hospitalized psychiatric patients. Prog Neuropsychopharmacol Biol Psychiatry 29(6):357–363
13. Ranceva N, Ashraf W, Odelola D (2010) Antipsychotic polypharmacy in outpatients at Birch Hill Hospital: incidence and adherence to guidelines. J Clin Pharmacol 50:699–704
14. Tapp A, Wood AE, Secrets L et al (2003) Combination antipsychotic therapy in clinical practice. Psychiatr Serv 54:55–59
15. Paton C, Lelliot P, Harrington M (2003) Patterns of antipsychotic and anticholinergic prescribing for hospital inpatients. J Psychopharmacol 17:223–229
16. Sim K, Su A, Senta F et al (2004) Antipsychotic polypharmacy in patients with schizophrenia: a multicentre comparative study in East Asia. Br J Clin Pharmacol 58:178–183
17. Alessi Severini S, Biscontri RG, Collins DM et al (2008) Utilization and costs of antipsychotic agents: a Canadian population-based study, 1996–2006. Psychiatr Serv 59:547–553
18. Loosbrock DL, Zhao Z, Johnstone BM et al (2003) Antipsychotic medication use patterns and associated costs of care for individuals with schizophrenia. J Ment Health Policy Econ 6:67–75
19. Johnsen E, Svingen GF, Jorgensen HA (2004) Practice regarding antipsychotic therapy: a cross-sectional survey in two Norwegian hospitals. Nord J Psychiatry 58:313–317
20. Kreyenbuhl J, Valenstein M, McCarthy J et al (2007) Long-term antipsychotic polypharmacy in the VA Health System: patient characteristics and treatment patterns. Psychiatr Serv 58:489–495
21. Lelliot P, Paton C, Harrington M et al (2002) The influence of patient variables on polypharmacy and combined high dose of antipsychotic drugs prescribed for inpatient. Psychiatr Bull 26:411–414
22. Diaz FJ, de Leon J (2002) Excessive antipsychotic dosing in 2 U.S. State Hospitals. J Clin Psychiatry 63:998–1003
23. Walkup J, McAlpine D, Olfson M et al (2000) Patients with schizophrenia at risk for excessive antipsychotic dosing. J Clin Psychiatry 61:5
24. Piccinelli M, Politi P, Barale F (2002) Focus on psychiatry in Italy. Br J Psychiatry 181:538–544
25. De Girolamo G, Picardi A, Micciolo R et al (2002) Residential care in Italy: a national survey of non-hospital facilities. Br J Psychiatry 181:220–225
26. De Girolamo G, Picardi A, Santone G (2005) The severely mentally ill in residential facilities: a national survey in Italy. Psychol Med 35:421–431
27. De Girolamo G, Cappiello V (1993) Gli studi di drug-utilization in psichiatria: una review. Rivista di Psichiatria 28:133–142
28. Muscettola G, Bollini P, Pampallona S (1991) Pattern of neuroleptic drug use in Italian mental health services. DICP 25:296–301
29. Tibaldi G, Munizza C, Bollini P (1997) Utilization of neuroleptic drugs in Italian Mental Health Services: a survey in Piedmont. Psychiatr Serv 48:213–217
30. Tognoni G, Terzian E (2007) Epidemiologia dell'appropriatezza e della sicurezza dei trattamenti farmacologici nella pratica assistenziale dei Servizi Psichiatrici Territoriali. Rivista Sperimentale di Freniatria; 131:125–145

31. Santone G, Bellantuono C, Rucci P et al (2011) Patient characteristics and process factors associated with antipsychotic polypharmacy in a nationwide sample of psychiatric inpatients in Italy. Pharmacoepidemiol Drug Saf 20(5):441–449
32. Woods SW (2003) Chlorpromazine equivalent doses for the newer atypical antipsychotics. J Clin Psychiatry 64:663–667
33. Taylor D, Paton C, Kerwin R (2007) The Maudsley prescribing guidelines, 9th edn. Informa Healthcare, London
34. Barbui C, Nosè M, Mazzi MA et al (2006) Persistence with polypharmacy and excessive dosing in patients with schizophrenia treated in four European countries. Int Clin Psychopharmachol 21:355–362
35. Suzuki T, Uchida H, Tanaka KF et al (2004) Revising polypharmacy to a single antipsychotic regimen for patients with chronic schizophrenia. Int J Neuropsychopharmacol 7:1–10
36. Waddington JL, Youssef HA, Kinsella A (1998) Mortality in schizophrenia. Antipsychotic polypharmacy and absence of adjunctive anticholinergics over the course of a 10-years prospective study. Br J Psychiatry 173:325–329
37. Preti A, Rucci P, Gigantesco A (2009) Patterns of care in patients discharged from acute psychiatric inpatient facilities. Soc Psychiatry Psychiatr Epidemiol 44:767–776
38. Sernyak MJ, Rosenheck R (2004) Clinicians' reasons for antipsychotic coprescribing. J Clin Psychiatry 65:1597–1600
39. Veronese A, Vivenza V, Nosè M, Cipriani A, Tansella M, Barbui C (2008) Understanding antipsychotic non-classical prescriptions: a quantitative and qualitative approach. Epidemiol Psichiatr Soc 17:236–241
40. Klein DF (1993) Clinical psychopharmacological practice: the need for developing a research based. Arch Gen Psychiatry 50:491–494

Chapter 5
Antipsychotic Polypharmacy and Associated Phenomena in Patients with Schizophrenia: Rational or Irrational?

Yong K.H. Michael, Norman Sartorius, and Kang Sim

Abstract A review of the literature of psychopharmacological studies reveals that there are great discrepancies in reported rates of psychotropic drug utilization patterns. As newer psychotropic agents are being introduced into the market, it is necessary to assess the prescribing patterns within specific local contexts, clinical factors associated with their use and their change over time. In the first psychopharmacological study of antipsychotic prescription patterns for schizophrenia in six East Asian countries and regions in 2001 (REAP-I), it was found that the second-generation antipsychotics (SGA) were generally under-utilized and Japan had a relatively higher dose and antipsychotic polypharmacy whilst China had a higher prescription of clozapine. A second study (REAP-II) was undertaken in 2004 and trends of increasing SGA use with reciprocal decreasing use of first generation antipsychotics (FGA) among the East Asian countries were noted. The current study aims to examine prescription patterns of psychotropic drugs, relevant associated factors with antipsychotic polypharmacy (defined as prescription of two or more antipsychotics) and their inter-relationships with associated phenomena such as

Y.K.H. Michael, M.D., M.Med (Psychiatry)
Department of Psychological Medicine, Jurong Health
Alexandra Hospital, Singapore, Singapore
e-mail: michael_yong@juronghealth.com.sg

N. Sartorius, M.D., Ph.D.
Association for the Improvement of Mental Health Programmes,
14 Chemin Colladon, 1209 Geneva, Switzerland
e-mail: sartorius@normansartorius.com

K. Sim, M.B.B.S. (Melb), M.Med (Psychiatry), PG Dip Psychotherapy (Distinction) (✉)
Research at Institute of Mental Health (IMH), Singapore, Singapore

Yong Loo Lin School of Medicine, National University of Singapore,
Singapore, Singapore
e-mail: kang_sim@imh.com.sg

M.S. Ritsner (ed.), *Polypharmacy in Psychiatry Practice, Volume II: Use of Polypharmacy in the "Real World"*, DOI 10.1007/978-94-007-5799-8_5,

long acting antipsychotic use, prescription of FGA and SGA medications within a tertiary psychiatric hospital setting in Singapore.

We conducted a cross-sectional pharmaco-epidemiological survey of psychotropic prescription patterns for 100 hospitalized patients with schizophrenia. Data collection was performed using a standardized protocol which included patient's social and clinical characteristics, psychiatric symptoms, course of illness, and information about medications including types of drugs, dosages and adverse effects.

Antipsychotic polypharmacy (74% of subjects) was associated with greater prescription of long acting antipsychotic, FGA use, higher antipsychotic dose and lower Brief Psychotic Rating Scale scores. Use of long acting antipsychotic was associated with older age group, less likelihood of SGA use, greater likelihood of antipsychotic polypharmacy, anticholinergic use and use of higher dosage of antipsychotic. Prescription of FGAs was associated with older age, verbal aggression, a higher total daily chlorpromazine equivalent dosage, higher rates of antipsychotic polypharmacy and lesser use of SGA. SGA prescription was associated with younger age, less prescriptions of anticholinergic and long acting antipsychotic medications but not antipsychotic polypharmacy.

We observed significant rates of antipsychotic polypharmacy but also in the use of SGA and prescription of low antipsychotic doses. The importance having regular psychotropic prescription audits and follow up studies may allow evaluation of all patterns of antipsychotic use including polypharmacy, promote understanding of contextual prescription trends and encourage consideration of rational prescription practices including antipsychotic polypharmacy.

Abbreviations

BPRS	Brief Psychiatric Rating Scale
FGAs	First generation antipsychotics
GAF	Global Assessment of Functioning Scale
SGAs	Second generation antipsychotics

5.1 Introduction

A review of the literature on psychopharmacological studies revealed that there were great discrepancies of reported rates for psychotropic drug utilization patterns [1–3]. Prescription of psychotropic medications can be affected by a myriad of factors including patient, prescriber, medication factors and issues related to healthcare system such as cost of medications, accessibility, medication subsidy [4, 5]. As more and more newer psychotropic agents are being introduced into the market, it is thus necessary to assess the psychotropic prescribing patters, factors associated with their use and their changes over time [6]. Naturalistic pharmacoepidemiological studies can also allow examination of gaps between treatment recommendations and what is practiced on the ground as well as factors affecting the conformance patterns [7, 8].

Schizophrenia is a severe debilitating disorder that typically begins in the late adolescent or early adult. Antipsychotic drugs have been around since 1950s and can be more effective in the treatment of certain aspects of schizophrenia such as positive symptoms but less effective for negative symptoms and cognitive deficits [9], Two groups of antipsychotic drugs are currently used to treat schizophrenia, namely, the first generation antipsychotics (FGAs) such as chlorpromazine, trifluoperazine and the novel or atypical antipsychotics (second generation antipsychotics, SGAs) such as olanzapine, risperidone. The first generation antipsychotics are now relatively inexpensive, but could result in higher frequency of adverse effects such as extra-pyramidal side effects. Apart from cost burden, antipsychotic drug utilization data can also be influenced by medical and non medical considerations with different healthcare and financing systems [10]. Prescription patterns of antipsychotics vary across geographical regions and with time. Existing literature on antipsychotic drug utilization in schizophrenia documented some variations across Europe [11], America [12] and Asia [13]. Recent studies have also suggested prescribing trend changes in terms of diminishing use of high doses of the older FGA but increasing use of moderate dose of SGA and in combination with other psychotropic agents like mood stabilizers and hypnotics [14–17].

Data about psychotropic prescription patterns is more sparse in East Asia compared to the West. However, in the first pharmacoepidemiological study of antipsychotic prescription patterns for schizophrenia in six East Asian countries and regions in 2001 [13, 18], it was found that Japan had a relatively higher dose and antipsychotic polypharmacy, Singapore had a high utilization of depot injections while China had a higher prescription of clozapine. High prescription of clozapine was observed in China with relatively lower utilization of other FGAs which was likely related to their availability and costs. The cost of clozapine is approximately 40-fold higher in Singapore or Taiwan compared to China.

A follow up study was undertaken in 2004 [19] and trends of increasing SGA use with reciprocal decreasing use of FGAs among the East Asian countries were noted. The current study aims to examine prescription patterns of psychotropic drugs, relevant associated factors with antipsychotic polypharmacy (defined as prescription of two or more antipsychotics) and their inter-relationships with long acting antipsychotic use, prescription of FGA and SGA medications within a tertiary psychiatric hospital setting in Singapore.

5.2 Methods

This study is a cross-sectional pharmacoepidemiological study of psychotropic prescription patterns for hospitalized patients with schizophrenia. We recruited 100 patients who were admitted to the Institute of Mental Health from January to February, 2009, who had a clinical diagnosis of Schizophrenia according to the

WHO International Classification of Diseases (ICD-10) or Diagnostic and Statistical Manual of Mental Disorders (fourth edition: DSM-IV) and were able to give informed consent at the point of entry into the study. Patients with clinically significant medical conditions or active psychotic symptoms related to co-morbid substance use disorders were excluded from the study. Data collection was conducted via a face to face interview using a standardized protocol which included patient's social and clinical characteristics, psychiatric symptoms, course of illness, and information about medications including types of drugs, dosages and adverse effects. Daily doses of all drugs and antipsychotic doses were averaged and long acting intramuscular injection of antipsychotic medications within 30 days of admission were converted to approximate daily chlorpromazine-equivalents (CPZeq, mg/day) using standard guidelines [2, 20, 21]. Clinical variables which included socio-demographic details, current psychiatric medications, blood pressure and body mass index (BMI) were obtained from the medical records. Brief Psychiatric Rating Scale (BPRS) [22] and Global Assessment of Functioning Scale (GAF) were used to assess the severity of psychopathology and level of psychosocial functioning respectively. Both BPRS and GAF scales were administered after the patient was stabilized for their illness and prior to their discharge from the hospital. All study procedures were approved by the Institutional Review Boards of Institute of Mental and National Health Group.

5.3 Statistical Analysis

In this study, averages were reported as means ± standard deviation (SD), risk estimates were reported as odds ratios (OR) with their 95% confidence interval (CI). Analyses of data were done using the Statistical Package for Social Sciences (SPSS) version 17. Normality of distributions of continuous measures was checked using Kolmogorov-Smirnov one-sample test. Differences between groups were tested by ANOVA (t-test) for normally distributed data, non-parametric Mann Whitney U tests for non-normally distributed continuous data and by contingency table (χ^2) for categorical variables. Significance was taken to be $p<0.05$. For analysis, low dose antipsychotic was defined as those who received less than 300 CPZeq mg/day and non-low dose antipsychotic was defined as those who received equal to or greater than 300 CPZeq mg/day. This segregation was based on treatment recommendations including that of the Schizophrenia Patient Outcomes Research Team (PORT) [23–25].

5.4 Results

In this study of 100 patients, there was equal gender preponderance and the mean (SD) age was 42.89 ± 10.4 years, of whom 71 (71%) were single. More than half of the patients (67%) were unemployed. About 34% of the patients suffered a duration of illness between 10 and 20 years. With regards to ethnicity, the majority was

Table 5.1 Socio-demographic characteristics of the sample (N = 100)

Factors	Mean	SD or percent
Age (± SD, years)	42.9	10.4
Years of education(± SD, years)	9.95	3.34
Weight (± SD, kg)	61.8	13.7
Sex (n, %)		
Male	50	50.0
Female	50	50.0
Ethnicity (n, %)		
Chinese	82	82.0
Malay	10	10.0
Indian	8	8.0
Marital status (n, %)		
Single	71	71.0
Married	23	23.0
Divorce/separated	6	6.0
Occupation (n, %)		
Employed	19	19.0
Unemployed	67	67.0
Others (student, homemaker)	14	14.0
Duration of illness (n, %)		
3–6 months	3	3.0
6 months–1 year	2	2.0
1–5 years	16	16.0
5–10 years	27	27.0
10–20 years	34	34.0
>20 years	18	18.0

Abbreviation: *SD* standard deviation

Chinese (82%) with Malays and Indian constituting 10 and 8% respectively of the study population (Table 5.1). The mean daily chlorpromazine equivalent dose of antipsychotic agents was 397.38 ± 323.34 mg/day. Patients received either 1(26%), 2(62%) or 3(12%) antipsychotics given during this study period, hence antipsychotic polypharmacy was observed in 74% of the subjects. The number of patients who were receiving low dose antipsychotic was 53% while the remaining (47%) were on antipsychotic doses equal to or above 300 chlorpromazine mg equivalents per day. Concomitant use of antidepressants occurred in 22 (22%) patients and mood stabilizers in 28 (28%) patients. More than half of the patients in this study (67%) used anticholinergics. Long-acting antipsychotics were commonly used in patients (79%). First generation antipsychotics were used in 49% of the study patients, while 50% of the patients were on second generation antipsychotics.

Antipsychotic polypharmacy was found in 74% of the subjects (Table 5.2). Patients who received more than one antipsychotic were associated with lower BPRS scores (mean 20.9 ± 2.9) ($p = 0.04$) and higher total CPZeq mg/day (mean 496.1 ± 329.6 versus 207.7 ± 215.0) ($p < 0.001$). Antipsychotic polypharmacy

Table 5.2 Factors associated with antipsychotic polypharmacy

	Antipsychotic polypharmacy (use of >1 antipsychotic)					
Factors	Yes (n=74)	No (n=26)	Test statistic	*p*	OR	CI_{95}
Age	43.9±9.3	39.9±12.9	F=3.04	0.08	–	–
Total CPZ equivalents mg/day	496.1±329.6	207.7±215	F=13.64	<0.001	–	–
GAF total score	37.9±6.5	36.9±9.2	F=0.3	0.59	–	–
BPRS total score	20.9±2.9	22.5±4.4	F=4.06	0.04	–	–
FGA						
Yes	46 (62.2%)	3 (11.5%)	$\chi^2=19.7$	<0.001	12.6	3.5, 45.8
No	28 (37.8%)	23 (88.5%)				
Dosage of antipsychotic CPZ-eq mg/day						
Non-low (≥300)	43 (58.1%)	4 (15.4%)	$\chi^2=14.1$	<0.001	7.63	2.39, 24.36
Low (<300)	31 (41.9%)	22 (84.6%)				
Long-acting AP						
Yes	69 (93.2%)	10 (38.5%)	$\chi^2=34.8$	<0.001	22.1	6.6, 73.56
No	5 (6.8%)	16 (61.5%)				

Abbreviations: *CPZ-eq* chlorpromazine equivalents, *GAF* global assessment functioning, *BPRS* brief psychiatric rating scale, *FGA* first generation antipsychotic

was associated with the use of long acting antipsychotic (93.2%) compared to those receiving one antipsychotic (38.5%) (p<0.001). Patients on more than one antipsychotic were more likely to be receiving first generation antipsychotics (62.2%) than those who were on monotherapy antipsychotic prescription (11.5%) (p<0.001).

As a group, patients receiving long acting (depot) antipsychotics were significantly older (mean 44.3 years) (p=0.007) than those who were not receiving long acting antipsychotics. The proportion of patients who were on long acting antipsychotics and second generation oral antipsychotics were lower (43%) when compared to those who were on second generation oral antipsychotics but not on long acting antipsychotics (76.2%) (p=0.007). Patients on long acting antipsychotics were more likely (87.3%) to be prescribed more than one antipsychotic than those on purely oral medications (23.8%) (p<0.001). There were more patients on long acting antipsychotics (74.7%) that were prescribed on anticholinergics than those who were on oral medications (38.1%) (p=0.002). Patients who were receiving long acting antipsychotics also received higher dosages of antipsychotics compared to those who were not on long acting antipsychotics (53.2% versus 23.8%) (p=0.017; Table 5.3).

In terms of use of FGA, patients who were receiving FGA were older compared to those not receiving FGA (mean age 45.7 versus 40.2 years) (p=0.008). The group of patients on first generation antipsychotics had higher total daily chlorpromazine equivalent dosage (496.4±358.4 mg/day) when compared with those who were not on FGA (302.2±254.6 mg/day) (p=0.002). Verbal aggression was seen more frequently in patients who were on FGA (38.8%) when compared with those who

Table 5.3 Prescription of long-acting antipsychotic and associated factors

	Long-acting antipsychotic use					
Factors	Yes (n=79)	No (n=21)	Test statistic	*p*	OR	CI_{95}
Age, years	44.3±9.2	37.5±13.1	F=7.47	0.007	–	–
Total CPZ equivalents mg/day	421.8±326.3	305.7±301.8	F=2.16	0.145	–	–
GAF total score	37.8±6.9	36.8±8.5	F=0.28	0.600	–	–
BPRS total score	21.2±3.3	21.9±4.0	F=0.78	0.379	–	–
Use of SGA						
Yes	34 (43.0%)	16 (76.2%)	χ^2=7.29	0.007	0.24	0.08, 0.71
No	45 (57.0%)	5 (23.8%)				
Polypharmacy						
Yes	69 (87.3%)	5 (23.8%)	χ^2=34.80	<0.001	22.08	6.63, 73.6
No	10 (12.7%)	16 (76.2%)				
Use of anticholinergics						
Yes	59 (74.7%)	8 (38.1%)	χ^2=10.05	0.002	4.79	1.74, 13.3
No	20 (25.3%)	3 (61.9%)				
Dosage of antipsychotic CPZ mg eq/day						
Low (<300)	37 (46.8%)	16 (76.2%)	χ^2=5.74	0.017	3.63	1.21, 10.9
Non-Low(>300)	42 (53.2%)	5 (23.8%)				

Abbreviations: *CPZ-eq* chlorpromazine equivalents, *GAF* global assessment functioning, *BPRS* brief psychiatric rating scale, *SGA* second generation antipsychotic

are not receiving FGA (19.6%) [odds ratio 2.6, 95% confidence interval 1.06, 6.38, p=0.035]. Patients on FGA (18.4%) were less likely to be in receipt of SGA (p<0.001) and in receipt of more than one antipsychotic (p<0.001). There was no significant association between the use of first generation antipsychotics and prescription of anticholinergics [p=0.076]. Patients receiving first generation antipsychotics tend to be in the category of taking higher dose of medications (61.2%) compared to patients not receiving first generation antipsychotics (33.3%) (p=0.005; Table 5.4).

In terms of SGA use, prescription of SGA was associated with younger age (mean 39.4 years versus 46.4 years) (p=0.001) compared to those subjects receiving FGA. There was a smaller proportion of patients receiving SGA who were given anticholinergics (56%) compared to those not on SGA (78%) (p=0.019). Patients on SGA were less likely to be receiving long acting antipsychotic (68%) when compared with patients not taking SGA (90%) (p=0.007; Table 5.5).

Patients who received low dose of antipsychotics were less likely to be associated with disorganized speech (15.1%) compared to those taking higher dose antipsychotic (38.3%) (p=0.008; Table 5.6). Patients who were on low dose antipsychotics also had less verbal aggression (18.9%) compared to those receiving higher doses of antipsychotics (40.4%) (p=0.018). Patients who were receiving higher doses of antipsychotics had significant side effect problems like galactorrhea, amenorrhea

Table 5.4 Prescription of first generation antipsychotic and associated factors

Factors	First-generation antipsychotic use Yes (n=49)	No (n=51)	Test statistic	p	OR	CI_{95}
Age	45.7±8.7	40.2±11.3	F=7.25	0.008	–	–
Total CPZ equivalents mg/day	496.4±358.4	302.2±254.6	F=9.82	0.002	–	–
GAF total score	37.7±6.9	37.4±7.6	F=0.038	0.847	–	–
BPRS total score	20.9±3.1	21.8±3.7	F=1.78	0.185	–	–
Polypharmacy						
Yes	46 (93.9%)	28 (54.9%)	χ^2=19.73	<0.001	12.6	3.46, 45.8
No	3 (6.1%)	23 (45.1%)				
Use of anticholinergics						
Yes	37 (75.5%)	30 (58.8%)	χ^2=3.15	0.076	2.16	0.92, 5.1
No	12 (24.5%)	21 (41.2%)				
Dosage of antipsychotic CPZ-eq mg/day						
Non-low (≥300)	30 (61.2%)	17 (33.3%)	χ^2=7.80	0.005	3.16	1.39, 7.16
Low (<300)	19 (38.8%)	34 (66.7%)				
Verbal aggression						
Yes	19 (38.8%)	10 (19.6%)	χ^2=4.46	0.035	2.6	1.06, 6.38
No	30 (61.2%)	41 (80.4%)				
SGA						
Yes	9 (18.4%)	41 (80.4%)	χ^2=38.46	<0.001	0.06	0.02, 0.15
No	40 (81.6%)	10 (19.6%)				

Abbreviations: *CPZ-eq* chlorpromazine equivalents, *GAF* global assessment functioning, *BPRS* brief psychiatric rating scale, *SGA* second generation antipsychotic

Table 5.5 Prescriptions of second generation antipsychotic and associated factors

Factors	Second-generation antipsychotic use Yes (n=50)	No (n=50)	Test statistic	p	OR	CI_{95}
Age	39.4±10.8	46.4±8.9	F=12.61	0.001	–	–
Total CPZ equivalents mg/day	368.8±286.8	425.9±356.8	F=0.78	0.38	–	–
GAF total score	37.3±6.9	37.8±7.6	F=0.12	0.73	–	–
BPRS total score	21.3±3.3	21.3±3.6	F=0.00	1	–	–
Use of anticholinergics						
Yes	28 (56%)	39 (78%)	χ^2=5.47	0.019	0.36	0.15, 0.86
No	22 (44%)	11 (22%)				
FGA						
Yes	9 (18%)	40 (80%)	χ^2=38.46	<0.001	0.06	0.02, 0.15
No	41 (82%)	10 (20%)				
Long-acting AP						
Yes	34 (68%)	45 (90%)	χ^2=7.29	0.007	0.24	0.08, 0.71
No	16 (32%)	5 (10%)				

Abbreviations: *CPZ-eq* chlorpromazine equivalents, *GAF* global assessment functioning, *BPRS* brief psychiatric rating scale

Table 5.6 Use of low dose (<300 CPZ mg eq/day) versus higher dose antipsychotic (>300 CPZ mg eq/day) and associated factors

	Dosages of antipsychotic					
Factors	Low dose (n=53)	Non-low dose (n=47)	Test statistic	*p*	OR	CI_{95}
Disorganized speech						
Yes	8 (15.1%)	18 (38.3%)	χ^2=6.97	0.008	3.49	1.34, 9.07
No	45 (84.9)	29 (61.7%)				
Hyperprolactinemia related (galactorrhea, amenorrhea, gynecomastia)						
Yes	0 (0%)	4 (8.5%)	χ^2=4.7	0.03	1.09	1, 1.2
No	53 (100%)	43 (91.5%)				
Long-acting antipsychotic						
Yes	37 (69.8%)	42 (89.4%)	χ^2=5.74	0.017	3.63	1.2, 10.9
No	16 (30.2%)	5 (10.6%)				
Verbal aggression						
Yes	10 (18.9%)	19 (40.4%)	χ^2=5.62	0.018	2.92	1.18, 7.19
No	43 (81.1%)	28 (59.6%)				
>1 antipsychotic						
Yes	31 (58.5%)	43 (91.5%)	χ^2=14.1	<0.001	7.63	2.39, 24.4
No	22 (41.5%)	4 (8.5%)				
Mood stabilizer						
Yes	9 (17%)	19 (40.4%)	χ^2=6.79	0.009	3.32	1.3, 8.36
No	44 (83%)	28 (59.6%)				

Abbreviation: *CPZ-eq* chlorpromazine equivalents

and gynecomastia compared to those on lower doses (p=0.03). Prescription of higher doses of antipsychotics was more likely associated with mood stabilizers use (p=0.009). High dose antipsychotic use was associated with prescription of long acting antipsychotics (p=0.017) and antipsychotic polypharmacy compared to those patients receiving low dose antipsychotic (p<0.001).

In terms of administration of concomitant psychotropic medications, mood stabilizer use was less likely to be associated with antidepressant use (p=0.025) but more likely to be associated with use of higher dose of antipsychotics (p=0.009). Patients receiving anticholinergics were more likely to be associated with prescription of long acting antipsychotics (p=0.002) but less likely associated with use of SGA (p=0.019).

5.5 Discussion

There were several main findings in this study. First, long acting antipsychotic use was associated with greater likelihood of antipsychotic polypharmacy and anticholinergic use, older age, less likelihood of SGA use and use of higher dosages of antipsychotics. Second, antipsychotic polypharmacy was associated with prescription of long acting antipsychotic, FGA use, higher dosages of antipsychotics used and lower BPRS scores. Third, FGA prescription was associated with older age, higher antipsychotic dosage, polypharmacy and verbal aggression. Fourth, SGA prescription was associated with younger age, less likelihood of anticholinergic and long acting antipsychotic use.

A previous study across six East Asian countries which examined the prevalence of depot antipsychotic use and its clinical correlates concluded that there was a wide variation in the prevalence of depot antipsychotic prescription and suggested that these practices may be less guided by specific psychopharmacological principles and more determined by local traditions and prescription culture [26]. Clinicians' attitudes and knowledge about antipsychotic long acting antipsychotics are important and can interface and inter-relate with patient factors such as choice, reasoning and stigma in treatment. A cross-sectional study of consultant psychiatrists' attitudes and knowledge towards the prescription of long acting antipsychotics in North West England [27] showed a 50% decrease in long acting antipsychotic prescription despite the findings that most clinicians in the study regarded long acting as being associated with better adherence. It was thought that whilst most of the clinicians' attitudes and knowledge have remained stable, concerns with regards to stigma and patients' acceptance associated with long acting antipsychotic use might influence the type and mode of delivery of particular antipsychotic medication being offered and actually administered to patients.

The association of use of long acting antipsychotics with older age may be related to the fact that the patients had been ill for a longer period of time as it was noted that more than two thirds of the patients in this study had duration of illness of more than 5 years. It was observed that compliance with medication also interact with the chronicity of illness [28]. A review of compliance with maintenance regimens of medical conditions like rheumatic fever prophylaxis, glaucoma, isoniazid for tuberculosis, and self-administered insulin showed a mean non-compliance rate of about 54% [29], which is not too different from that found in patients with psychotic conditions [30, 31]. Clinicians may choose to use long acting antipsychotics in order to achieve stable drug therapeutic levels and thus enhance treatment adherence [2]. It is possible that they have been given FGA first in view of their longer duration of illness or be given more than one medication for stabilization of their symptoms over the years including a depot antipsychotic. Multiple or recurrent relapses secondary to non-compliance might have influenced clinician's decision to start long acting antipsychotics apart from the administration of more than one antipsychotic medication [27].

Patients on depot antipsychotic tend to be given higher dosages of antipsychotics and we found a modest negative correlation between age and daily antipsychotic dose in patients aged 45 years and older. This was in contrast to the study by Mamo [32] who did not find any correlation of age with total daily dose of antipsychotic medication. However, a systemic review of long acting antipsychotic use by Adams [33] showed that long acting antipsychotic is an effective maintenance therapy for schizophrenia, in that standard dose was more effective than placebo thus behooving the need to constantly review effective doses of depot antipsychotic over time following initiation.

The prescription of anticholinergics in patients receiving long acting antipsychotic needs to be better clarified [34]. Studies have shown that there was no convincing evidence that the range, nature or severity of adverse effects reported with depot treatment was significantly different from that seen with oral treatment [35]. Since older patients were more likely to develop extrapyramidal side effects when given an antipsychotic medication, clinicians might have chosen to add an anticholinergic as a prophylaxis to reduce the extrapyramidal side effects and ensure continual acceptance of therapy. Fenton [36] had suggested that in standard clinical settings, the individual patient's acceptance or rejection of the prescribed pharmacological regimens was often the single greatest determinant of the effectiveness of any treatment and adverse effects may lead to diminished acceptance of treatment with antipsychotic medications. Several previous studies have also shown that there was no significant difference in the efficacy of different types of depot antipsychotic [37–39]. Thus the choice of which depot antipsychotic to use must always take into account clinical judgment as well as the preferences of the recipients of care and their caregivers, and providing psycho education about the benefits and rationale for the administration of any depot antipsychotic [40, 41].

As patients with schizophrenia continues to grow older, this raises concerns regarding our choice of use of first generation long acting antipsychotic preparations such as haloperidol decanoate and flupenthixol decanoate, all of which can have side effects like tremor, bradykinesia, unsteadiness, and falls which the elderly are particularly vulnerable. The availability of second generation long acting antipsychotic like risperidone Consta could perhaps offer an alternative solution, in terms of reduction of positive and negative symptoms with minimization of extrapyramidal side-effects [42]. Similar precautions are required for older patients who are started on long acting risperidone injection in terms of monitoring of blood glucose and lipid function [43, 44]. The minimal use of second generation depot antipsychotic in this study could be a result of multiple factors including medication cost, preferences of patients and their caregivers, clinicians' attitudes towards long acting antipsychotic.

Antipsychotic polypharmacy is a prevalent phenomenon [13, 45–49] within clinical practice, with rates ranging from 5 to 18% in outpatient settings and up to 50% in inpatient context [46]. A survey of six Asian countries showed that antipsychotic polypharmacy was found in about half of sample of the patients [13].

Despite guidelines dissuading the practice of polypharmacy, antipsychotic polypharmacy for prolonged periods is not uncommonly observed [20, 50–53]. Current literatures have failed to show superior efficacy for polypharmacy over monotherapy [54–56] and Gardos [17] had suggested that the relative cost of antipsychotic polypharmacy might actually be higher than monotherapy.

In practice, there is a place for rational polypharmacy which is a reflection of the often unsatisfactory outcome of treatment with single antipsychotic [54], which may involve adding an oral antipsychotic to another oral antipsychotic or to a depot antipsychotic which can result in higher overall daily antipsychotic dose as was observed in this study. Interestingly, a study by Ito [49] revealed that polypharmacy and excessive dosing were influenced by the clinicians' skepticism towards the use of algorithms, nurses' requests for more drugs and the patient's clinical condition. Despite clinicians' attitude towards using algorithms and treatment guidelines, a local study by Chong et al. [57] which was conducted on a group of patients with early psychosis showed that the implementation of a treatment algorithm coupled with audit successfully reduced the rate of antipsychotic polypharmacy. The finding of lower BPRS scores may indicate that the symptoms were successfully ameliorated with the treatment regime or that interventions that improve adherence which included associated use of long acting antipsychotics may be effective in the reduction of psychotic symptomatology [35, 58].

Furthermore, diagnostic systems such as DSM-IV and ICD-10 adopt a hierarchical system and view disorders as categorical entities rather than affected domains of thought, speech, affect, behavior along a dimensional spectrum [59]. Thus patients presenting with a mixture of psychotic, affective symptoms or cognitive deficits may need treatment with more than one medication in warranted circumstances [60]. There is also non specificity of the targets of different classes of medications as they treat symptoms which may cut across different diagnostic categories rather than discrete disorders per se. To define what constitutes an adequate psychotropic drug prescription can be a complex task since it entails not only the consideration of clinical factors, pharmacological properties of the medications, past response, drug sensitivities, prescriber experience but also social, economic aspects including healthcare funding and subsidy structures [1]. This complexity probably contributes and interacts with myriad of factors to account for the observed variations in the type and quantities of psychotropic drugs prescribed within different hospitals and in different countries [13]. Most of the patients studied were prescribed two antipsychotics or less (88%) which may include a long acting antipsychotic. Additional psychotropic medication may involve the prescription of antidepressants and mood stabilizers used to treat co-morbid affective symptoms in our patients.

Ultimately, the reasons behind antipsychotic polypharmacy may be complex and comprised of the interplay of various factors including severity of psychopathology, adverse effects, tolerance of adverse effects and response to treatment. Antipsychotic polypharmacy can also occur in the context of cross-titration of two antipsychotic agents [61]. However, clinicians might have stopped cross-titration at the first sign of clinical improvement, with the result of two or more medications being prescribed. In addition, clinicians seeking more rapid responses may attempt antipsychotic polypharmacy with the hope of expediting improvement in their patients despite the understanding by clinicians that optimal responses to antipsychotic monotherapy can often take longer [62]. The pressure of getting patients well in a busy acute psychiatric ward with the increasing need to address the expectations of family members, may influence the prescription habits in order to hasten the recovery of the patient. Polypharmacy using a second antipsychotic might be unnecessary and could add to the cost of treatment. Within the clinical practice guidelines (CPG) from the local Ministry of Health [63], there is now recommendations for the use of lower dosage of antipsychotics for our patients as well as single antipsychotic during treatment as much as possible unless otherwise indicated such as during transitional periods of switching between antipsychotics or during augmentation of clozapine treatment. There is a paucity of studies about the feasibility and efficacy of reducing antipsychotic polypharmacy [64] and future studies may want to look at the utility and safety of these different antipsychotic combinations as well as better ways to reduce unnecessary antipsychotic polypharmacy within naturalistic treatment settings.

An obvious advantage of using FGA may relate to cost burden superficially and FGA are perceived to be associated with greater cost savings when compared with SGA [65–67]. We found that FGA use was associated with older age, higher daily antipsychotic dose, higher rates of polypharmacy and verbal aggression and less likelihood to be prescribed a second generation antipsychotic. Having a longer duration of illness and being in the era when SGA were just appearing in the market during their first break illness and cost considerations might have influenced clinicians' preference to choose FGA as their first line medication then. Paton and his colleague [68] showed that in a group of inpatients who were prescribed antipsychotics, 48% of whom were prescribed more than one medications and large doses of antipsychotics were frequently prescribed 'as required'. The higher doses required may be related to the use of more than one antipsychotic or in response to more intractable symptoms which may include verbal aggression as was found to be associated with FGA use. In this study, there was no significant association between the first generation antipsychotic and anticholinergic use or higher rates of reported extrapyramidal side effects. This is in contrast to a survey of inpatients with schizophrenia which found that anticholinergic use was highest in patients treated with FGA as compared with patients who received SGA or combination of FGA and SGA [69]. There is also data to suggest that antipsychotic polypharmacy can be associated with an increased rate of anticholinergic prescription [34, 70–72].

Although the costs of SGA were higher compared to the FGA, several published economic evaluations suggested that SGA may be more cost-effective compared with the FGA [73, 74]. Second generation antipsychotics are thought to be effective not only in treating positive symptoms but can be useful in treating the negative symptoms [59, 75] or improving the cognitive functioning of patients with schizophrenia [76] with an increasing trend of use worldwide [1, 3, 77, 78]. Our study found that second generation antipsychotic was associated with a younger age, less FGA, depot antipsychotic use and anticholinergic use. Second generation antipsychotics tend to have a lower risk of extrapyramidal side effects (EPS) including tardive dyskinesia compared with FGA [79]. In this regard, a recent review was conducted by the World Psychiatry Association Section on Pharmacopsychiatry which examined approximately 1,600 randomized controlled trials related to antipsychotic treatment and compared the effectiveness of different antipsychotic treatments for schizophrenia [80]. It was reported that despite the relative similar efficacy of antipsychotics in the treatment of positive symptoms, there were substantial differences amongst the first and second generation antipsychotic agents in terms of their propensity to cause extrapyramidal, metabolic and other adverse effects. The SGAs have a lower liability to cause extrapyramidal symptoms and tardive dyskinesia [80] and this could explain why clinicians prefer to use SGA for younger patients. However, clinicians need to be aware about the possible onset of metabolic syndromes especially in younger patients receiving SGA longitudinally [81, 82].

In terms of the dosages of antipsychotics that were observed in this study, low dose antipsychotic use was associated with less disorganized speech, less verbal aggression, absence of hyperprolactinemia related adverse events such as galactorrhea, amenorrhea and gynecomastia, less use of mood stabilizers, less likelihood to be associated with long acting antipsychotic and antipsychotic polypharmacy. A study by Sim et al. [19] noted that over time in Asia, there was a trend of greater prescription of low dose antipsychotic suggesting that conservative dosing of antipsychotics is increasingly prevalent in East Asia, and which may be related to relevant clinical and patient characteristics. The use of high dose of antipsychotic is thought to have little added therapeutic advantage beyond the dose range of 375 mg daily CPZ equivalents [14]. High dose antipsychotic use especially in association with FGA use has an increased rate of adverse events [80, 83]. It was possible that patients receiving lower antipsychotic doses may be less ill as observed by the association with less disorganized speech and verbal aggression or that they denote a group of patients inherently requiring lower antipsychotic dose. Furthermore, there is less need to combine antipsychotics or prescribe another class of psychotropic medications such as mood stabilizers in such instances. The association with oral rather than depot antipsychotic is consistent with earlier data from Asia indicating that those who were not receiving depot antipsychotic drugs had less aggression and lower dose of antipsychotic [26]. In terms of pharmacokinetic and pharmacodynamic profiles, it is possible that our patients may require lower dose of antipsychotics compared with the West. This is supported by earlier data [84–86] which highlighted that Asian patients required significantly lower antipsychotic dose for optimal clinical response as well as the onset of extrapyramidal symptoms.

We found that the majority of the subjects were not given either an antidepressant or mood stabilizer or a combination of both antidepressant and mood stabilizer. The higher percentage of patients on a mood stabilizer without any antidepressant could represent our clinicians' preference in using a mood stabilizer either as an adjunctive medication with the antipsychotic or to help in the management of aggressive behavior in our patients. To date, most data on the augmentation strategies with anticonvulsants except valproic acid were uncontrolled and most reported adverse effects [87]. Our study showed similar findings in that higher dose antipsychotic use was associated with the prescription of mood stabilizer which calls for better rationalization of the different aspects of psychotropic polypharmacy [88]. One possible explanation why anticholinergic use was found to be higher with the use of long-acting antipsychotic could be that the patients were receiving first generation long acting antipsychotic. This was previously shown to be associated with antipsychotic polypharmacy and in higher doses, which could in turn result in greater tendency towards the onset of extrapyramidal side effects. A study in Hong Kong which looked at the clinical and social determinants of prescribing anticholinergic medication for Chinese patients with schizophrenia showed that anticholinergic use was associated with higher doses of antipsychotics and less frequent use of SGA [89]. While socio-cultural and economical factors as well as traditions of psychiatric practice were also important factors in determining the use of anticholinergic medication [89], the protracted use of anticholinergic medication is not without long term complications. A previous study [90] observed that long-term prophylactic administration of anticholinergic medication may be unnecessary in the treatment of the majority of Chinese patients with chronic schizophrenia and that anticholinergic withdrawal can be accomplished without adverse mental or motor effects.

Additionally, clozapine use was found to be low (7%) in this study. Clozapine has been proven to be efficacious and could even reduce antipsychotic polypharmacy [75, 80, 91]. While most treatment guidelines advocated the use clozapine [20, 50, 52, 53] in patients who are treatment resistant, many clinicians may be still hesitant about the initiation of treatment with clozapine. One major reason may relate to the tedious blood monitoring which may not be tolerated or preferred by some patients or their family members and the concern about its impact on adherence with regular reviews and hematological monitoring. Most official guidelines on recommendations of the use of psychotropic drugs are mainly based on randomized controlled trial findings under pristine controlled conditions, while prescribing practices principally occur on the at the clinics and wards and must take into consideration factors such as efficacy, effectiveness of antipsychotic agent in patients with often comorbid conditions, as well as tolerability and cost [4]. It is known that differences do exist between the conditions of pre-marketing clinical trials and those of the actual practice several years into the market life of a pharmaceutical product [7]. In pre-marketing clinical trial, a small sample of people was selected from the source population by inclusion and non-inclusion criteria in order to reduce inter-individual variability. These people are usually treated with a fixed protocol, specifying dosage, duration and concomitant medications [8]. In actual clinical practice, however, clinicians may accept different indications for therapy (off-label use) and often use drugs in populations that often deviate from those studied in pre- or post-marketing trials. Thus considerations for rational prescribing practices including antipsychotic polypharmacy would have to balance evidence base medicine principles with treatment based evidence on the ground.

There are several limitations in this study. First, the number of subjects surveyed is small compared with some of the other studies. This is part of a larger international study and the Singapore portion limits itself to examining the prescription patterns of inpatients with schizophrenia and in this case within a tertiary psychiatric centre, and may not be generalizable to all patients with schizophrenia including those in the community or who are not hospitalized. Second, one can understand association but not attribute causality in cross sectional studies such as in this study. Third, the fact that these subjects were recruited from a tertiary specialist centre might have represented a more ill group as compared to the psychiatric patients from other general hospitals or the community in Singapore, thus this must be borne in mind when generalizing the findings to patients in other contexts. Third, we did not investigate related pharmaco-economic factors as these elements would be relevant and can interact with clinical considerations in influencing prescription practices.

Fourth, we start with cross sectional observations and would extend these observations prospectively in the future to better understand psychotropic prescription patterns in our local context and in appreciating how these trends may change over time [92].

5.6 Conclusions and Future Directions

There is a need for appropriate rationalization of psychotropic drug prescription based on evidence as well as practical considerations. We found that antipsychotic polypharmacy is not uncommon and patients were more likely to receive first generation antipsychotics as well as higher dosages of antipsychotic. Patients who were given long acting antipsychotic received higher antipsychotic dosages, were less likely to be on second generation antipsychotic and had a greater likelihood of antipsychotic polypharmacy and anticholinergic use. First generation antipsychotic prescription was associated with older age, higher antipsychotic dosage, polypharmacy and verbal aggression. Patients who received SGA were younger and were less likely to receive long acting antipsychotic and anticholinergics. Future studies may want to focus on examining out-patient psychotropic prescribing patterns and trends over time. Although trends such as antipsychotic polypharmacy may stay with the treatment of often highly complex cases of schizophrenia with other co-morbidities within tertiary hospital settings, further studies are needed to understand changes in prescribing patterns and how they relate to extant recommendations or guidelines based on evidence based medicine principles.

Acknowledgements We would like to thank all the patients who participated in the study as well as all the hospital staff that supported this project.

References

1. Bitter I, Chou JC, Ungvari GS et al (2003) Prescribing for inpatients with schizophrenia: an international multi-center comparative study. Pharmacopsychiatry 36(4):143–149
2. Kane JM, Leucht S, Carpenter D et al (2003) The expert consensus guideline series. Optimizing pharmacologic treatment of psychotic disorders. Introduction: methods, commentary, and summary. J Clin Psychiatry 64(Suppl 12):5–19
3. Suarez D, Haro JM (2008) Overview of the findings from the European SOHO study. Expert Rev Neurother 8(6):873–880
4. Parish PA (1973) Drug prescribing – the concern of all. R Soc Health J 93(4):213–217
5. Hemminki E (1975) Review of literature on the factors affecting drug prescribing. Soc Sci Med 9(2):111–116
6. Parish PA (1973) What influences have led to increased prescribing of psychotropic drugs? J R Coll Gen Pract 23(Suppl 2):49–58
7. Martin K, Begaud B, Latry P et al (2004) Differences between clinical trials and postmarketing use. Br J Clin Pharmacol 57(1):86–92
8. Verdoux H, Tournier M, Cougnard A et al (2006) Pharmacoepidemiology of psychotropic medication: utilisation and impact in real-life conditions. Therapie 61(1):17–22

9. Kane JM, Freeman HL (1994) Towards more effective antipsychotic treatment. Br J Psychiatry Suppl 25:22–31
10. Committee WE (1977) The selection of essential drugs (Technical report series 615). World Health Organization, Geneva
11. Bowers L, Callaghan P, Clark N et al (2004) Comparisons of psychotropic drug prescribing patterns in acute psychiatric wards across Europe. Eur J Clin Pharmacol 60(1):29–35
12. Rothbard AB, Kuno E, Foley K (2003) Trends in the rate and type of antipsychotic medications prescribed to persons with schizophrenia. Schizophr Bull 29(3):531–540
13. Sim K, Su A, Fujii S et al (2004) Antipsychotic polypharmacy in patients with schizophrenia: a multicentre comparative study in East Asia. Br J Clin Pharmacol 58(2):178–183
14. Bollini P, Pampallona S, Orza MJ et al (1994) Antipsychotic drugs: is more worse? A meta-analysis of the published randomized control trials. Psychol Med 24(2):307–316
15. Faries D, Ascher-Svanum H, Zhu B et al (2005) Antipsychotic monotherapy and polypharmacy in the naturalistic treatment of schizophrenia with atypical antipsychotics. BMC Psychiatry 5:26
16. Freudenreich O, Goff DC (2002) Antipsychotic combination therapy in schizophrenia. A review of efficacy and risks of current combinations. Acta Psychiatr Scand 106(5):323–330
17. Gardos G (2005) Antipsychotic polypharmacy or monotherapy? Neuropsychopharmacol Hung 7(2):72–77
18. Sim K, Su A, Chan YH et al (2004) Clinical correlates of antipsychotic polytherapy in patients with schizophrenia in Singapore. Psychiatry Clin Neurosci 58(3):324–329
19. Sim K, Su HC, Fujii S (2009) Low doses of antipsychotic drugs for hospitalized schizophrenia patients in East Asia: 2004 vs. 2001. Int J Neuropsychopharmacol 12(1):117–123
20. American Psychiatric Association (2004) Practice guidelines for the treatment of patients with schizophrenia, Secondth edn. American Psychiatric Press, Washington, DC
21. Inagaki A (1999) Equivalent doses of psychotropics. Seiwa Shoten, Tokyo
22. Overall JE (1962) The brief psychiatric rating scale. Psychol Rep 10:799–812
23. Buchanan RW, Kreyenbuhl J, Zito JM et al (2002) The schizophrenia PORT pharmacological treatment recommendations: conformance and implications for symptoms and functional outcome. Schizophr Bull 28(1):63–73
24. Lehman AF, Steinwachs DM (1998) Patterns of usual care for schizophrenia: initial results from the schizophrenia patient outcomes research team (PORT) client survey. Schizophr Bull 24(1):11–20, discussion 20–32
25. Lehman AF, Steinwachs DM (1998) Translating research into practice: the Schizophrenia Patient Outcomes Research Team (PORT) treatment recommendations. Schizophr Bull 24(1):1–10
26. Sim K, Su A, Ungvari GS et al (2004) Depot antipsychotic use in schizophrenia: an East Asian perspective. Hum Psychopharmacol 19(2):103–109
27. Patel MX, Haddad PM, Chaudhry IB et al (2010) Psychiatrists' use, knowledge and attitudes to first- and second-generation antipsychotic long-acting injections: comparisons over 5 years. J Psychopharmacol 24(10):1473–1482
28. Blackwell B (1973) Drug therapy: patient compliance. N Engl J Med 289(5):249–252
29. Sacket DL (1978) Patients and therapies: getting the two together. N Engl J Med 298(5): 278–279
30. Hogan TP, Awad AG, Eastwood R (1983) A self-report scale predictive of drug compliance in schizophrenics: reliability and discriminative validity. Psychol Med 13(1):177–183
31. Awad AG, Voruganti LN (2004) New antipsychotics, compliance, quality of life, and subjective tolerability – are patients better off? Can J Psychiatry 49(5):297–302
32. Mamo DC, Sweet RA, Chengappa KN et al (2002) The effect of age on the pharmacological management of ambulatory patients treated with depot neuroleptic medications for schizophrenia and related psychotic disorders. Int J Geriatr Psychiatry 17(11):1012–1017
33. Adams CE, Fenton MK, Quraishi S et al (2001) Systematic meta-review of depot antipsychotic drugs for people with schizophrenia. Br J Psychiatry 179:290–299

34. Chong SA, Sachdev P, Mahendran R et al (2000) Neuroleptic and anticholinergic drug use in Chinese patients with schizophrenia resident in a state psychiatric hospital in Singapore. Aust N Z J Psychiatry 34(6):988–991
35. Barnes TR, Curson DA (1994) Long-term depot antipsychotics. A risk-benefit assessment. Drug Saf 10(6):464–479
36. Fenton WS, Blyler CR, Heinssen RK (1997) Determinants of medication compliance in schizophrenia: empirical and clinical findings. Schizophr Bull 23(4):637–651
37. Coutinho E, Fenton M, Quraishi S (2009) Zuclopenthixol decanoate for schizophrenia and other serious mental illnesses. Cochrane Database Syst Rev 2000(2):CD001164
38. Kane JM (2006) Utilization of long-acting antipsychotic medication in patient care. CNS Spectr 11(12 Suppl 14):1–7, quiz 7–8
39. Messer T, Glaser T, Landen H et al (2009) Long-term treatment with flupentixol results of a post-marketing surveillance study. J Psychopharmacol 23(7):805–813
40. Patel MX, De Zoysa N, Bernadt M et al (2009) Depot and oral antipsychotics: patient preferences and attitudes are not the same thing. J Psychopharmacol 23(7):789–796
41. Patel MX, de Zoysa N, Bernadt M et al (2008) A cross-sectional study of patients' perspectives on adherence to antipsychotic medication: depot versus oral. J Clin Psychiatry 69(10): 1548–1556
42. Masand PS, Gupta S (2003) Long-acting injectable antipsychotics in the elderly: guidelines for effective use. Drugs Aging 20(15):1099–1110
43. Lasser RA, Bossie C, Gharabawi G et al (2004) Patients with schizophrenia previously stabilized on conventional depot antipsychotics experience significant clinical improvements following treatment with long-acting risperidone. Eur Psychiatry 19(4):219–225
44. Singh D, O'Connor DW (2007) Depot risperidone in elderly patients: the experience of an Australian aged psychiatry service. Int Psychogeriatr 19(4):789–792
45. Messer T, Tiltscher C, Schmauss M (2006) Polypharmacy in the treatment of schizophrenia. Fortschr Neurol Psychiatr 74(7):377–391
46. Lerma-Carrillo I, de Pablo Bruhlmann S, del Pozo ML et al (2008) Antipsychotic polypharmacy in patients with schizophrenia in a brief hospitalization unit. Clin Neuropharmacol 31(6):319–332
47. Kreyenbuhl JA, Valenstein M, McCarthy JF et al (2007) Long-term antipsychotic polypharmacy in the VA health system: patient characteristics and treatment patterns. Psychiatr Serv 58(4):489–495
48. Jaffe AB, Levine J (2003) Antipsychotic medication co prescribing in a large state hospital system. Pharmacoepidemiol Drug Saf 12(1):41–48
49. Ito H, Koyama A, Higuchi T (2005) Polypharmacy and excessive dosing: psychiatrists' perceptions of antipsychotic drug prescription. Br J Psychiatry 187:243–247
50. (1999) The expert consensus guideline series. Treatment of schizophrenia. J Clin Psychiatry 60(Suppl 11): 3–80
51. Lehman AF, Steinwachs DM (2003) Evidence-based psychosocial treatment practices in schizophrenia: lessons from the patient outcomes research team (PORT) project. J Am Acad Psychoanal Dyn Psychiatry 31(1):141–154
52. Miller AL, Chiles JA, Chiles JK et al (1999) The Texas Medication Algorithm Project (TMAP) schizophrenia algorithms. J Clin Psychiatry 60(10):649–657
53. National Institute for Clinical Excellence (2002) Guidance on the use of newer (atypical) antipsychotic drugs for the treatment of Schizophrenia. Technology appraisal guidance. National Institute for Clinical Excellence, London
54. Goodwin G, Fleischhacker W, Arango C et al (2009) Advantages and disadvantages of combination treatment with antipsychotics ECNP Consensus Meeting, March 2008, Nice. Eur Neuropsychopharmacol 19(7):520–532
55. Goren JL, Parks JJ, Ghinassi FA et al (2008) When is antipsychotic polypharmacy supported by research evidence? Implications for QI. Jt Comm J Qual Patient Saf 34(10):571–582

56. Glick ID, Pham D, Davis JM (2006) Concomitant medications may not improve outcome of antipsychotic monotherapy for stabilized patients with nonacute schizophrenia. J Clin Psychiatry 67(8):1261–1265
57. Chong SA, Ravichandran N, Poon LY et al (2006) Reducing polypharmacy through the introduction of a treatment algorithm: use of a treatment algorithm on the impact on polypharmacy. Ann Acad Med Singapore 35(7):457–460
58. Kane JM (2006) Review of treatments that can ameliorate nonadherence in patients with schizophrenia. J Clin Psychiatry 67(Suppl 5):9–14
59. Kendell R, Jablensky A (2003) Distinguishing between the validity and utility of psychiatric diagnoses. Am J Psychiatry 160(1):4–12
60. Rittmannsberger H (2002) The use of drug monotherapy in psychiatric inpatient treatment. Prog Neuropsychopharmacol Biol Psychiatry 26(3):547–551
61. Stahl SM (1999) Antipsychotic polypharmacy, part 2: tips on use and misuse. J Clin Psychiatry 60(8):506–507
62. Lieberman JA, Koreen AR, Chakos M et al (1996) Factors influencing treatment response and outcome of first-episode schizophrenia: implications for understanding the pathophysiology of schizophrenia. J Clin Psychiatry 57(Suppl 9):5–9
63. Ministry of Health (2011) Clinical practice guidelines: schizophrenia. Ministry of Health, Singapore
64. Tranulis C, Skalli L, Lalonde P et al (2008) Benefits and risks of antipsychotic polypharmacy: an evidence-based review of the literature. Drug Saf 31(1):7–20
65. Davies L, Lewis S (2000) Antipsychotic medication for people with schizophrenia: an exploratory economic analysis of alternative treatment algorithms. University of York, Centre for Health Economics, York
66. Bagnall A-M, Jones L, Ginnelly L et al (2003) A systematic review of atypical antipsychotic drugs in schizophrenia. Health Technol Assess 7(13):1–193
67. Davies LM, Jones PB, Barnes TRE et al (2007) Cost-effectiveness of first- v. second-generation antipsychotic drugs: results from a randomised controlled trial in schizophrenia responding poorly to previous therapy. Br J Psychiatry 191:14–22
68. Paton C, Lelliott P, Harrington M et al (2003) Patterns of antipsychotic and anticholinergic prescribing for hospital inpatients. J Psychopharmacol 17(2):223–229
69. De Hert M, Wampers M, van Winkel R et al (2007) Anticholinergic use in hospitalised schizophrenic patients in Belgium. Psychiatry Res 152(2–3):165–172
70. Acquaviva E, Gasquet I, Falissard B (2007) Antipsychotics dosage and antiparkinsonian prescriptions. Clin Pract Epidemiol Ment Health 3:14
71. Clark RE, Bartels SJ, Mellman TA et al (2002) Recent trends in antipsychotic combination therapy of schizophrenia and schizoaffective disorder: implications for state mental health policy. Schizophr Bull 28(1):75–84
72. Magliano L, Fiorillo A, Guarneri M et al (2004) Prescription of psychotropic drugs to patients with schizophrenia: an Italian national survey. Eur J Clin Pharmacol 60(7):513–522
73. Almond S, O'Donnell O (2000) Cost analysis of the treatment of schizophrenia in the UK. A simulation model comparing olanzapine, risperidone and haloperidol. Pharmacoeconomics 17(4):383–389
74. Lewis M, McCrone P, Frangou S (2001) Service use and costs of treating schizophrenia with atypical antipsychotics. J Clin Psychiatry 62(10):749–756
75. Lieberman JA, Stroup TS, McEvoy JP et al (2005) Effectiveness of antipsychotic drugs in patients with chronic schizophrenia. N Engl J Med 353(12):1209–1223
76. Keefe RS, Silva SG, Perkins DO et al (1999) The effects of atypical antipsychotic drugs on neurocognitive impairment in schizophrenia: a review and meta-analysis. Schizophr Bull 25(2):201–222
77. Weissman EM (2002) Antipsychotic prescribing practices in the veterans healthcare administration–New York metropolitan region. Schizophr Bull 28(1):31–42

78. Bret P, Bret MC, Queuille E (2009) Prescribing patterns of antipsychotics in 13 French psychiatric hospitals. Encéphale 35(2):129–138
79. Lieberman JA III (2004) Managing anticholinergic side effects. Prim Care Companion J Clin Psychiatry 6(Suppl 2):20–23
80. Tandon R, Belmaker RH, Gattaz WF et al (2008) World Psychiatric Association Pharmacopsychiatry Section statement on comparative effectiveness of antipsychotics in the treatment of schizophrenia. Schizophr Res 100(1–3):20–38
81. Lieberman JA III (2004) Metabolic changes associated with antipsychotic use. Prim Care Companion J Clin Psychiatry 6(Suppl 2):8–13
82. Baptista T, Kin NM, Beaulieu S et al (2002) Obesity and related metabolic abnormalities during antipsychotic drug administration: mechanisms, management and research perspectives. Pharmacopsychiatry 35(6):205–219
83. Tandon R (2006) Comparing antipsychotic efficacy. Am J Psychiatry 163(9):1645
84. Lin KM, Finder E (1983) Neuroleptic dosage for Asians. Am J Psychiatry 140(4):490–491
85. Lin KM, Poland RE, Nuccio I et al (1989) A longitudinal assessment of haloperidol doses and serum concentrations in Asian and Caucasian schizophrenic patients. Am J Psychiatry 146(10):1307–1311
86. Lin KM, Shen WW (1991) Pharmacotherapy for southeast Asian psychiatric patients. J Nerv Ment Dis 179(6):346–350
87. Stahl SM, Grady MM (2004) A critical review of atypical antipsychotic utilization: comparing monotherapy with polypharmacy and augmentation. Curr Med Chem 11(3):313–327
88. Chen H, Kennedy WK, Dorfman JH et al (2007) The effect of adjunctive mood stabilizers on antipsychotic utilization pattern and health resource utilization for Medicaid enrollees with schizophrenia. Curr Med Res Opin 23(6):1351–1365
89. Xiang YT, Weng YZ, Leung CM et al (2007) Exploring the clinical and social determinants of prescribing anticholinergic medication for Chinese patients with schizophrenia. Hum Psychopharmacol 22(3):173–180
90. Ungvari GS, Chiu HF, Lam LC et al (1999) Gradual withdrawal of long-term anticholinergic antiparkinson medication in Chinese patients with chronic schizophrenia. J Clin Psychopharmacol 19(2):141–148
91. Jones PB, Barnes TR, Davies L et al (2006) Randomized controlled trial of the effect on quality of life of second- vs first-generation antipsychotic drugs in schizophrenia: Cost Utility of the Latest Antipsychotic Drugs in Schizophrenia Study (CUtLASS 1). Arch Gen Psychiatry 63(10):1079–1087
92. Gilbody S, Wahlbeck K, Adams C (2002) Randomized controlled trials in schizophrenia: a critical perspective on the literature. Acta Psychiatr Scand 105(4):243–251

Chapter 6
Antipsychotic Polypharmacy in Schizophrenia. How to Counteract This Common Practice?

Takefumi Suzuki, Hiroyuki Uchida, Koichiro Watanabe, and Masaru Mimura

Abstract Antipsychotic polypharmacy (using multiple antipsychotics simultaneously) in schizophrenia appears to be a common practice in the real world. However, it has been a practice with substantial debate for its possible pros and cons. In this section, we systematically review clinical evidence on antipsychotic polypharmacy in schizophrenia. We first focus on the prevalence of antipsychotic polypharmacy in schizophrenia in the real-world clinical settings, to highlight the fact that it is becoming a frequent reality. Next, we discuss potential mechanisms that lead to such a controversial practice. Then, meta-analyses and systematic reviews that addressed the usefulness of antipsychotic polypharmacy in schizophrenia are qualitatively assessed.

The results of this critical appraisal on the currently available evidence indicate that usefulness of antipsychotic polypharmacy in schizophrenia has been a focus of extensive research. However, there are practically too many possible combinations to be evaluated with each antipsychotic dosage also in mind. Evidence on antipsychotic polypharmacy currently remains equivocal at best even for polypharmacy involving clozapine; it is all the more questionable for other mode of antipsychotic combination therapy. Moreover, there has been no study that evaluated antipsychotic polypharmacy in reference with other various augmentation strategies that may potentially be effective.

T. Suzuki, M.D., Ph.D. (✉)
Department of Neuropsychiatry, Keio University School of Medicine, Tokyo, Japan

Inokashira Hospital, Tokyo, Japan
e-mail: takefumi@oak.dti.ne.jp

H. Uchida, M.D., Ph.D. • M. Mimura, M.D., Ph.D.
Department of Neuropsychiatry, Keio University School of Medicine, Tokyo, Japan
e-mail: mcn41320@biglobe.ne.jp; mimura@a7.keio.jp

K. Watanabe, M.D., Ph.D.
Department of Neuropsychiatry, Kyorin University School of Medicine, Tokyo, Japan
e-mail: koichiro@tke.att.ne.jp

M.S. Ritsner (ed.), *Polypharmacy in Psychiatry Practice, Volume II: Use of Polypharmacy in the "Real World"*, DOI 10.1007/978-94-007-5799-8_6,

While a possibility cannot be denied for clinical usefulness of some mode of antipsychotic combination therapy in schizophrenia in general (e.g., combining prolactin-raising or metabolically problematic antipsychotics with more benign agents) or on an individual basis (i.e., for treatment-resistant schizophrenia), the currently available evidence supports the notion that prescribers should remain very conservative in resorting to antipsychotic polypharmacy. In other words, physicians should keep in mind the very basic of pharmacotherapy in every field of medicine; medications should be simple at least at early stages of treatment unless evidence unequivocally points to the contrary.

An effort will be made to synthesize the currently available evidence to be translated into future directions on this critically relevant topic. Further, potential strategies to counteract antipsychotic polypharmacy in schizophrenia are discussed in detail. More work is clearly indicated for this important issue that will remain a matter of hot debate for the years to come.

Abbreviations

BPRS	Brief Psychiatric Rating Scale
CGI	Clinical Global Impression
EPS	Extrapyramidal symptoms
FGAs	First-generation antipsychotics
GAF	Global Assessment of Functioning
PANSS	Positive and Negative Syndrome Scale
SGAs	Second-generation antipsychotics
TRS	Treatment resistant schizophrenia

6.1 Introduction

The basic rule of antipsychotic treatment in schizophrenia is to use a single medication at the lowest possible dose. However, many patients remain unresponsive to a series of trials with the currently available antipsychotic agents [1]. In the treatment guidelines, a trial of clozapine, the gold standard antipsychotic for treatment resistant schizophrenia (TRS), is recommended after a failure to respond to at least two trials with different antipsychotics at an adequate dosage for an adequate duration [2, 3]. Still, a sizeable proportion of patients remain refractory to clozapine, and there has been no consensus on how best to treat these difficult patients.

One strategy in an effort to derive better response may include a usage of antipsychotic polypharmacy in which multiple antipsychotics are administered simultaneously. Nonetheless, antipsychotic polypharmacy appears to have been resorted to too frequently without compelling evidence, and potential risks are not negligible. In this chapter, we review the prevalence of antipsychotic polypharmacy in the real-world clinical settings, and critically appraise previous studies of antipsychotic polypharmacy in schizophrenia. We then go on to evaluate strategies to counteract antipsychotic polypharmacy and finally present future directions regarding this common but highly controversial practice.

While the use of multiple psychotropic medications in schizophrenia may at times be effective and represents another pertinent but debatable topic (based on a hypothetical notion that such combination of agents with different psychopharmacological mechanisms of action could be effective), we do not discuss augmentation of antipsychotics with other psychotropics (or psychotropic polypharmacy) in detail in this manuscript.

6.2 How Prevalent Is Antipsychotic Polypharmacy in the Real-World?

A PubMed search was conducted using the keyword "antipsychotic polypharmacy" to identify reports on the prevalence of antipsychotic polypharmacy that was supplemented with cross-referencing of the identified articles published during the previous 4 years (2008–2011). The results are summarized in Table 6.1.

As is clearly seen, the rate of antipsychotic polypharmacy has been staying high across countries (from 8.1% to as frequent as 79%) [4–29]. Recent prescription data indicate a remarkable predominance of second-generation antipsychotics (SGAs) over first-generation antipsychotics (FGAs), which appears to reflect treatment recommendations. However, some recent evidence form large-scale pragmatic trials casts some doubts regarding a relative superiority of SGAs over FGAs [30, 31], and such a skepticism might be translated into the fact that a recent prescription survey from Canada showed an increase in the rate of recommendation for FGAs that was larger than SGAs [32].

The most significant limitation of these reports on the prevalence of antipsychotic polypharmacy lies in the fact that they are mostly cross-sectional or retrospective. This makes it difficult to shed light on a dynamic process of prospective antipsychotic switching versus an ongoing augmentation, although some studies defined a specific period in an effort to filter out transient cases of polypharmacy. For instance, Procyshyn et al. [14] used a cutoff of 90 days or more, Ahn et al. [22] 60 days, and Nielsen et al. [13] 4 months. Further, some studies [10] investigated the prevalence over multiple timelines, but data on the same original cohort at different timelines have been rarely found [20]. Another major issue is a limited sample size, raising a concern on the representativeness of the study sample. A lack of information on the actual status of the patients, such as illness severity, psychopathology and functioning, poses another problem that needs to be addressed. Information on cost-effectiveness is generally lacking.

In this context, several findings are worthy of comment. First, the use of polypharmacy has been understandably associated with increased antipsychotic dosage in at least some of the studies [10, 14, 16, 19]. This is highly relevant in light of

Table 6.1 Prevalence of antipsychotic polypharmacy in studies published over the last 4 years (2008–2011)

References	Country	Study sample	Rate of polypharmacy	Comments
Bolstad et al.[4]	Norway	329 patients with schizophrenia	30.7%	Cross-sectional study. Increasing number of hospital admissions (strongest predictor), low GAF scores and high PANSS scores were significantly associated with APP. 92.7% received SGAs and 7.3% FGAs.
Dolder and McKinsey [5]	USA	416 patients admitted to an inpatient geriatric psychiatry ward	12.5% (at admission); 7.9% (at discharge)	Retrospective study. Mean age 74.8 ± 9.7 y.o., dementia 73.1%, schizophrenia 18.5%. Patients residing in an assisted facility and with a severe mental illness were significantly more likely to receive APP.
Li et al. [6]	USA	1,898 office-based visits for antipsychotic prescription	8.9% (weighted estimate)	Cross-sectional study. Obese patients were less likely to receive antipsychotics with high or medium risk of causing metabolic abnormalities, but having preexisting metabolic conditions had little effect on drug choice.
Misawa et al. [7]	Japan	334 outpatients with schizophrenia, schizotypal or delusional disorders	50.0%	Cross-sectional survey. Pre-metabolic syndrome was significantly associated with APP (adjusted OR: 2.348; 95% CI: 1.181–4.668), but metabolic syndrome was not.
Santone et al. [8]	Italy	1,022 psychiatric patients to be discharged from acute inpatient facilities (schizophrenia n = 468)	32.6%	SGAs + FGAs: 178/333 cases; FGAs + FGAs: 80/333 cases. Patients with schizophrenia and poorer insight into illness at admission were significantly more likely to receive APP.
Wu et al. [9]	Taiwan	3,690 patients with schizophrenia	40.1%	The rate was 20.7% for benzodiazepine nonusers, 40.3% for short-term users and 48.0% for long-term users (≥180 days of cumulated prescription in 1 year). One-year prevalence rate of benzodiazepine use was 79.2%.
Xiang et al. [10]	9 Asian countries	6,761 inpatients with schizophrenia (2399/2136/2226 in 2001/2004/2009)	46.8% in 2001; 38.3% in 2004; 43.4% in 2009	Three-point cross-sectional survey. Rate varied from 13.2 to 78.6%. Patients treated with APP were younger, had a higher dose of antipsychotics, had more severe positive and negative symptoms, and were more likely to receive depot and FGAs.

An et al. [11]	China	1,123 inpatients with schizophrenia (605 in 1999; 518 in 2008)	10.7% in 1999; 12% in 2008	Two-point cross-sectional survey. The proportion of patients on mood stabilizers/antidepressants rose from 3.3%/4.3% in 1999 to 18%/9.5% in 2008. Use of electroconvulsive therapy increased from 0.5 to 5.6%, and use of benzodiazepines decreased from 47.8 to 37.6%.
Constantine et al. [12]	USA	51,756 Florida Medicaid enrollees (schizophrenia/schizoaffective disorder n = 19,587)	21.0%	Retrospective longitudinal analysis. The rate in schizophrenia/schioaffective disorder: 24.8–28.5%; in other diagnoses: 9.9–11.2%. The prevalence consistently increased until Florida's APP quality improvement program and then steadily declined.
Nielsen et al. [13]	Denmark	13,600 first-episode schizophrenia patients	33.3–56.2%	Observational cohort study. Long-term (>4 m) APP: 16.7–37.1%. DDD of antipsychotics doubled. Inpatient days decreased and outpatient contacts doubled. Use of antidepressants and antiepiletics increased significantly from 1996 to 2005. Use of SGAs increased and anticholinergics decreased.
Procyshyn et al. [14]	Canada	435 outpatients (schizophrenia n = 164; schizoaffective disorder n = 83)	25.7% (≥90 days)	Cross-sectional study. The rate in schizoaffective disorder: 33.7%; schizophrenia: 31.7%. AAP was associated with higher DDD compared to monotherapy (1.94 ± 0.12 versus 0.94 ± 0.04, $p < 0.005$).
Ramos-Rios et al. [15]	Spain	171 inpatients with schizophrenia	79%	Cross-sectional survey. After controlling for significant variables, APP as well as dose and type of antipsychotics did not significantly influence the mean QTc interval.
Ranceva et al. [16]	UK	196 outpatients (schizophrenia n = 80; bipolar affective disorder n = 37)	17.4%	Cross-sectional study. APP was associated with high-dose antipsychotic prescribing and also with long-term sedative and hypnotic use.

(continued)

Table 6.1 (continued)

References	Country	Study sample	Rate of polypharmacy	Comments
Kroken et al. [17]	Norway	412 patients with schizo phrenia discharged from emergency inpatient treatment (486 discharges)	35.6%	Cross-sectional study. Younger age, previous inpatient treatment in the previous 12 months, and comorbid personality disorder or mental retardation were predictors for APP.
Huang et al. [18]	Taiwan	650 patients with schizophrenia or schizoaffective disorder from community rehabilitation institutions	20.2%	Cross-sectional survey. APP had a marginally significant association with metabolic syndrome (OR: 1.6; 95% CI: 1.0–2.6; $p=0.06$).
McKean and Vella-Brincat [19]	New Zealand	201 inpatients	31%	Cross-sectional survey. The average CPZ equivalent dose for APP was 838 mg, while that for monotherapy was 373 mg ($p<0.0001$).
Wheeler [20]	New Zealand	794 outpatients with schizophrenia and schizoaffective disorder	10.6% (cross-sectionally); 6.2% (of the original sample at 10 months)	Two-step survey. All but two APP cases included an SGA at 10-month survey. The average duration of APP was 35.8 months and CPZ eq. dose was 699 mg/day. 46.9% of APP cases lacked justification while 32.7% were well-justified.
Yu et al. [21]	USA	2,321 pairs of patients with schizophrenia treated with OLZ or QTP (Pennsylvania Medicaid claim database)	9.8%/15.7% (for OLZ/QTP at 3 months); 12.5%/18.6% (at 6 months)	12-month observational study using propensity matching. Patients treated with OLZ were less likely to have APP during the course of treatment compared to those treated with QTP.
Ahn et al. [22]	USA	36,195 California Medicaid enrolees with schizophrenia	8.1% (≥60 days)	Latent class analysis for 1-year follow-up data. 14.8% were adherent, 20.7% partially adherent and 64.5% nonadherent. Patients treated with APP were more likely to be classified into partial adherence group.
Connoly and Taylor [23]	UK	255 inpatients	25.7% (White patients) 31.1% (Black patients)	Cross-sectional study. APP was more likely to be used in Black patients (adjusted OR: 3.05; 95% CI: 1.44–6.46; $p=0.004$) but this was primarily driven by site differences.

Koen et al. [24]	South Africa	510 patients with schizophrenia or schizo-affective disorder	28.6%	Cross-sectional study. Some discrepancies in antipsychotic prescribing patterns were noted within the country.
Lass et al. [25]	Estonia	142 inpatients with schizophrenia, schizotypal or delusional disorders	9.9% (≥3 days)	Retrospective case note review. APP resulted in a total antipsychotic amount exceeding the maximum recommended dose in 2 of 14 cases, while 9 of 142 were treated with such a dose.
Lerma-Carrillo et al. [26]	Spain	209 inpatients to a brief psychiatric unit with schizophrenia or schizo-affective disorder	55.5% (at discharge)	Retrospective chart review. Patients were given a mean of 3.06 psychotropics and 1.61 antipsychotics at discharge. The most prevalent combination was long-acting RIS plus an SGA and AMI was the most frequently used adjunctive antipsychotic.
Pickar et al. [27]	USA	200 outpatients with schizophrenia or schizoaffective disorder	42.5%	Cross-sectional survey. SGA use was far more prevalent than FGA (88% vs. 21.5%). The most frequent drug class combination was an antipsychotic plus an off-label mood stabilizer (25.5% of the sample).
Taylor et al. [28]	UK	400 patients with schizo phrenia or related psychosis newly started on an antipsychotic	35% (AMI); 3% (CLZ); 40% (OLZ); 20% (QTP); 12% (RIS)	Retrospective chart review. CLZ was the least likely to be combined with other agents, while there were no significant differences in coprescription rate among other SGAs. Discontinuation rate was significantly lower for CLZ.
Wheeler et al. [29]	New Zealand	4,742 outpatients with schizophrenia (2,236 in 2000; 2,506 in 2004)	13.6–26.6%	Two-point cross-sectional survey. Monotherapy rates increased slightly (2.7–12.2%) over 4.5 years in various ethnic groups. Use of SGAs including CLZ increased while use of depot and FGAs decreased.

Abbreviations: *AMI* amisulpiride, *APP* antipsychotic polypharmacy, *CI* confidence interval, *CLZ* clozapine, *DDD* defined daily dose, *FGA* first-generation antipsychotic, *GAF* global assessment of functioning, *OLZ* olanzapine, *OR* odds ratio, *PANSS* positive and negative syndrome scale, *QTP* quetiapine, *RIS* risperidone, *SGA* second-generation antipsychotic dose-dependent, problematic adverse effects of antipsychotics. Second, the use of adjunctive psychotropic medications is not so uncommon [9, 11, 26, 27]. This turned out to be true in the real-world despite a lack of unequivocal evidence to support a specific mode of augmentation strategy in schizophrenia [33]. Third, there is some indication that the need to resort to polypharmacy may vary according to the antipsychotics in question [21, 28]. These observations need to be interpreted also in consideration of the findings from many randomized comparative trials of antipsychotics and meta-analyses. Fourth, the use of antipsychotic polypharmacy appears not confined to patients with schizophrenia and/or schizoaffective disorder [6, 12], in spite of an essential absence of evidence on antipsychotic polypharmacy in other psychiatric populations. Fifth, antipsychotic polypharmacy might be associated with metabolic disturbances [7, 18], which is critically pertinent considering the necessity of long-term maintenance treatment in schizophrenia. Sixth, the rate of polypharmacy appears to vary across the countries [10], within the country [24] or according to the ethnicity [23]. Finally, there is a plausible indication that antipsychotic polypharmacy may be more likely utilized for those with more severe illness or challenging presentations [4, 5, 10, 17], while Wheeler on the other hand indicated that about a half of instances of polypharmacy lacked justification [20].

6.3 Why Is Antipsychotic Polypharmacy Becoming Common in the Real-World Clinical Practice?

While the evidence base to support the use of antipsychotic polypharmacy has been far from adequate (see the next section), the rate of use has been staying high (see the previous section) [34]. Some investigations shed light on the cause of polypharmacy. In the Danish study, Baandrup et al. [35] found that treatment settings with low use of antipsychotic polypharmacy were characterized by better knowledge/awareness of local antipsychotic treatment guidelines. Among physicians, these settings were also characterized by an elevated confidence in the guidelines, frequent local educational activities and increased recent involvement in research activities. Among nurses, a perception of overwhelming work-load and time pressure and belief in the benefit of antipsychotic polypharmacy were significantly more prevalent in treatment settings with high use.

According to the study by Correll et al. [36], 44 prescribers reported the use of antipsychotic polypharmacy in $17.0 \pm 10.0\%$ of antipsychotic-treated patients. Cross-titration, failed clozapine trial, evidence from randomized controlled trials and clozapine intolerance were likely to be considered as justifiable instances of antipsychotic polypharmacy. On the other hand, Tsutsumi et al. [37] reported a hasty tendency to move to polypharmacy. Of 208 patients who started antipsychotic monotherapy, 34.1% gave up and moved to antipsychotic switch (27.4%) and/or polypharmacy (17.8%) within 2 years. In a subgroup of 100 patients who started as antipsychotic-free, 2-year prevalence rates of antipsychotic switching and polypharmacy were 27.0 and 18.0%, respectively. In addition, polypharmacy was resorted to after a median of one antipsychotic had been tried for a median of 84 days, implying polypharmacy begins without a series of tenacious monotherapy in this Japanese sample.

Kreyenbuhl et al. [38] explored the reasons for addition of antipsychotic versus switching by surveying 209 psychiatrists and reported that compared with patients whose antipsychotic medications were switched, those treated with antipsychotic polypharmacy were more likely to be female, to have received care from the same psychiatrist for more than 2 years, and to have been recently prescribed an antidepressant. Compared with psychiatrists who switched antipsychotic prescriptions, those who added an antipsychotic reported that the change was less likely to reduce positive symptoms, improve functioning, and prevent hospitalization, indicating that psychiatrists perceive antipsychotic polypharmacy to be a generally ineffective strategy. The finding should also be appreciated in the context of possible adverse consequences of antipsychotic polypharmacy such as increased healthcare costs [39], increased likelihood of receiving various psychotropic [40] and increased risk of diabetes mellitus [41] as well as increased antipsychotic dosage.

6.4 Meta-Analyses and Systematic Reviews of Antipsychotic Polypharmacy in Schizophrenia

Because of a relative abundance of the studies (interested readers are advised to go over the reference list of each meta-analysis in Table 6.2), space limitation and our main focus on counteractions against polypharmacy, this section will briefly comment on usefulness of antipsychotic polypharmacy by taking a "review of meta-analyses" approach [42], while individual studies of interest will be presented for further discussion. An exhaustive review on this topic can also be found elsewhere [43, 44]. Because of a unique standing of clozapine, antipsychotic polypharmacy is dichotomized to one that involves clozapine and not.

6.4.1 Meta-Analyses of Antipsychotic Polypharmacy Involving Clozapine

Table 6.2 lists meta-analyses of the studies on clozapine polypharmacy in schizophrenia.

As is seen, evidence on using another antipsychotic with clozapine has been equivocal overall and the effects appear to be modest at best. Moreover, the quality of included studies and the study number as well as the sample size are usually limited to draw a firm conclusion. Likewise, evidence is scarce to sufficiently evaluate the relative effectiveness of a specific combination of antipsychotics (possibly with

Table 6.2 Meta-analysis of polypharmacy involving clozapine in schizophrenia

References	Comparison	Study sample	Main findings	Comments
Porcelli et al. [45]	CLZ+placebo versus CLZ+RIS	5 DBRCTs (6–16 weeks, n=24–68); 227 patients with schizophrenia or schizoaffective disorder	RIS augmentation of CLZ was not superior to placebo (mean score change in the PANSS or BPRS: z=0.14; p=0.89; I(2): 33%) (meta-regression not performed due to the small number of studies).	6 of 11 studies on this specific combination reported a positive effect. There was some evidence for CLZ augmentation with APZ (5 of 6 positive studies) or AMI (5 of 5 positive studies).
Taylor et al. [46]	CLZ+placebo versus CLZ+8 different antippsychotics	14 DBRCTs (6–16 weeks except for 1 study lasting 24 weeks, n=10–207); 734 patients with schizophrenia	CLZ augmentation with a second antipsychotic resulted in a small benefit over placebo (ES=standardized difference in mean of the PANSS or BPRS scores: –0.239; 95% CI: –0.452 to –0.02); p=0.028; I(2): 40.1%). Meta-regression of the effect of treatment duration on ES showed no relationship.	Updated analysis of Ref. [51]. Which antipsychotic is the best to use with CLZ and longer-term effectiveness as well as safety remain unknown.
Wang et al. [47]	CLZ+placebo versus CLZ+SLP	4 RCTs (8–12 weeks except for 1 study lasting 3 years, n=28–105); 221 patients with schizophrenia	Patients treated with CLZ plus SLP were more likely to show clinically important response (4 trials; RR: 0.56; 95% CI 0.36–0.88; NNT: 8; 95% CI 6–29; I(2): 0%). They also had less incidence of hypersalivation (3 trials; RR: 0.49; 95% CI: 0.29–0.83).	Limited number of studies and suboptimal study quality preclude to draw a firm conclusion on this particular combination.

Barbui et al. [48]	CLZ +/– placebo versus CLZ+5 different antippsychotics	21 RCTs (3–12 weeks except for 2 studies (24 and 96 weeks), n=24–215); 1,291 patients with schizophrenia	14 open studies significantly favored CLZ polypharmacy on mean difference the PANSS or BPRS (random effect SMD: –0.80; 95% CI: –1.14 to –0.46; I(2): 85.1%). However, data from 6 double-blind studies did not show a statistically significant positive effect (SMD: –0.12; 95% CI: –0.57 to 0.32; I(2): 63.1%), making the evidence of polypharmacy modest to absent.	15 of 21 studies were Chinese trials and there were concerns regarding study quality. CLZ dose was comparable in double-blind studies (488 mg vs. 498 mg) but lower among patients allocated to the augmentation arm in open studies (299 mg vs. 488 mg).
Cipriani et al. [49]	CLZ+an antipsy chotic versus CLZ+another antippsychotic	3 RCTs (6–8 weeks, n=28–60); 144 patients with schizophrenia	Methodological quality of the studies was low to allow for meta-analytic approach to draw conclusions.	Which antipsychotic is relatively better (or the best) to use with CLZ remains unknown.
Correll et al. [50]	antipsychotic monotherapy versus polypharmacy	19 RCTs (4–12 weeks except for 3 studies (32, 52 weeks and follow-up up to 152 week), n=17–233); 1,229 p atients with schizophrenia	28 monotherapy and 19 polypharmacy arms. Patients treated with APP were less likely to show inefficacy (as defined by the study) (22 trials; n=1,202; RR: 0.76; 95% CI: 0.63–0.90; p=0.002; NNT: 7; 95% CI: 4–17; p=0.0008; I(2): 78.9%) and all-cause discontinuation (20 trials; n=1052; RR: 0.65; 95% CI: 0.54–0.78; p<0.00001; I(2): 0%).	12 studies involved CLZ (n=701). Various combinations and heterogeneity across the studies make study interpretation complicated.

(continued)

Table 6.2 (continued)

References	Comparison	Study sample	Main findings	Comments
Taylor and Smith [51]	CLZ+placebo versus CLZ+6 different antippsychotics	10 DBRCTs (6–16 weeks, n=10–207); 522 patients with schizophrenia	CLZ polypharmacy showed significant benefit on the PANSS or BPRS scores (mean ES: –0.180; 95% CI: –0.356 to –0.004; I(2): 33.50%), but did not show advantage on withdrawals from trials (RR 1.261; 95% CI: 0.679–2.345; I(2): 0.0%) or on the CGI scores (ES –0.661; 95% CI: –1.475 to 0.151; I(2): 78.23%). Meta-regression analysis showed ES was not associated with study duration.	Various inclusion criteria make study interpretation complicated. ES of polypharmacy was small and its clinical significance equivocal.
Paton et al. [52]	CLZ+placebo versus CLZ plus RIS (n=3) or SLP (n=1)	4 DBRCTs (6–12 weeks, n=28–68); 166 patients with schizophrenia	The 2 studies lasting ≥10 weeks produced an estimate favoring clozapine polypharmacy (response rates (≥20% decrease in the PANSS or BPRS) 42% vs. 9%; mean (weighted) RR: 4.41; 95% CI: 1.38–14.07), whereas the 2 studies of <10 weeks' duration did not (26% vs. 27%; RR: 0.59; 95% CI: 0.27–1.30).	In 5 open studies of ≥10 weeks' duration, response rates ranged from 50 to 78%. Of 3 open studies lasting <10 weeks, 2 did not report any responders whereas 83% responded in one study (n=6–33).

Also see Table 6.1 for abbreviations: *APZ* aripiprazole, *BPRS* brief psychiatric rating scale, *DBRCT* double-blind randomized controlled trial, *ES* effect size, *NNT* number needed to treat, *RCT* randomized controlled trial, *RR* relative risk, *SLP* sulpiride, *SMD* standardized mean difference an exception of risperidone for which polypharmacy with clozapine is not reported to yield a differential compared to placebo [45]), and "clozapine plus antipsychotic X versus clozapine plus antipsychotic Y" approach has been surprisingly rare [49, 53]. Further, study duration is frequently too short to evaluate long-term effectiveness or safety. Finally, the use of blood clozapine levels for optimal dose titration and the duration of clozapine pretreatment before resorting to polypharmacy are frequently unclear although both perspectives are highly critical in optimizing response to clozapine [54].

6.4.2 *Systematic Reviews of Antipsychotic Polypharmacy Not Involving Clozapine*

In contrast to clozapine polypharmacy in the previous part, studies on antipsychotic polypharmacy not involving clozapine have been rather limited both in the number and the scope. In fact, dominance of case reports/series and retrospective reports renders meta-analytic approach difficult [43, 55, 56]. This lack of systematic studies translates into an essential absence of a specific recommendation in the guidelines regarding antipsychotic polypharmacy not involving clozapine. In other words, clozapine is usually considered as the third-line antipsychotic. When clozapine is ineffective, augmentation of clozapine is generally indicated, until which stage the flow of antipsychotic treatment in the guideline appears relatively straightforward [2]. However, there has been eventually no good evidence on what to do after an augmentation strategy of clozapine fails. Further, the fact is although sequential antipsychotic trials are recommended [2], only few studies systematically evaluated antipsychotic polypharmacy after failure to respond to a series of monotherapy trials [1, 57].

6.4.3 *Possibility of Rational Antipsychotic Polypharmacy?*

Although the evidence on antipsychotic polypharmacy has been equivocal and only modest at best, this does not rule out a possibility that some individual patients will only preferentially respond to polypharmacy in some instances of TRS. In other cases, adverse events of some specific antipsychotics may be diminished by concomitantly taking the second antipsychotic. For example, there have been some studies on clozapine and aripiprazole polypharmacy. Henderson et al. [58] noted a significant improvement in weight, total cholesterol and triglyceride in ten patients. Ziegenbein et al. [59] reported on 11 patients and there was a 63.6% decrease in the Brief Psychiatric Rating Scale (BPRS) score in 7 patients. Karunakaran et al. [60] also reported on favorable changes in symptoms, functioning, weight and HDL cholesterol among 24 patients.

Chang et al. [61] conducted a double-blind study (n=62, 8 weeks) and found that prolactin and triglyceride levels were significantly lower and improvements in the BPRS negative subscale were better with aripiprazole combination therapy. Fleischhacker et al. [62] conducted a large double-blind study (n=207, 16 weeks with 12-week extension) and reported favorable changes in body mass index, waist circumference, and total as well as LDL cholesterol. Finally, in the recent double-blind study by Muscatello et al. [63], there were improvements in symptoms but not in cognition with polypharmacy (n=40, 31 evaluable, 24 weeks).

In these instances of clozapine plus aripiprazole polypharmacy, the rationale and the motivation appear relatively simple; weight gain and metabolic disturbances are well-known notorious adverse effects of clozapine while aripiprazole is known to be relatively benign in this respect [64], although it is important to note that this antipsychotic is still associated with due risks of weight gain [65]. Combining these antipsychotics could therefore yield favorable changes in metabolic parameters, which has in fact been mostly the case. Further, some but not all studies reported some positive changes in symptoms as well.

Another example may be to complement relatively weak dopamine D_2 blockade of clozapine with D_2 selective antagonists such as amisulpiride. Potential effectiveness of this strategy has been reported in the literature [66], and interestingly, this combination may be useful to counteract clozapine-induced sialorrhea [67]. Nevertheless, longer-term effectiveness and safety of such combinations are still far from clear. Whether clozapine polypharmacy allows its dosage to be reduced is another important topic that needs be systematically addressed [66].

6.5 How to Counteract Antipsychotic Polypharmacy in Schizophrenia?

There have been several studies that evaluated usefulness of antipsychotic polypharmacy for those who did not show adequate response to monotherapy, usually by comparing antipsychotic plus placebo (monotherapy) versus antipsychotic plus another antipsychotic (polypharmacy) (see Table 6.2). On the other hand, only a few studies thus far have evaluated usefulness of antipsychotic polypharmacy through switching to antipsychotic monotherapy.

6.5.1 Studies of Switching from Polytherapy to Monotherapy

Godlesky et al. [68] studied 14 chronic inpatients (12 with schizophrenia, 10 male patients). Participants had a duration of the illness of more than 10 years with a current hospitalization lasting at least 1 year. The average age of the study sample was 36.3 year-old with a total of 5.1 years of hospitalization. Patients had been refractory to five antipsychotic medications as well as to lithium and carbamazepine. At baseline, all patients had been treated with two FGAs, and one of them was tapered by roughly 10% every 1–2 weeks. A decision on which to discontinue was guided by such factors as relative dosage and patient preference.

The results showed that, at the completion of 12-month study period, 6 of 14 patients were successful in conversion to antipsychotic monotherapy, while such a switching was unsuccessful in the rest of 8 patients. In the successful group, a conversion to monotherapy was completed in 15.7±6.3 weeks, and chlorpromazine equivalent dosage was reduced from 2,553±1,809 to 1,883±412 mg. One patient needed additional lorazepam and another valproate. Relatively severe patients who were successful in switching to monotherapy in this study did not improve further but simply did not deteriorate.

Suzuki et al. [69] studied 47 patients with chronic schizophrenia who had been treated with the same antipsychotic polypharmacy regimen for more than 6 months before entry. There were 33 male patients and 27 inpatients, and the mean age was 51.0 year-old with the illness duration of 24.1 years. Which antipsychotics to discontinue was guided by the relative dosage, and it was aimed to roughly maintain the total chlorpromazine equivalent amount in a process of cross-titration. Conversion to monotherapy was conducted slowly in response to clinical status that was assessed with the Clinical Global Impression (CGI) and Global Assessment of Functioning (GAF), and doses of as low as about chlorpromazine 25 mg or its equivalent were allowed to continue as an aid to hypnotics. No addition of other psychotropics was permitted, however.

The results indicated that, at the completion of 24-week follow up period with monotherapy, 10 of 44 evaluable patients improved by converting antipsychotic polypharmacy to monotherapy, 24 remained stable, while such a switching was unsuccessful in the rest of 10 patients. The number of antipsychotics in the successful (better plus stable) patients was significantly reduced from 3.0 to 1.4 ($p<0.0001$) over the average period of 4.8 weeks. In this group of patients, 22 were successful in a complete conversion to monotherapy while 12 needed a continuation of low-dose low-potency antipsychotics. Overall, the GAF score stayed at 35.5 and the CGI-improvement was 4.05, indicating no change. Those who did not succeed in conversion to monotherapy had been hospitalized for a longer period of time ($p<0.01$) and exhibited a lower GAF score ($p<0.05$) at baseline.

This study had several limitations. Only FGAs were studied with an exception of risperidone because of the availability at the time of the study. The assessment was confined to global impression and functioning, and the study was open-label. Further, chlorpromazine equivalent dose of antipsychotics in the successful patents was significantly reduced from 1,171 to 951 mg ($p<0.0001$) in the end, mainly in response to keep the degree of extrapyramidal symptoms (EPS) around its baseline status. Since high-potency conventional antipsychotics, rather than low-potency ones, were more likely selected as the main antipsychotic to be converted to in this study, the results indicate that a blinded reliance on antipsychotic dose equivalence is risky, especially when the original dosage is high. Another viewpoint is that this study might be interpreted in a context of very modest dose reduction of antipsychotics. The average number of antipsychotics of 2.91 at baseline is also a complicating factor, since evidence is almost absent for using three or more antipsychotics in schizophrenia.

More recently, Essock et al. [70] reported on the systematic results regarding this issue. They evaluated effectiveness of antipsychotic polypharmacy in patients with schizophrenia by comparing continuation of two antipsychotics (polypharmacy group) versus switching to monotherapy (monotherapy group) in an open-label trial with blinded raters. They recruited patients 18 years or older for whom a change of antipsychotics is clinically considered but excluded patients with very severe presentation as well as those with an exacerbation of psychiatric symptoms within the past 3 months that resulted in significant interventions such as psychiatric emergency visits.

Which one of the two antipsychotics to discontinue was decided through the best clinical judgment, and conversion was to be completed in 30 days. There were no restrictions on the antipsychotic dosage as well as adjunctive psychotropic medications. The study lasted for 6 months plus an additional 6-month follow-up, and the assessments included time to discontinuation as well as the Positive and Negative Syndrome Scale (PANSS) and adverse events including EPS. The study sample consisted of 127 patients from 19 sites (84 male patients). Quetiapine plus risperidone (n=25), quetiapine plus an FGA (n=25), risperidone plus an FGA (n=23) and olanzapine plus an FGA (n=22) were the common combinations at baseline.

The results showed that in monotherapy group, 21% discontinued quetiapine, 17% risperidone, 15% olanzapine and 14% haloperidol. Time to all-cause discontinuation from treatment (the primary endpoint) was shorter in monotherapy group, and 86% of patients in monotherapy group versus 69% in polypharmacy group were still taking the same antipsychotics at 6 months. On the other hand, the PANSS score that was moderate originally at about 72 did not change appreciably in both groups without a difference. Further, weight control was better with monotherapy (0.50 decrease in body mass index versus 0.29 increase for polypharmacy over the 6 months, with body mass index being about 32 at baseline). The authors reasonably concluded that switching antipsychotic polypharmacy to monotherapy represents a viable option, a notion compatible with the above-mentioned study, provided that a return to polypharmacy is secured upon worsening.

Regarding this important work, the following information would have contributed to interpretation of the findings. First, how long the participants had been maintained on polypharmacy before entry is a pertinent consideration as long-term users of polypharmacy could be different from recent users. Second, although the protocol specified that the switch be commenced in 30 days, more detailed information on how one antipsychotic was converted to another (such as 25% biweekly decrease [71]) would be clinically relevant. Third, while the baseline dose was modest at approximately 360 mg chlorpromazine equivalent/day, the end dose of antipsychotics is another relevant information, especially to make sure that the dose was not significantly changed (or increased) in the monotherapy group. Fourth, data on adjunctive psychotropic medications that were clinically indicated in this study are important since some mode of augmentation therapy may be effective in schizophrenia [72].

These studies taken together, a conversion from polypharmacy to monotherapy warrants a serious case-by-case consideration. If worsening happens, it may be generally addressed by switching back to the original regimen. Nevertheless, given a paucity of data, more work is clearly indicated that will investigate a switch from polypharmacy to monotherapy in schizophrenia.

6.5.2 Systematic Interventions to Counteract Polypharmacy

Thompson et al. [73] conducted a cluster randomized controlled trial (The DEBIT trial) to investigate the effectiveness of a multifaceted intervention that comprised of an educational/cognitive behavioral workbook, an educational visit to consultants and a reminder system on medication charts. This relatively labor-intensive intervention resulted in a lower likelihood of using antipsychotic polypharmacy compared with guideline dissemination alone (adjusted odds ratio 0.43, 95% confidence interval 0.21–0.90, $p=0.028$). However, a considerable between-unit variation in polypharmacy rates was noted and the change in the rates was also variable between baseline and follow-up at 5 months. This suggests a complex role of local political and cultural issues in prescribing habits, in spite of the fact that the workbook indeed appeared to change staff beliefs about antipsychotic polypharmacy to a right direction.

Mistler et al. [74] evaluated an algorithm-based approach to optimize treatment with a single medication in 12 patients and found that, in comparison with 12 controls who were treated as usual, the former patients were discharged on significantly fewer medications while symptom reduction and length of stay did not differ significantly. Goh et al. [75] reported that the average number and the dose of antipsychotics for inpatients with chronic schizophrenia were reduced from 2.9 to 2.3 and 1,523 to 1,246 mg, respectively, in the absence of relapse for 6 months, as a result of implementing a clinical practice improvement program. As early as in 1980, Laska et al. [76] reported on a computerized drug review system for the purpose of both reviewing drug orders and notifying clinicians of orders that were considered exceptions to some clinical guidelines. The impact of this system in a psychiatric center (with about 40 psychiatrists) was examined in terms of the reduction in the percentage of polypharmacy or dose-range exceptions. The results showed a substantial reduction in the rate of polypharmacy or dose-range exceptions from 0.34 to 0.10 as a result of the implementation of the system. Hazra and the coauthors, in a single treatment setting, found that an active feedback by the pharmacist to the prescribers dramatically reduced the prevalence of antipsychotic polypharmacy from 18.3 to 6.6% in a 3-year span (prescriptions for a total of 648 patients were examined in 2006 and 778 in 2008) ($p<0.001$) [77]. The results of these preliminary reports need to be replicated in larger systematic studies.

From a system-wide viewpoint, Tucker reported on the introduction of the Psychiatric Clinical Knowledge Enhancement System (PSYCKES) in the New York State Office of Mental Health [78]. It allows physicians to visualize the medication history of their patients as well as of their colleagues' patients as a way of making better-informed decisions and supporting recovery of patients by simplifying antipsychotic regimens, and its introduction resulted in a decrease in antipsychotic polypharmacy of nearly 15% within 6 months at the most successful of the 26 hospitals. In a retrospective longitudinal analysis of the prevalence of antipsychotic polypharmacy from 2002 to 2006 in the Florida's Medicaid program, Constantine et al. [12] found that a statewide quality improvement program resulted in a prevalence that increased from January 2003 to December 2004 and then declined for four successive 6-month periods beginning in the January 2005 through June 2005 period when the program began.

However, not all studies that aimed to counteract polypharmacy yielded an unequivocally positive result. For instance, Robst [79] recently reported on the implementation of Prepaid Mental Health Plans (PMHPs) in Florida Medicaid and found that while a short-run change in the rate of polypharmacy improved from 7.7 to 7.0%, adherence rate on the other hand worsened with no change in the likelihood of prescriptions being written within recommended dosage ranges. In a controlled quasi-experimental study, Baandrup et al. evaluated the effect of a multifaceted educational intervention on the frequency of antipsychotic polypharmacy in adult outpatients with schizophrenia. The intervention consisted of 1-day of didactic lectures, six 3-h educational outreach visits and an electronic reminder during drug prescribing. The results showed that the prevalence of polypharmacy after 1 year was not different in the intervention group in comparison with the control group, highlighting an importance of organizational barriers [80]. Only a modest (although statistically significant) change in antipsychotic polypharmacy prescribing was noted with a usage of workbook in the DEBIT trial, implicating that an achievement of substantial changes in clinician behavior may require further exploration of other factors important in complex prescribing issues [81].

More system-wide PSYCKES data indicated a rebound of polypharmacy rate at follow-up, although the rate remained well below the starting point [82]. Finally, it is important to point out that, apart from a modest effect of audit-based quality improvement programs, a marked variation across and within healthcare organizations has been revealed in the level of compliance with evidence-based clinical practice standards [83].

6.6 Summary and Conclusions

The results from this review clearly show that evidence on antipsychotic polypharmacy thus far is modest at best. While it is well possible that some difficult patients may have good response with polypharmacy on an individual basis, the likelihood of overall response, who indeed can enjoy favorable outcomes and a possibility that the patient could have responded to other modes of therapy (such as augmentation of antipsychotics with other psychotropics), and long-term risks with polypharmacy all remain far from clear. Moreover, drug interactions are likely to be a source of concern [84].

In this context, it may be a case that antipsychotic polypharmacy is excessively used in the absence of compelling evidence. In fact, recent systematic review indicates a median rate of 19.6% with regional differences remaining unaccounted for [85]. It has been shown that at least a proportion of patients treated with antipsychotic polypharmacy could be converted to antipsychotic monotherapy. Systematic approaches to counteract polypharmacy can be effective although potentially labor-extensive efforts may translate into effects that are only modest in a limited setting. It is important to be aware of a possibility, however, that even a modest change found in one setting can sum up to make a significant difference if successful strategies penetrate to be adopted nationwide or even worldwide across many treatment settings.

It would be practically impossible to evaluate every possible antipsychotic combination with dose also in mind [86]. It is also highly likely that the number of available antipsychotics will increase rather than decrease, making the number of possible combinations to be tested even greater. Combinations may be guided by a hypothesis (e.g., combination of tight and loose D_2 blockers) or established evidence (e.g., combination of a metabolically problematic antipsychotic with a relatively benign one) but they should be interpreted in comparison with other reasonable strategies (e.g., lower-dose treatment [87]). Many questions still remain unaddressed and more work is clearly indicated with the following factors (see the next section) in mind on this controversial but notoriously common clinical practice.

6.7 Future Directions

A number of issues need to be carefully taken into account for future studies of antipsychotic polypharmacy in schizophrenia. They are briefly discussed in a point-by-point manner.

6.7.1 Treatment Duration

While a majority of patients with schizophrenia require long-term antipsychotic treatment, studies are usually too short to discern any positive or adverse effects in a long run. This is also the case for studies on antipsychotic polypharmacy that usually lasted for weeks to months rather than years to decades. Response may happen relatively early (in weeks) [88] but this is clearly not the case for every patient. Observational rather than strictly regulated interventional studies should provide more useful information in this respect.

6.7.2 Relevant Outcome Measures

Past studies of antipsychotic treatment for schizophrenia usually adopted the representative rating scales, most notably the PANSS, as an important outcome measure. And treatment response has mostly been driven by an improvement in classical symptoms (such as 20% or more decrease in the PANSS in case of TRS) [3]. Recently, more pragmatic outcomes, such as time to discontinuation from the allocated medication or relapse/rehospitalization, have been adopted in an effort to capture real-world effectiveness rather than efficacy [30, 31, 89, 90].

However, assessment for schizophrenia is not confined to classical (positive and negative) psychopathological evaluation but extends well to motor and non-extrapyramidal adverse effects, cognition, subjective perspectives, adherence, psychosocial circumstances and functioning [91]. How to incorporate these issues as the "main outcome of interest" in a study is an important consideration in order to better interpret the study results [92]. Nonetheless, it is also important to keep in mind that the greater number of the outcome measures (evaluated with the rating scales), the higher the chance of rater disagreement and the more difficult to find unequivocal differences (with actual study conduct being made rather complicated) [93, 94].

6.7.3 Cost Effectiveness

Although only a few studies evaluated cost-effectiveness of antipsychotic polypharmacy versus monotherapy in particular [39] and the cost may vary across antipsychotics [95], antipsychotic polypharmacy has intuitively been linked to higher costs [96]. Nevertheless, it remains to be seen whether added drug acquisition cost of antipsychotic polypharmacy or potentially pronounced adverse consequences (e.g., added cost to treat metabolic disturbances) could be offset by other critical cost-saving factors such as prevention of relapse or hospitalization. This question is critical but would likely be a challenging topic to address in a randomized trial.

6.7.4 Stay, Increase, Switch or Go to Antipsychotic Polypharmacy?

One important question is when some antipsychotic agent is not effective enough, it remains unclear about which is better to stay with the same agent (in favor of a probable delayed onset of action of antipsychotics), increase the dosage of the same agent (possibly favoring a dose response relationship of antipsychotics, and with anticholinergics to mitigate EPS if this occurs), or switch to another antipsychotic (believing potential differential effectiveness across antipsychotics), before resorting to antipsychotic polypharmacy [97]. However, only a few studies addressed this issue and it is implicated that practitioners may be rather hasty to resort to antipsychotic polypharmacy [37].

6.7.5 *Target Multiple Receptors or Stick to Dopamine D_2 Receptors?*

While dopamine D_2 receptors have been implicated and all antipsychotics on the market act on these receptors [98], pathophysiology of schizophrenia has been far from understood and other multiple receptors (such as serotonin 5-HT_2 receptors amongst others) and neurotransmitters (such as glutamatergic systems) are presumed to be involved. One notion may be to use of multiple antipsychotics so that multiple neurotransmitter systems could be modified. Another possibility may be to offer stronger (or tight and long-lasting) D_2 receptor antagonism to augment relatively weaker (or loose and transient) binding with some antipsychotics such as quetiapine and clozapine. However, it should also be noted that higher D_2 occupancy may be achievable with even higher dosage of these medications at least transiently. How optimal modification of multiple neurotransmitters could be achieved with a certain combination therapy that takes into account the variety as well as dosage of antipsychotics still remains completely elusive.

Another related issue is whether or not it is necessary to provide continuous D_2 antagonism throughout the day, especially in the maintenance phase of antipsychotic treatment [99–102].

6.7.6 *Proceed or Stop When Patients Get Better?*

Antipsychotic polypharmacy is inevitable when a switch from one to another antipsychotics is being performed (i.e., cross-titration to better avoid withdrawal effects) and treatment guidelines also make note on this since an abrupt discontinuation of antipsychotics is not without risks. The question is, when patients get better in the process or switching, which is better to go on with switching completely anyway or stay in the middle that results in polypharmacy? Although guidelines usually appear to endorse the former idea, there has not been adequate evidence in this respect [103].

6.7.7 *Antipsychotic Polypharmacy Versus Augmentation of an Antipsychotic with Other Psychotropics?*

While a detailed discussion of antipsychotic augmentation strategies (or psychotropic polypharmacy) is beyond the scope of this manuscript, there are a number of reports regarding augmentation treatment of antipsychotics [33]. Indeed, prescription surveys have shown that some adjunctive psychotropic medications such as benzodiazepines, antidepressants or mood stabilizers are frequently utilized in reality in addition to antipsychotics [85]. The role of antiparkinsonian medications is much less explicit in the era of SGAs that are, as a rule albeit controversial [104], more benign in terms of EPS. However, despite substantial efforts, there has not been compelling evidence to support a specific mode of augmentation strategy, either in general or in a specific situation. Moreover, there appear to have been no studies to compare a relative effectiveness of antipsychotic augmentation therapy with psychotropics versus antipsychotic polypharmacy in a reasonably well-defined resistant population [92].

6.7.8 Clozapine

Clozapine has been the gold standard medication for TRS and is seriously considered after failing to respond to at least two adequate trials with different antipsychotics, apparently making its position straightforward [2]. However, it has been reported that an initiation of clozapine is frequently delayed and some patients indeed need to discontinue clozapine for various reasons [105]. It appears true that weight and other metabolic issues plausibly influence the choice of antipsychotics [6], but how these parameters are affected by utilizing clozapine polypharmacy versus clozapine monopharmacy in a long run remains an important problem. Another important question is whether its dose could be reduced by adding another antipsychotic, which potentially results in less adverse effects burden of clozapine. All the issues discussed above are also relevant with this specific antipsychotic, and clozapine polypharmacy indeed appears common in the real-world [106]. Nevertheless, we need to be keenly aware of some systematic studies of clozapine polypharmacy that were found to be negative [107, 108].

To finalize, critical appraisal of the currently available evidence indicates that antipsychotic polypharmacy, as a rule, should be exceptional. Nonetheless, antipsychotic polypharmacy has been (probably too) often used in general [85] and recent data regarding the elderly are provocative for serious concern [109]. Moreover, antipsychotic polypharmacy involving long-acting formulations may also be frequent [110]. More work is clearly necessary to investigate the effectiveness and safety of antipsychotic polypharmacy in schizophrenia that remains highly controversial but very common in the real-world. Confronted with a reality that antipsychotic polypharmacy is not an infrequent clinical practice, our urgent challenge now is, instead of simply saying no, to well characterize patients who are likely to benefit from antipsychotic polypharmacy [57, 111] and to identify those who could successfully be converted to monotherapy [112].

References

1. Suzuki T, Uchida H, Watanabe K et al (2007) How effective is it to sequentially switch among Olanzapine, Quetiapine and Risperidone?—a randomized, open-label study of algorithm-based antipsychotic treatment to patients with symptomatic schizophrenia in the real-world clinical setting. Psychopharmacology (Berl) 195(2):285–295

2. Moore TA, Buchanan RW, Buckley PF et al (2007) The Texas medication algorithm project antipsychotic algorithm for schizophrenia: 2006 update. J Clin Psychiatry 68(11):1751–1762
3. Suzuki T, Remington G, Mulsant BH et al (2011) Treatment resistant schizophrenia and response to antipsychotics: a review. Schizophr Res 133(1–3):54–62
4. Bolstad A, Andreassen OA, Røssberg JI et al (2011) Previous hospital admissions and disease severity predict the use of antipsychotic combination treatment in patients with schizophrenia. BMC Psychiatry 11:126
5. Dolder CR, McKinsey J (2011) Antipsychotic polypharmacy among patients admitted to a geriatric psychiatry unit. J Psychiatr Pract 17(5):368–374
6. Li C, Mittal D, Owen RR (2011) Impact of patients' preexisting metabolic risk factors on the choice of antipsychotics by office-based physicians. Psychiatr Serv 62(12):1477–1484
7. Misawa F, Shimizu K, Fujii Y et al (2011) Is antipsychotic polypharmacy associated with metabolic syndrome even after adjustment for lifestyle effects?: a cross-sectional study. BMC Psychiatry 11:118
8. Santone G, Bellantuono C, Rucci P et al (2011) Patient characteristics and process factors associated with antipsychotic polypharmacy in a nationwide sample of psychiatric inpatients in Italy. Pharmacoepidemiol Drug Saf 20(5):441–449
9. Wu CS, Lin YJ, Liu SK (2011) Benzodiazepine use among patients with schizophrenia in Taiwan: a nationwide population-based survey. Psychiatr Serv 62(8):908–914
10. Xiang YT, Wang CY, Si TM et al (2012) Antipsychotic polypharmacy in inpatients with schizophrenia in Asia (2001–2009). Pharmacopsychiatry 45(1):7–12
11. An FR, Xiang YT, Wang CY et al (2010) Change of psychotropic drug prescription for schizophrenia in a psychiatric institution in Beijing, China between 1999 and 2008. Int J Clin Pharmacol Ther 48(4):270–274
12. Constantine RJ, Andel R, Tandon R (2010) Trends in adult antipsychotic polypharmacy: progress and challenges in Florida's Medicaid program. Community Ment Health J 46(6):523–530
13. Nielsen J, le Quach P, Emborg C et al (2010) 10-year trends in the treatment and outcomes of patients with first-episode schizophrenia. Acta Psychiatr Scand 122(5):356–366
14. Procyshyn RM, Honer WG, Wu TK et al (2010) Persistent antipsychotic polypharmacy and excessive dosing in the community psychiatric treatment setting: a review of medication profiles in 435 Canadian outpatients. J Clin Psychiatry 71(5):566–573
15. Ramos-Ríos R, Arrojo-Romero M, Paz-Silva E et al (2010) QTc interval in a sample of long-term schizophrenia inpatients. Schizophr Res 116(1):35–43
16. Ranceva N, Ashraf W, Odelola D (2010) Antipsychotic polypharmacy in outpatients at Birch Hill Hospital: incidence and adherence to guidelines. J Clin Pharmacol 50(6):699–704
17. Kroken RA, Johnsen E, Ruud T et al (2009) Treatment of schizophrenia with antipsychotics in Norwegian emergency wards, a cross-sectional national study. BMC Psychiatry 9:24
18. Huang MC, Lu ML, Tsai CJ et al (2009) Prevalence of metabolic syndrome among patients with schizophrenia or schizoaffective disorder in Taiwan. Acta Psychiatr Scand 120(4):274–280
19. McKean A, Vella-Brincat J (2009) Audit of antipsychotic polypharmacy in Christchurch. Australas Psychiatry 17(4):336–337
20. Wheeler A (2009) Explicit versus implicit review to explore combination antipsychotic prescribing. J Eval Clin Pract 15(4):685–691
21. Yu AP, Ben-Hamadi R, Birnbaum HG et al (2009) Comparing the treatment patterns of patients with schizophrenia treated with olanzapine and quetiapine in the Pennsylvania Medicaid population. Curr Med Res Opin 25(3):755–764
22. Ahn J, McCombs JS, Jung C et al (2008) Classifying patients by antipsychotic adherence patterns using latent class analysis: characteristics of nonadherent groups in the California Medicaid (Medi-Cal) program. Value Health 11(1):48–56
23. Connolly A, Taylor D (2008) Ethnicity and quality of antipsychotic prescribing among in-patients in south London. Br J Psychiatry 193(2):161–162
24. Koen L, Magni P, Niehaus DJ, le Roux A (2008) Antipsychotic prescription patterns in Xhosa patients with schizophrenia or schizoaffective disorder. Afr J Psychiatry (Johannesbg) 11(4):287–290

25. Lass J, Männik A, Bell JS (2008) Pharmacotherapy of first episode psychosis in Estonia: comparison with national and international treatment guidelines. J Clin Pharm Ther 33(2):165–173
26. Lerma-Carrillo I, de Pablo Brühlmann S, del Pozo ML et al (2008) Antipsychotic polypharmacy in patients with schizophrenia in a brief hospitalization unit. Clin Neuropharmacol 31(6):319–332
27. Pickar D, Vinik J, Bartko JJ (2008) Pharmacotherapy of schizophrenic patients: preponderance of off-label drug use. PLoS One 3(9):e3150
28. Taylor M, Shajahan P, Lawrie SM (2008) Comparing the use and discontinuation of antipsychotics in clinical practice: an observational study. J Clin Psychiatry 69(2):240–245
29. Wheeler A, Humberstone V, Robinson E (2008) Ethnic comparisons of antipsychotic use in schizophrenia. Aust N Z J Psychiatry 42(10):863–873
30. Lieberman JA, Stroup TS, McEvoy JP et al (2005) Effectiveness of antipsychotic drugs in patients with chronic schizophrenia. N Engl J Med 353(12):1209–1223
31. Kahn RS, Fleischhacker WW, Boter H et al (2008) Effectiveness of antipsychotic drugs in first-episode schizophrenia and schizophreniform disorder: an open randomized clinical trial. Lancet 371(9618):1085–1097
32. Pringsheim T, Lam D, Tano DS et al (2011) The pharmacoepidemiology of antipsychotics for adults with schizophrenia in Canada, 2005 to 2009. Can J Psychiatry 56(10):630–634
33. Remington G, Saha A, Chong SA et al (2005) Augmentation strategies in clozapine-resistant schizophrenia. CNS Drugs 19(10):843–872
34. Mojtabai R, Olfson M (2010) National trends in psychotropic medication polypharmacy in office-based psychiatry. Arch Gen Psychiatry 67(1):26–36
35. Baandrup L, Allerup P, Nordentoft M et al (2010) Exploring regional variation in antipsychotic coprescribing practice: a Danish questionnaire survey. J Clin Psychiatry 71(11):1457–1464
36. Correll CU, Shaikh L, Gallego JA et al (2011) Antipsychotic polypharmacy: a survey study of prescriber attitudes, knowledge and behavior. Schizophr Res 131(1–3):58–62
37. Tsutsumi C, Uchida H, Suzuki T et al (2011) The evolution of antipsychotic switch and polypharmacy in natural practice—a longitudinal perspective. Schizophr Res 130(1–3):40–46
38. Kreyenbuhl J, Marcus SC, West JC et al (2007) Adding or switching antipsychotic medications in treatment-refractory schizophrenia. Psychiatr Serv 58(7):983–990
39. Baandrup L, Sørensen J, Lublin H, Nordentoft M, Glenthoj B (2012) Association of antipsychotic polypharmacy with health service cost: a register-based cost analysis. Eur J Health Econ 13(3):355–363
40. Kreyenbuhl JA, Valenstein M, McCarthy JF et al (2007) Long-term antipsychotic polypharmacy in the VA health system: patient characteristics and treatment patterns. Psychiatr Serv 58(4):489–495
41. Kessing LV, Thomsen AF, Mogensen UB et al (2010) Treatment with antipsychotics and the risk of diabetes in clinical practice. Br J Psychiatry 197(4):266–271
42. Citrome L (2012) A systematic review of meta-analyses of the efficacy of oral atypical antipsychotics for the treatment of adult patients with schizophrenia. Expert Opin Pharmacother 13(11):1545-1573. doi:10.1517/14656566.2011.626769
43. Pandurangi AK, Dalkilic A (2008) Polypharmacy with second-generation antipsychotics: a review of evidence. J Psychiatr Pract 14(6):345–367
44. Stahl SM, Grady MM (2004) A critical review of atypical antipsychotic utilization: comparing monotherapy with polypharmacy and augmentation. Curr Med Chem 11(3):313–327
45. Porcelli S, Balzarro B, Serretti A (2012) Clozapine resistance: augmentation strategies. Eur Neuropsychopharmacol 22(3):165–182
46. Taylor DM, Smith L, Gee SH, Nielsen J (2012) Augmentation of clozapine with a second antipsychotic – a meta-analysis. Acta Psychiatr Scand 125(1):15–24. doi:10.1111/j.1600-0447.2011.01792.x
47. Wang J, Omori IM, Fenton M, Soares B (2010) Sulpiride augmentation for schizophrenia. Cochrane Database Syst Rev doi:10.1002/14651858.CD008125.pub2
48. Barbui C, Signoretti A, Mulè S et al (2009) Does the addition of a second antipsychotic drug improve clozapine treatment? Schizophr Bull 35(2):458–468

49. Cipriani A, Boso M, Barbui C (2009) Clozapine combined with different antipsychotic drugs for treatment resistant schizophrenia. Cochrane Database Syst Rev doi:10.1002/14651858. CD006324.pub2
50. Correll CU, Rummel-Kluge C, Corves C et al (2009) Antipsychotic combinations vs. monotherapy in schizophrenia: a meta-analysis of randomized controlled trials. Schizophr Bull 35(2):443–457
51. Taylor DM, Smith L (2009) Augmentation of clozapine with a second antipsychotic—a meta-analysis of randomized, placebo-controlled studies. Acta Psychiatr Scand 119(6):419–425
52. Paton C, Whittington C, Barnes TR (2007) Augmentation with a second antipsychotic in patients with schizophrenia who partially respond to clozapine: a meta-analysis. J Clin Psychopharmacol 27(2):198–204
53. Barbui C, Accordini S, Nosè M et al (2011) Aripiprazole versus haloperidol in combination with clozapine for treatment-resistant schizophrenia in routine clinical care: a randomized, controlled trial. J Clin Psychopharmacol 31(3):266–273
54. Suzuki T, Uchida H, Watanabe K et al (2011) Factors associated with response to clozapine in schizophrenia: a review. Psychopharmacol Bull 44(1):32–60
55. Chan J, Sweeting M (2007) Review: combination therapy with non-clozapine atypical antipsychotic medication: a review of current evidence. J Psychopharmacol 21(6):657–664
56. Zink M (2005) Augmentation of olanzapine in treatment-resistant schizophrenia. J Psychiatry Neurosci 30(6):409–415
57. Suzuki T, Uchida H, Watanabe K et al (2008) Effectiveness of antipsychotic polypharmacy for patients with treatment refractory schizophrenia: an open-label trial of olanzapine plus risperidone for those who failed to respond to a sequential treatment with olanzapine, quetiapine and risperidone. Hum Psychopharmacol 23(6):455–463
58. Henderson DC, Kunkel L, Nguyen DD et al (2006) An exploratory open-label trial of aripiprazole as an adjuvant to clozapine therapy in chronic schizophrenia. Acta Psychiatr Scand 113(2):142–147
59. Ziegenbein M, Wittmann G, Kropp S (2006) Aripiprazole augmentation of clozapine in treatment-resistant schizophrenia: a clinical observation. Clin Drug Invest 26(3):117–124
60. Karunakaran K, Tungaraza TE, Harborne GC (2007) Is clozapine-aripiprazole combination a useful regime in the management of treatment-resistant schizophrenia? J Psychopharmacol 21(4):453–456
61. Chang JS, Ahn YM, Park HJ et al (2008) Aripiprazole augmentation in clozapine-treated patients with refractory schizophrenia: an 8-week, randomized, double-blind, placebo-controlled trial. J Clin Psychiatry 69(5):720–731
62. Fleischhacker WW, Heikkinen ME, Olié JP et al (2010) Effects of adjunctive treatment with aripiprazole on body weight and clinical efficacy in schizophrenia patients treated with clozapine: a randomized, double-blind, placebo-controlled trial. Int J Neuropsychopharmacol 13(8):1115–1125
63. Muscatello MR, Bruno A, Pandolfo G et al (2011) Effect of aripiprazole augmentation of clozapine in schizophrenia: a double-blind, placebo-controlled study. Schizophr Res 127(1–3):93–99
64. Tschoner A, Engl J, Laimer M et al (2007) Metabolic side effects of antipsychotic medication. Int J Clin Pract 61(8):1356–1370
65. Klemp M, Tvete IF, Skomedal T et al (2011) A review and bayesian meta-analysis of clinical efficacy and adverse effects of 4 atypical neuroleptic drugs compared with haloperidol and placebo. J Clin Psychopharmacol 31(6):698–704
66. Zink M, Knopf U, Henn FA et al (2004) Combination of clozapine and amisulpride in treatment-resistant schizophrenia—case reports and review of the literature. Pharmacopsychiatry 37(1):26–31
67. Kreinin A, Novitski D, Weizman A (2006) Amisulpride treatment of clozapine-induced hyper salivation in schizophrenia patients: a randomized, double-blind, placebo-controlled cross-over study. Int Clin Psychopharmacol 21(2):99–103

68. Godleski LS, Kerler R, Barber JW et al (1989) Multiple versus single antipsychotic drug treatment in chronic psychosis. J Nerv Ment Dis 177(11):686–689
69. Suzuki T, Uchida H, Tanaka KF et al (2004) Revising polypharmacy to a single antipsychotic regimen for patients with chronic schizophrenia. Int J Neuropsychopharmacol 7(2):133–142
70. Essock SM, Schooler NR, Stroup TS et al (2011) Effectiveness of switching from antipsychotic polypharmacy to monotherapy. Am J Psychiatry 168(7):702–708
71. Takeuchi H, Suzuki T, Uchida H et al (2008) A randomized, open-label comparison of 2 switching strategies to aripiprazole treatment in patients with schizophrenia: add-on, wait, and tapering of previous antipsychotics versus add-on and simultaneous tapering. J Clin Psychopharmacol 28(5):540–543
72. Suzuki T, Uchida H, Takeuchi H et al (2009) Augmentation of atypical antipsychotics with valproic acid. An open-label study for most difficult patients with schizophrenia. Hum Psychopharmacol 24(8):628–638
73. Thompson A, Sullivan SA, Barley M et al (2008) The DEBIT trial: an intervention to reduce antipsychotic polypharmacy prescribing in adult psychiatry wards—a cluster randomized controlled trial. Psychol Med 38(5):705–715
74. Mistler LA, Mellman TA, Drake RE (2009) A pilot study testing a medication algorithm to reduce polypharmacy. Qual Saf Health Care 18(1):55–58
75. Goh YL, Seng KH, Chuan AS et al (2011) Reducing antipsychotic polypharmacy among psychogeriatric and adult patients with chronic schizophrenia. Perm J 15(2):52–56
76. Laska E, Siegel C, Simpson G (1980) Automated review system for orders of psychotropic drugs. Arch Gen Psychiatry 37(7):824–827
77. Hazra M, Uchida H, Sproule B et al (2011) Impact of feedback from pharmacists in reducing antipsychotic polypharmacy in schizophrenia. Psychiatry Clin Neurosci 65(7):676–678
78. Tucker WM (2007) When less is more: reducing the incidence of antipsychotic polypharmacy. J Psychiatr Pract 13(3):202–204
79. Robst J (2012) Changes in antipsychotic medication use after implementation of a Medicaid mental health carve-out in the US. PharmacoEconomics 30(5):387–396
80. Baandrup L, Allerup P, Lublin H et al (2010) Evaluation of a multifaceted intervention to limit excessive antipsychotic co-prescribing in schizophrenia out-patients. Acta Psychiatr Scand 122(5):367–374
81. Thompson A, Sullivan S, Barley M et al (2010) Effectiveness of a cognitive behavioral workbook for changing beliefs about antipsychotic polypharmacy: analysis from a cluster randomized controlled trial. J Eval Clin Pract 16(3):520–528
82. Finnerty MT, Kealey E, Leckman-Westin E et al (2011) Long-term impact of web-based tools, leadership feedback, and policies on inpatient antipsychotic polypharmacy. Psychiatr Serv 62(10):1124–1126
83. Barnes TR, Paton C (2011) Improving prescribing practice in psychiatry: the experience of the Prescribing Observatory for Mental Health (POMH-UK). Int Rev Psychiatry 23(4):328–335
84. Bebawy M, Chetty M (2008) Differential pharmacological regulation of drug efflux and pharmacoresistant schizophrenia. Bioessays 30(2):183–188
85. Gallego JA, Bonetti J, Zhang J, Kane JM, Correll CU (2012) Prevalence and correlates of antipsychotic polypharmacy: a systematic review and meta-regression of global and regional trends from the 1970s to 2009. Schizophr Res 138(1):18–28. doi:10.1016/j.schres.2012.03.018
86. Suzuki T (2011) An importance of dose in antipsychotic combination therapy for schizophrenia. J Clin Psychopharmacol 31(3):399
87. Uchida H, Suzuki T, Takeuchi H et al (2011) Low dose vs. standard dose of antipsychotics for relapse prevention in schizophrenia: meta-analysis. Schizophr Bull 37(4):788–799
88. Suzuki T, Remington G, Arenovich T et al (2011) Time course of improvement with antipsychotic medication in treatment-resistant schizophrenia. Br J Psychiatry 199(4):275–280
89. Csernansky JG, Mahmoud R, Brenner R et al (2002) A comparison of risperidone and haloperidol for the prevention of relapse in patients with schizophrenia. N Engl J Med 346(1):16–22
90. Rosenheck RA, Krystal JH, Lew R et al (2011) Long-acting risperidone and oral antipsychotics in unstable schizophrenia. N Engl J Med 364(9):842–851

91. Suzuki T (2011) Which rating scales are regarded as 'the standard' in clinical trials for schizophrenia? A critical review. Psychopharmacol Bull 44(1):18–31
92. Suzuki T, Remington G, Mulsant BH et al (2012) Defining treatment-resistant schizophrenia and response to antipsychotics: a review and recommendation. Psychiatry Res 197(1-2):1–6
93. Stern RG, Schmeidler J, Davidson M (1997) Limitations of controlled augmentation trials in schizophrenia. Biol Psychiatry 42(2):138–143
94. Suzuki T, Takeuchi H, Nakajima S et al (2010) Magnitude of rater differences in assessment scales for schizophrenia. J Clin Psychopharmacol 30(5):607–611
95. Zhu B, Ascher-Svanum H, Faries DE et al (2008) Cost of antipsychotic polypharmacy in the treatment of schizophrenia. BMC Psychiatry 8:19
96. Stahl SM, Grady MM (2006) High-cost use of second-generation antipsychotics under California's Medicaid program. Psychiatr Serv 57(1):127–129
97. Kinon BJ, Kane JM, Johns C et al (1993) Treatment of neuroleptic-resistant schizophrenic relapse. Psychopharmacol Bull 29(2):309–314
98. Seeman P (2011) All roads to schizophrenia lead to dopamine super sensitivity and elevated dopamine D2(high) receptors. CNS Neurosci Ther 17(2):118–132
99. Remington G, Seeman P, Feingold A et al (2011) "Extended" antipsychotic dosing in the maintenance treatment of schizophrenia: a double-blind, placebo-controlled trial. J Clin Psychiatry 72(8):1042–1048
100. Mizuno Y, Bies RR, Remington G et al (2012) Dopamine D2 receptor occupancy with risperidone or olanzapine during maintenance treatment of schizophrenia: a cross-sectional study. Prog Neuropsychopharmacol Biol Psychiatry 37(1):182–187. doi:10.1016/j.pnpbp.2011.12.013
101. Suzuki T, Uchida H, Takeuchi H et al (2005) Simplifying psychotropic medication regimen into a single night dosage and reducing the dose for patients with chronic schizophrenia. Psychopharmacology (Berl) 181(3):566–575
102. Moriguchi S, Bies RR, Remington G et al (In Press) Estimated Dopamine D2 Receptor Occupancy and Remission in Schizophrenia: Analysis of the CATIE Data. J Clin Psychopharmacol
103. Takeuchi H, Suzuki T, Uchida H et al (2012) Antipsychotic treatment for schizophrenia in the maintenance phase: a systematic review of the guidelines and algorithms. Schizophr Res 134(2–3):219–225
104. Fischer-Barnicol D, Lanquillon S, Haen E et al (2008) Typical and atypical antipsychotics—the misleading dichotomy. Results from the Working Group 'Drugs in Psychiatry' (AGATE). Neuropsychobiology 57(1–2):80–87
105. Krivoy A, Malka L, Fischel T et al (2011) Predictors of clozapine discontinuation in patients with schizophrenia. Int Clin Psychopharmacol 26(6):311–315
106. Pai NB, Laidlaw M, Vella SC (2012) Augmentation of clozapine with another pharmacological agent: treatment for refractory schizophrenia in the 'real world'. Acta Psychiatr Scand Mar 20. doi:10.1111/j.1600-0447.2012.01854.x. [Epub ahead of print]
107. Honer WG, Thornton AE, Chen EY et al (2006) Clozapine alone versus clozapine and risperidone with refractory schizophrenia. N Engl J Med 354(5):472–482
108. Friedman JI, Lindenmayer JP, Alcantara F et al (2011) Pimozide augmentation of clozapine in patients with schizophrenia and schizoaffective disorder unresponsive to clozapine monotherapy. Neuropsychopharmacology 36(6):1289–1295
109. López de Torre A, Lertxundi U, Hernández R, Medrano J (2012) Antipsychotic polypharmacy: a needle in a haystack? Gen Hosp Psychiatry 34(4):423–432
110. Aggarwal NK, Sernyak MJ, Rosenheck RA (2012) Prevalence of concomitant oral antipsychotic drug use among patients treated with long-acting, intramuscular, antipsychotic medications. J Clin Psychopharmacol 32(3):323–328
111. Stahl SM (2012) Antipsychotic polypharmacy: never say never, but never say always. Acta Psychiatr Scand 125(5):349–351
112. Tani H, Uchida H, Suzuki T, Fujii Y, Mimura M (In Press) Interventions to reduce antipsychotic polypharmacy: A systematic review. Schizophr Res

Chapter 7
Clozapine Combinations in Treatment-Resistant Schizophrenia Patients

Vladimir Lerner and Chanoch Miodownik

Abstract Schizophrenia is a severe disabling mental illness affecting about 1% of the population throughout the world. Antipsychotic medications (conventional and atypical antipsychotics) are the pharmacological basis for the cure of schizophrenia and schizoaffective patients, however not all patients are positively affected by this treatment. One fifth to one third of people suffering from schizophrenia is considered as treatment resistant. In other words, these people have persistent psychotic symptoms and poor functioning despite adequate treatment with conventional or novel antipsychotics.

To date one of the most effective medications is clozapine, which produces clinically significant improvement of symptoms in 30–50% of patients receiving it. However, from one-third to two thirds of schizophrenia patients still have persistent 'positive' symptoms despite adequate dosage and duration of clozapine monotherapy.

Among treatment-resistant schizophrenia patients with poor response to an adequate trial of clozapine monotherapy, 30–50% are treated with a combination of clozapine and second psychotropic medication.

Clinicians usually prescribe a combination of antipsychotics, in order to reach a greater or more rapid therapeutic response than has been achieved with antipsychotic monotherapy.

In this chapter, we present a summary of the literature concerning the combination of clozapine with different psychotropic medications or procedure in management of resistant schizophrenia and schizoaffective patients.

V. Lerner, M.D., Ph.D. (✉) • C. Miodownik, M.D.
Ministry of Health, Faculty of Health Sciences, Ben Gurion University of the Negev and Be'er Sheva Mental Health Center, Be'er-Sheva, Israel
e-mail: proflernervld@gmail.com; lernervld@yahoo.com; lernerv@bgu.ac.il; chanoch_m@yahoo.com

M.S. Ritsner (ed.), *Polypharmacy in Psychiatry Practice, Volume II: Use of Polypharmacy in the "Real World"*, DOI 10.1007/978-94-007-5799-8_7,

Abbreviations

bid	Twice a day
BMI	Body mass index
BPRS	Brief psychiatric rating scale
CIS	Clozapine-induced hypersalivation
CYP1A2	Cytochrome P450 1A2
ECT	Electroconvulsive therapy
EEG	Electroencephalography
EPS	Extrapyramidal symptoms
FACT-Sz	Functional assessment for comprehensive treatment of schizophrenia
FGAs	First-generation antipsychotics
GABA	Gamma aminobutiric acid
GAS	Global assessment scale
HoNOS-Rome	Health of the nation outcome scales (a new Italian version of the HoNOS)
HDL	High-density lipoprotein
HRSD	Hamilton rating scale for depression
LDL	Low-density lipoprotein
MMSE	Mini-mental status examination
MRI	Magnetic resonance imaging
NMDA	N-Methyl-D-aspartate
NMDAR	N-Methyl-D-aspartate receptor
PANSS	Positive and negative syndrome scale
PSP	Personal and social performance scale
RCT	Randomized controlled study
SANS	Scale for the assessment of negative symptoms
SAPS	Scale for the assessment of positive symptoms
SGAs	Second-generation antipsychotics
SSRI	Selective serotonin re-uptake inhibitor
TRS	Treatment-resistant schizophrenia
WBC	White blood cells

Psychiatry is an absolutely exact science—the number of opinions is equal the number of psychiatrists. ... but psychopharmacology is not an exact science.

(From a conversation between a psychiatrist and mathematician)

The treatment of schizophrenia has been changed dramatically with the ongoing development of pharmacologic agents and better evidence of the effectiveness of several psychosocial treatments. Despite progress in treatment of mental disturbances, schizophrenia is still remained one of the disabling disorders. It is among the ten leading causes of disability in the age group of 15–44 [1]. Antipsychotic medications (conventional and atypical antipsychotics) are a pharmacological basis for the therapeutic care of schizophrenia and schizoaffective patients, although it is obvious that not all patients have positive results from this intervention. Ten to thirty percents of patients have a little or no benefit from treatment with all kinds of antipsychotics using adequate dosages and duration [2]. Additional 30% of patients have only partial response to treatment [3]. Treatment resistance may be an enduring feature for some patients, however more commonly it is developed over the course of the illness [4].

Treatment of these patients has remained a persistent public health problem since medication-resistant patients are often highly symptomatic, have a significant quality of life reduction, and need extensive periods of institutional care [5]. The proportion of patients with treatment resistant schizophrenia have been consistent over time since the introduction of conventional antipsychotics, or first-generation ("typical") antipsychotics (FGA) at 1952 [6].

Despite recent advances and increasing treatment options after appearance of second-generation antipsychotics (SGA) such as amisulpiride, aripiprazole clozapine, olanzapine, quetiapine, risperidone, sulpiride, and ziprasidone, many schizophrenia patients remain symptomatic even with this treatment. It should be mentioned that new drugs have new side effects in addition to its expensiveness.

This chapter reviews and summarizes the publications concerning treatment strategies for those patients who do not respond or only partially respond to clozapine. For this aim, we performed a systematic literature search in the MEDLINE database for the years ranging from 1970 to March 2012 to identify all publications dealing with assessment of efficacy and safety of adjunctive agents in clozapine-resistant schizophrenic or schizoaffective patients. For this search, we used the keywords of "schizophrenia", "schizoaffective", "resistant/refractory schizophrenia", "clozapine-resistant", "combination", "augmentation", "add-on", "addition", "additive", "adjunctive", "co-administration", "clozapine", "clozaril", "leponex", and the names of the particular pharmacological components used for augmentation.

7.1 Definitions of Treatment Resistance or Partially Respond in Schizophrenia

Concerning those patients who are medically treated, there are two kinds of patients who are not well react to medications. The first group is partial responders (incomplete), while the other group is defined as treatment resistant.

The definition of partial response is based on the following criteria: (1) a history of residual positive and/or negative symptoms after at least a 6-week trial of a therapeutic dose of a neuroleptic agent, (2) at least a minimum level of positive and/or negative symptoms at the time of evaluation for the study, and (3) at least a minimum level of positive and/or negative symptoms after a prospective trial of at least 2 weeks of fluphenazine, 20 mg/day (with dose adjustments between 10 and 30 mg/day allowed in order to optimize outcome). The minimum positive symptom level was a total score of at least eight for the four Brief Psychiatric Rating Scale (BPRS) positive symptom items (conceptual disorganization, hallucinations, unusual thought content, and suspiciousness). The minimum negative symptom level was a total score on the Scale for the Assessment of Negative Symptoms (SANS) of at least 20 [7].

Various definitions of the criteria for treatment resistant schizophrenia have been presented to date. Treatment resistance may be presented even from the first episode of psychosis. Although most patients at the onset of the psychotic phase of schizophrenia respond well to neuroleptics in terms of delusions and hallucinations, and remain responsive except for occasional relapses, 5–20% of patients have persistent positive symptoms during the first episode [8]. Definitions of 'treatment resistance' acquired new meaning with the evolution of different kinds of therapeutic interventions. A narrow definition of treatment resistant schizophrenia was introduced by Kane et al. in 1988 [9]. The criteria included the aspects of patient's clinical history, cross-sectional measures and prospective assessments.

Recently Suzuki and colleagues [10] proposed improved criteria require both a score of ≥4 on the Clinical Global Impression (CGI)-Severity and a score of ≤49 on the Functional Assessment for Comprehensive Treatment of Schizophrenia (FACT-Sz) [11] or ≤50 on the Global Assessment of Functioning (GAF) scales to define treatment resistant schizophrenia (TRS). The authors proposed that when TRS is established, subsequent treatment response be defined based on a CGI-Change score of ≤2, a ≥20% decrease on the total PANSS or Brief Psychiatric Rating Scale (BPRS) scores, and an increase of ≥20 points on the FACT-Sz or GAF.

Treatment resistance is usually permanent. True treatment resistance should be distinguished from a breakthrough of positive symptoms or increasing severity of negative symptoms despite being compliant with pharmacotherapy [12].

Treatment resistance once referred to the positive symptoms, such as hallucinations and delusions that would persist despite reasonable trials of antipsychotic medicine. However, along the time, the concept of nonresponders was re-conceptualized. The recent attitude concerns it as a multidimensional mean. According to this idea, resistance may refer not only to positive symptoms, but also to negative, cognitive, excitement, or depressive symptom domains [13]. Even if a patient's positive symptoms respond or remit with an antipsychotic agent, residual negative and cognitive symptoms often persist [3].

Before making a decision that a patient is treatment-resistant, the clinician should define the patient as drug compliant. Covert or partial noncompliance is the most frequent causes for lack of clinical improvement. This situation can easily be missed and the physician should be aware of it. A trial with depot antipsychotic agents can be helpful for better compliance. Although therapeutic levels of most typical and atypical antipsychotics can be measured and may help to determine whether a patient is a rapid metabolizer (or noncompliant), but usually it is not practical. As drug blood level is influenced by multiple factors and there is a large variation among different patients even in the same patient under different conditions with similar doses of medications.

Though various authors have used varied definitions of treatment resistant schizophrenia, according to Meltzer [12], the most common definition denotes patients who despite at least two adequate trials of classical neuroleptic drugs have persistent moderate to severe, positive, or disorganization, or negative symptoms together with poor social and work function over a prolonged period of time. Approximately 30% of schizophrenic patients (10–45%) meet these criteria. This definition may be inadequate for few patients whose positive symptoms respond adequately to neuroleptics, but have clinically significant negative symptoms, poor social and work functions, cognitive dysfunctions, poor quality of life and who constitute a significant burden to the family and society. In addition, this definition does not consider suicidality (suicidal thoughts or attempts) of the patient [12].

Treatment resistance or failure of another type also can be determined by examining relapse rates for patients on going therapy. Lehman et al. defined treatment-resistant schizophrenia in a more quantitative way. According to these researchers, the definition can be based on little or no symptomatic response to multiple (at least 2) antipsychotic trials of an adequate duration (of at least 6 weeks) and at a therapeutic dose range [3]. A 4–6 week neuroleptics trial of 400–600 mg/day of chlorpromazine equivalent is now accepted as a standard for an adequate trial [14, 15].

Using the term 'treatment resistance' may lead to a pessimistic conclusion that this is the endpoint for these patients. Some clinicians are skeptic about it and suggest replacing this term into 'incomplete recovery' [13].

When encountered by what appears to be treatment resistance, the clinician should review the diagnosis, check for another psychiatric disorder or substance abuse co-morbidity, rule out medical co-morbidities, and assess the adequacy of past and present pharmacotherapy (duration/dosage/compliance). Unfortunately, such data gathering is often difficult to be performed due to poor history from the patient and a fragmented system leading to a problem in accessing medical records. Treatment resistance may be related to suboptimal dosing of the antipsychotic, poor adherence with the prescribed medication regimen, ineffectiveness of the antipsychotic, or substance abuse [3]. Once treatment resistance is established, the origin of the non-responding pattern should be identified. The psychiatrist should develop a sequential, systematic treatment plan; determine the duration of each trial; and use standardized rating scales such as the Brief Psychiatric Rating Scale (BPRS) or the Positive and Negative Syndrome Scale (PANSS) to monitor response. Research protocols should define an inadequate response such as scores above a certain level on the assessment scales and/or an insufficient decrease in the score after a defined course of treatment.

The clinician should also identify defined target symptoms, consider that inadequate psychosocial treatment may create the appearance of treatment resistance, and maintain a positive therapeutic attitude [2].

7.2 Possible Factors Associated with Treatment Resistance

Until now the pathophysiology of schizophrenia remains unclear and some researchers assume that this disease has the status of a clinical syndrome and may comprise a number of specific disease entities [16–18].

Different factors and mechanisms may be responsible for treatment resistance. The most frequently mentioned factors associated with treatment resistance are: clinical, biological, brain morphological features, and pharmacological factors [19]. The clinical factors contain male gender, illness onset before age of 20 years, negative symptoms, severity of illness, low grade of pre-morbidity, social and work adjustment, residual symptoms after first psychotic episode, and neurological soft signs. Biological factors contain low plasma level of homovanillic acid and alpha activity changes on EEG. Brain morphological features: brain abnormalities demonstrated by computerized tomography or magnetic resonance imaging, or abnormalities of central dopamine D_2 functions. Pharmacological factors: responding failure to standard antipsychotic initial treatment, late start of medication, concurrent agents such as anticholinergic medications, extrapyramidal adverse effects, smoking or alcohol.

Until standard defining criteria became available, research into the neurobiological substrate of treatment resistance was restricted [20]. Recently, some objective criteria for distinguishing treatment resistant from nonresistant patients appeared. Lawrie et al. found that treatment-resistant schizophrenic patients showed a tendency to greater cerebral atrophy than those who were treatment responsive [21]. Furthermore, it was demonstrated that the patients with a poor outcome had greater lateral ventricular enlargement over time than patients with good outcome [22]. Other researchers found that during neuroleptic treatment, negative schizophrenia symptoms were significantly diminished in patients without cortical atrophy, than in subjects with cortical atrophy demonstrated in MRI. It attributes especially to the severity of emotional blunting [23]. However, more researches dealing with neurological correlates of treatment resistance are required.

7.3 Treatment

Poor treatment response in patients with schizophrenia is an important clinical issue. Traditionally, the recommendations for management of treatment-resistant patients were (a) increasing the neuroleptics dose; (b) switching from existing (conventional) antipsychotic to an alternative conventional agent from a different chemical class; (c) using augmentation effect by adding another psychotropic drug such as benzodiazepines, lithium, anticonvulsive agents, or to combine high and low potency antipsychotic medications; and finally (d) electroconvulsive therapy.

This chapter deals only with one method of treatment for these patients: combinations of clozapine with other psychotropic drugs (polypharmacy).

Polypharmacy was first described in the psychiatric literature in 1969 [24]. From that time, antipsychotic combinations became a relatively common and growing practice. Although polypharmacy is successfully applied in some clinical settings (for example, stabilization of mood disorders, controlling violence and so on), the evidence-based benefits for treatment-resistant schizophrenia is less clear. This idea is consisted with the fact that there is no specific combination emerged among all prescribers points to a lack of definite theoretical, evidence-based or pragmatic guidelines for antipsychotic polypharmacy.

There is no consensus concerning polypharmacy. Some guidelines clearly state that antipsychotics combination should be avoided. Other researchers abstain of any recommendations while others do not negate it [25–27]. Combinations can be justified in certain clinical circumstances such as switching one antipsychotic to another, or when it is necessary to augment clozapine in treatment-resistant patients [28, 29]. The reason for including combinations, according to Miller's recommendations, as a final option in treating resistant schizophrenia patients is to give clinicians reasonable choices for treating all their patients, even those who respond poorly to the best evidence-based medication treatments, while conveying the message that combining antipsychotics is a last resort [30].

Recent evidences demonstrate that practically more than 20% of patients are taking two or more drugs [31]. To date, the possible concurrent antipsychotic prescriptions of antipsychotic drug regimens are numerous. Antipsychotic combination therapy is widespread in many countries. For example, in Europe it fluctuates from 25% to almost 70% of psychotropic drugs prescriptions [25, 32–43]. In Australia antipsychotic polypharmacy reaches up to 15% [44, 45] and according to Pai et al., even 84.5% [46], in Canada 27.5% [47]. In China and East Asia it varies from 45.7 to 66% [48, 49], in Japan 90% [50, 51], in Mexico 48% [52]. The prevalence of antipsychotic polypharmacy in the United States varies from 7% to approximately 50%, while most studies find prevalence rates of between 10 and 30% [53–58].

7.4 Clinical Efficacy of Clozapine

Clozapine is the first prototypic atypical antipsychotic agent, which was patented in 1960. It appears to be more effective than conventional antipsychotics for schizophrenia patients, who are severely psychotic and poorly responsive to the first generation of antipsychotic drugs. Unlike any of the typical agents at the time, it was not associated with extrapyramidal symptoms (EPS). Clozapine is effective on a broad range of psychopathology including both positive and negative symptoms in 30–50% of patients receiving treatment [59]. It can reduce violence and persistent aggression in patients with schizophrenia and other psychiatric disorders [60].

The exact neurochemical mechanism by which clozapine exerts its atypical effect is unknown. It has complex receptor pharmacology, including antagonist activity at dopaminergic (D_1, D_2); serotonergic ($5\text{-}HT_2a$, $5\text{-}HT_2c$, $5\text{-}HT_3$); adrenergic ($alpha_1$, $alpha_2$); histaminergic (H_1); and muscarinic (M1) receptors Meltzer, 1999 #301}.

After being approved in Europe in 1972, it was withdrawn from the market in 1975 due to reports of deaths from agranulocytosis. Problems with other side effects, including hypersalivation, seizures, hypotension, and excessive sedation, limited the general utility of the agent. Although clozapine was not clinically available in the US from 1975 until 1990, it continued to be used in this period in other parts of the world (Europe and China). The cumulative experience from these countries demonstrated that clozapine is an effective antipsychotic without or with a small number of extrapyramidal symptoms (EPS). Although, it was found that clozapine treatment is associated with a 0.7% risk of agranulocytosis and death, however when patients are carefully monitored, clozapine could be administered safely [61].

7.5 Clozapine Dosing Considerations

The usual target range for clozapine is about 400–700 mg/day, and it is generally given in a divided dose schedule. Notably, the average European dose range is approximately one-half its US counterpart. This difference more than likely reflects the US practice of reserving clozapine for the most densely unresponsive of schizophrenic syndromes. Such subjects typically, and predictably, require higher doses than more responsive patients. Since clozapine has pronounced α_1 blockade (inducing a marked decrease in peripheral vascular resistance with a reflex increase in cardiac output and possible clinically significant orthostatic hypotension) and H_1 blockade (sedation inducing), it must be titrated very slowly over several weeks to this target dose range. In general, patients should be started at 12.5 mg bid, with gradual titration to approximately 500 mg/day by no more than 50-mg increments every 2 days. In addition to the required weekly monitoring of WBC counts, patient's vital signs (with orthostatic changes) should be measured daily during the first week of titration. Patients who demonstrate cardiovascular intolerance to the clozapine-induced decrease in peripheral vascular resistance (persistent, subjectively distressing orthostatic hypotension) should be titrated with extreme caution [62].

Clozapine dosage can be a relatively complicated issue. Standard dose of clozapine is from 251 to 600 mg/day. High dose of clozapine is from 601 to 900 mg/day, and very high the clozapine dose is 901 mg/day or above [63]. In particular, there is no meaningful relationship between clozapine plasma level and its clinical response. However, there is a consensus in the literature that a plasma level of about 350–450 ng/ml has to be attained before the patient is considered to be non-respondent to clozapine [64, 65].

There is an increasing amount of researches examining a number of other possible treatment options based on our new understanding of the pathophysiology of schizophrenia. The current best accepted strategy for neuroleptic-resistant schizophrenia patients is to use clozapine. Although clozapine is more effective in overcoming treatment-resistant, approximately from 40 to 70% of these patients despite clozapine monotherapy in adequate dose and duration do not respond to it [9]. Some researchers suppose that the treatment-resistant schizophrenia patients represent a specific subgroup, united by the same biological substrate [66].

Poor treatment response in patients with schizophrenia who do not have an optimal response to clozapine has been cited as the most common reason for concurrent treatment with two or more antipsychotic drugs [67]. This strategy has received little empirical evaluation, although published case studies and expert opinions have suggested some therapeutic possibilities.

The benefits of clozapine augmentation with other antipsychotics have been questioned. Some authors pointed out that it should not be used during the first 3–6 months of treatment with clozapine [68].

A number of augmentation strategies have been suggested for patients who were not improved with clozapine, but most guidelines and recommendations suggest clozapine as the "last therapeutic line". In fact, there is no definite consensus on the treatment for an inadequate response to multiple previous antipsychotic trials, including clozapine [69]. For that, clinicians should keep in mind that no guidelines can address the complexities involved in the care of each individual patient and that sound clinical judgment based on clinical experience should be used in applying these recommendations [70].

Unfortunately, there are only few controlled studies in this area. Most of them include small numbers of patients with various definitions of partial response, and are open-label.

Despite the disappointing results from the recent meta-analyses [71–73], some partial clozapine responders may benefit from augmentation with an antipsychotic drug, and because the evidence-based alternatives are sparse, augmentation may be worth trying [74, 75]. To date augmentation with antipsychotics is a common procedure although the literature does not favor any particular antipsychotic agent as an augmenting drug of choice [68]. After a failure of clozapine treatment as monotherapy, its augmentation with a second antipsychotic medication is relatively common in clinical practice [76–78] that fluctuates from 18 to 44% [67, 79]. Besides the use of antipsychotics, other augmentation strategies include addition of antidepressants, various mood stabilizers, medications from different chemical groups such as clonidine, glycine, d-cycloserine, donepezil, omega-3, ginkgo biloba, and ECT are applied [18, 80–99].

In this chapter, we define polypharmacy as the use of clozapine with another medication for treatment of the same condition. In contrast to this, a combination of two drugs or more in order to treat different illnesses or conditions, for example, combination of clozapine and metformin for diabetic schizophrenic patient or clozapine and amisulpride for clozapine-induced hypersalivation, would not be considered as a polypharmacy. We also would not consider as polypharmacy the addition of another medication to treat side effects, such as the use of anticholinergic drugs in order to treat EPS.

Here we present a summary of the literature dealing with the combination of clozapine with different medications in management of resistant schizophrenia and schizoaffective patients. This theme is a "hot topic" in the current professional journals.

7.6 Clozapine Combinations with Antipsychotics

7.6.1 Clozapine in a Combination with First Generation Antipsychotic Drugs

There are some few publications concerning the combination of clozapine with first generation antipsychotics. One of the first publications was an open clinical trial described a combination of clozapine with chlorpromazine [100].

Potter and coworkers compared the efficacies of chlorpromazine monotherapy, clozapine monotherapy, and clozapine-chlorpromazine combination therapy in a double-blind, flexible-dose study. Monotherapy treated patients could receive doses up to 600 mg/day of each agent, while those in the combination group (n = 20) could receive doses up to 400 mg/day of each agent. There were no differences between the three groups for total BPRS. The combination group showed a significant improvement in comparison to the chlorpromazine group, but not to the clozapine group. This improvement was demonstrated on the withdrawal, conceptual disorganization, unusual thoughts, and hostility items at the BPRS. There were no notable side effects [100].

Loxapine was added to seven chronic schizophrenia or schizoaffective disorder patients who remained stabilized for at least 9 months on clozapine. The study lasted from 18 to 50 weeks. Severity of symptoms was assessed with the BPRS. On this combination, all patients were improved at least slightly and two improved remarkably. The authors noted that in four cases in which assessment was made, loxapine had no apparent effect on plasma clozapine levels. They suggest that adjunctive treatment with typical neuroleptics for patients with an incomplete response to clozapine merits further investigations [101].

We found two publications about a combination of clozapine with pimozide. One study was an open-label that provided promising data in support of a larger controlled trial [102]. In a 14 years, one of the authors repeated this combination in a double-blind, placebo-controlled, parallel-designed 12-week trial in 53 patients with schizophrenia and schizoaffective disorder partially or completely unresponsive to clozapine monotherapy. The researchers found that a combination of pimozide in average dose of 6.48 mg/day with clozapine was not better than placebo at reducing PANSS total, positive, negative, and general psychopathology scores [103].

Nine publications (case reports, open and double-blind studies) dealt with a combination of clozapine-sulpiride (a selective D_2 dopaminergic antagonist) [104–112]. Of these studies one was a randomized, double-blind, placebo-controlled trial [104] and in the other the researchers compared influence of sulpiride-clozapine and clomipramine-clozapine combinations on negative symptoms of schizophrenia patients [111]. In the first trial was found that the clozapine-sulpiride group exhibited substantially greater and significant improvements in positive and negative psychotic symptoms. However, this research had some methodological limitations such as the small size sample and the short duration of the trial. Moreover, the major issue was represented by the fact that complete nonresponders to clozapine were excluded from the trial (only a subgroup of partial responders to clozapine was selected to participate in this study). The second one did not demonstrate difference between these combinations. Three open studies and case report [105, 106, 108, 112] demonstrated that the addition of sulpiride to clozapine, resulted in significant clinical improvement in some patients assessed with BPRS, Scale for the Assessment of Positive Symptoms (SAPS), SANS, and Hamilton Rating Scale for Depression (HRSD). The rest publications demonstrated only implicit changes in mental condition of the patients [107, 109, 110]. According to Cochrane review, the sulpiride-clozapine combination is probably more effective than clozapine alone in producing clinical improvement in some people whose illness has been resistant to other antipsychotic drugs including clozapine [113].

Co-administration of clozapine and zuclopenthixol demonstrated a good tolerance of this combination in a patient susceptible to development of EPS. According to authors' opinion, the combined treatment presented in this case report might be an optional intervention for patients with refractory schizophrenia [114].

According to another report, three patients partial responder to clozapine were treated with fluphenazine or haloperidol in long-acting forms additionally to clozapine. All patients demonstrated significant improvement without new or worsening side effects [115]. In opposite, Mossaheb et al. in a double-blind placebo controlled study did not find any difference between combinations of clozapine-haloperidol versus clozapine-placebo [116].

Another combination of clozapine and pipothiazine in tablet and depot forms did not demonstrate any improvement in mental state of patients assessed by BPRS [117, 118].

Three other publications (case reports) regarding the combination of clozapine with other conventional antipsychotic medications (perphenazine, haloperidol) describe adverse effects [119–121], including death [120, 121].

As can be seen, the results of these scientific reports are not consistent. Most trials are based on small numbers of patients with various definitions of partial response or resistance, and most of them are open-label. These combinations should be performed as new studies in double-blind placebo controlled mode.

7.6.2 Clozapine in a Combination with Second-Generation Antipsychotics

Since advent of the SGAs as a new option to manage schizophrenia, a number of publications concerning a combination of clozapine with these medications are significantly more than with FGAs, and their quantity is increasing over last years. Along with case reports and open label studies, many double-blind placebo controlled trials and even few meta-analyses concerning clozapine combinations were performed [71, 72, 122–124].

7.7 Augmentation with Aripiprazole

The clozapine-aripiprazole combination is a relatively frequent issue in the psychiatric literature during last years. We found at least 12 publications on this topic. Aripiprazole has been described as the prototype of a new generation of antipsychotic agents. Its function is dopamine-serotonin system stabilizing, since it is a partial agonist of D_2 and 5-HT_{1A} receptors, and agonist of 5-HT_2 receptors [125]. Partial agonism may be a beneficial property by allowing optimal neurotransmission. For instance, it acts as an antagonist in areas where there is an abundance of dopamine causing psychosis while acting as an agonist at receptor sites where low dopaminergic tone would produce adverse effects such as EPS or hyperprolactinemia [126, 127]. Adverse effects associated with this drug such as somnolence, headache, lightheadedness, and gastrointestinal upset may be explained by its affinity for several other receptors including D_3, D_4, 5-HT_{2C}, 5-HT_7, α_1, and H_1.

Some case reports and case series described that adjunctive therapy with aripiprazole can ameliorate positive as well as negative symptoms in clozapine resistant schizophrenia patients [128–134].

Mitsonis and coworkers [135] for 16 weeks investigated whether augmentation of clozapine with aripiprazole improves clinically significant residual symptoms in 27 stabilized outpatients with chronic schizophrenia. The authors found that aripiprazole augmentation in these patients treated with clozapine led to a substantial improvement in clinically significant residual symptoms, such as negative-depressive symptoms, cognitive impairment and quality of life, without worsening the side effect burden.

In a retrospective study of 24 treatment-resistant schizophrenia patients treated with clozapine-aripiprazole combination was found that it was associated with 22% reduction of clozapine dose. Eighteen of 24 patients (75%) have lost a mean weight of 5.05 kg. There was improvement in positive and negative symptoms, social functions, weight loss and a moderate increase in high-density lipoprotein (HDL). The authors suggest that clozapine-aripiprazole is a safe and tolerable combination, however, control trials are needed [136]. Augmentation of clozapine with aripiprazole was found as safe and effective in a retrospective trial with seven participants suffered from severe psychotic schizoaffective and bipolar disorders, who failed to respond to atypical antipsychotics [137].

However, double blind placebo-controlled studied do not show definitive results. Millar et al. performed a double-blind, randomized the 16 week study [138]. The authors found that clozapine-aripiprazole combination was associated with a significant decrease in mean weight compared with placebo (aripiprazole 2.53 kg, placebo 0.018 kg; $P<0.001$) and waist circumference (aripiprazole −2.00 cm, placebo 0 cm; $P<0.001$). Both treatment groups showed similar improvement in the GAF.

Fleischhacker et al. performed a 16-week double-blind placebo controlled trial in order to evaluate the influence of aripiprazole-clozapine combination on patients' weight, PANSS and lipid profile [139]. Clinically relevant weight loss from baseline was seen in 13% of those who previously were in the placebo group and in 21% of those who were taking aripiprazole for 28 weeks. There were no significant differences in PANSS scores between the two groups. It was reported that switch from placebo to aripiprazole led to reduction of total cholesterol, low-density lipoprotein (LDL) cholesterol, and triglycerides at week 12.

A multisite study was conducted by Barbui and colleagues in order to compare the efficacy and tolerability of clozapine plus aripiprazole combination versus clozapine plus haloperidol in patients with schizophrenia who did not have an optimal response to clozapine [140]. Patients continued to take clozapine and were randomly assigned to receive daily augmentation with aripiprazole or haloperidol.

After 3 months, the authors found no difference in the proportion of patients who discontinued treatment between the aripiprazole and haloperidol groups. The 3-month change of the BPRS total score was similar in the aripiprazole and haloperidol groups, but EPS were seen more prominently in the haloperidol group. These results suggest that augmentation of clozapine with aripiprazole offers no benefit regarding to treatment withdrawal and overall symptoms in schizophrenia compared to haloperidol augmentation. However, diminishing EPS could elevated the subjective well-being feeling [140].

In another 24-week double-blind, randomized, placebo-controlled trial demonstrated that 15 mg/day of aripiprazole added to stable clozapine treatment lead to a beneficial effect on the positive and general psychopathological symptoms in a sample of treatment-resistant schizophrenia patients in comparison to placebo [74].

Chang et al. [141] in a 8-week double-blind placebo controlled study found that improvement was significantly greater with aripiprazole treatment than with placebo for negative symptoms assessed by both the BPRS negative symptom sub-scale and the SANS total score but not for positive symptoms. Prolactin and triglyceride levels were significantly lower in the aripiprazole group than in the placebo group. No significant differences between the two groups were observed in adverse effects, including extrapyramidal symptoms and serum glucose levels. The authors concluded that although aripiprazole-clozapine combination did not lead to a significant improvement of total symptom severity in schizophrenia, a favorable change in the negative symptom domain was observed.

De Risio and colleagues [142] investigated the change in BPRS scores and metabolic features like BMI, fasting glucose, total and LDL cholesterol, triglycerides, functional outcome Health of the Nation Outcome Scales (HoNOS-Rome) and Personal and Social Performance Scale (PSP) scores after aripiprazole augmentation in 16 persons with treatment-resistant schizophrenia who were already treated with clozapine for 6 weeks. The results demonstrated a statistically significant improvement in metabolic indices, psychopathology and functional outcome measures from baseline to endpoint after augmentation with aripiprazole. Statistically significant correlations were observed between psychopathological and behavioral measures at baseline and at endpoint.

7.8 Augmentation with Risperidone

Clozapine and risperidone were by far the most studied antipsychotics combination, with 50% of all available random clinical trials (RCTs).

Since clozapine has a broad-spectrum receptor activity, but a weak dopamine D_2 blockade, it was hypothesized that risperidone (a significantly stronger D_2-antagonist agent) could enhance the therapeutic effects of clozapine non-responders [143]. Risperidone was probably favored over other D_2 antagonists because of its better EPS profile at its conventional therapeutic window (dosages lower than 6 mg/day) [144]. Until writing this chapter, there were performed three randomized clinical trials [143, 145, 146]. One of them was positive [143] and two others were negative. The positive study was longer and lasted for 12 weeks while the other lasted for 6–8 weeks [145, 146]. The positive results' study demonstrated improvement in positive and negative symptoms. It should be noted that during 6 weeks of treatment, the between-group difference was insignificant. The superiority of clozapine plus risperidone clearly appears later and was significant at 12 weeks. Both positive and negative symptoms decreased significantly from baseline to week 12.

In two others randomized, placebo-controlled, double-blind studies did not demonstrate significant improvement of psychopathology in patients with poor or incomplete response to clozapine monotherapy. They lasted only for 6 [145] and 8 [146] weeks. In the placebo and treatment groups, both positive and negative symptoms decreased significantly from baseline to the end in these two studies. Honer and coworkers found that working memory showed a small decline in the risperidone group, and a small improvement in the placebo group. Furthermore, they also observed some evidence for higher fasting serum glucose in the risperidone augmentation group [146].

In order to exclude the possibility that risperidone addition needs more than 8 weeks to show any benefit, Honer et al. [147] extended the study for 18 weeks in the open-label mode. There were no significant benefits during this extension, and even placebo effect was higher.

Furthermore, three prospective open studies [148–150] were performed. Two [149, 150] were positive and reported a significant improvement in the BPRS and the PANSS positive and negative subscale scores. By contrast, in the third trial, none of the enrolled patients responded [148]. Some case studies reported about significant clinical improvement in patients treated with clozapine plus risperidone [151–156]. Others reported adverse effects such as neuroleptic malignant syndrome [157, 158], neutropenia [159], agranulocytosis [160], oculogyric crisis [161], exacerbation of hoarding disorder [162], and atrial ectopics [163].

In summary, although this combination has been extensively studied, proof of efficacy has been elusive. There is still significant uncertainty regarding long-term safety.

7.9 Augmentation with Amisulpride

Amisulpride is a relatively novel antipsychotic medication and is not yet available in the USA. Anyway, we have found 13 publications concerning the combination of clozapine-amisulpride, 4 double blind and most other are open studies and case reports [164–176].

Assion et al. performed a double-blind placebo-controlled trial including 16 patients with chronic schizophrenia and partially responsive to clozapine participated. The researchers compared 6 weeks augmentation of clozapine with 400–600 mg/day of amisulpride or placebo. They found that amisulpride was more beneficial in a higher dose. No severe side-effects occurred, but tremor, bradykinesia, akathisia and elevated prolactin levels were recorded [166].

Genc and colleagues [169] in double-blind study, compared during 6 weeks the effectiveness and tolerability of the amisulpride-clozapine combination with the combination of quetiapine and clozapine in 56 patients who were only partially responsive to clozapine monotherapy. The authors concluded that amisulpride seems to be effective and well tolerated for augmentation purposes in clozapine-resistant patients.

The combination of clozapine and amisulpride was studied in two other double-blind RCT protocols [172, 173] with primary goal of reducing clozapine-induced hypersalivation (CIS). In the first study [173] amisulpride addition was effective in diminishing hypersalivation after 3 weeks of treatment, but failed to show any efficacy on primary psychotic symptoms, and in 95% of subjects was found prolactinemia. No extrapyramidal adverse effects were identified. This randomized, controlled trial did not confirm the previous positive case reports relating to clozapine augmentation by amisulpride [164, 170, 171]. In the second study [172] the primary goal was also reducing CIS, but in this trial amisulpride augmentation compared with moclobemide addition. Both medications were safe and effective as treatment of CIS. Although moclobemide exceeded amisulpride in antisalivation activity, treatment of CIS with amisulpride leads to improvement in psychotic symptoms.

Other studies have suggested that addition of amisulpride allows clozapine dose to be reduced [167, 168, 176]. A support for the efficacy of this combination comes from an open study of 33 patients with suboptimal response to clozapine treatment [175]. Twenty-eight subjects completed the 6-month study, showing statistically significant improvements on PANSS, SANS and GAS (Global Assessment Scale).

In another open retrospective study, 15 patients with resistant schizophrenia were treated with amisulpride in combination with other novel antipsychotics. Five of them received amisulpride-clozapine combination. The mean amisulpride dose was 693.3 ± 279.6 mg/day. The mental state of all this subgroup patients was improved [174].

Some case reports also described that this combination significantly improves schizophrenia symptoms after a relatively short time and may be considered as a therapeutic option [164, 165].

7.10 Augmentation with Olanzapine

We found only two reports concerning this combination. Both are case reports describing three patients suffered from resistant schizophrenia with partial effect to clozapine monotherapy. Addition of olanzapine was found effective in reduction of positive symptoms (auditory hallucinations and delusions) without any side effect [177, 178]. Unfortunately, no controlled trials were conducted in order to prove these findings.

7.11 Augmentation with Quetiapine

We found only one report regarding clozapine augmentation with quetiapine in schizophrenia patients with substantial response to clozapine monotherapy. This single-blind study compared two combinations: clozapine-amisulpride and clozapine-quetiapine. The amisulpride dose was up to 600 mg/day and maximum quetiapine dose was 900 mg/day, while clozapine was fixed. A substantial improvement occurred in both groups by the end of the eighth week; however, the improvement associated with amisulpride was significantly greater than that seen with quetiapine [169].

7.12 Augmentation with Sertindole

The combination of clozapine with sertindole was examined in only two studies [179, 180]. The first study [179] was a 12-week, double-blind, randomized, placebo-controlled trial including patients treated with clozapine for at least 6 months who had not achieved sufficient response. Patients were randomized to receive an add-on medications either sertindole 16 mg/day or placebo. Assessment was done at baseline and after 6 and 12 weeks. Clozapine augmentation with sertindole was not superior to placebo regarding total score or subscale score of the PANSS, CGI, World Health Organization Quality of Life Brief, and Drug Attitude Inventory. Four patients demonstrated a significant worsening of psychosis after sertindole addition, and 2 of them required psychiatric hospitalization. Metabolic parameters were unchanged during the study, but augmentation of clozapine with sertindole was associated with no significant increasing QTc prolongation (12 ± 20 ms compared with 0 ± 20 ms in the placebo group) [179].

In the second study the authors investigated effects of sertindole on cognition in clozapine-treated schizophrenia patients [180]. Participants were also randomized to receive 16 mg of sertindole or placebo as adjunctive treatment to clozapine in 12-week, double-blinded, randomized, placebo-controlled trial. Adding sertindole did not improve or worsen cognitive functioning, which is consisted with previous negative studies regarding influence of another antipsychotic drug on cognition disturbances induced by clozapine [180].

7.13 Augmentation with Ziprasidone

We found four case reports [181–184] regarding this combination describing overall 22 patients. According to these publications, mental state of all patients improved without any side effects.

There are four meta-analyses concerning the augmentation of clozapine treatment with another antipsychotic for people with an inadequate response to clozapine monotherapy [71–73, 122]. The largest meta-analysis was conducted by Barbui et al. [122]. The authors came into conclusion that the evidence considered for clozapine augmentation with another SGA antipsychotic medication is weak and observed benefits are moderate at best. On the other hand, Correll and coworkers performed a meta-analysis of 19 studies concerning co-treatment with clozapine. They found that generally antipsychotic combinations are more beneficial than monotherapy [72]. However, the variability of clozapine-resistance's definitions, outcome measures, dose and duration of pharmacological trials is a major limitation for definite conclusions.

7.14 Augmentation with Anticonvulsants

Glutamate hypofunction hypothesis of schizophrenia is the base for searching new directions trials in coping with resistant schizophrenia patients. This hypothesis consists on post-mortem brain studies and the lack of efficacy of glutamate agonists as antipsychotic drugs. Abnormalities in N-Methyl-D-aspartate (NMDA) receptor (NMDAR) function may contribute to these symptoms that are resistant to antipsychotic medications [185]. This assumption has also generated interest in the role of glutamate release inhibitors as clozapine augmenters and has led to performance of some studies.

7.14.1 Clozapine-Lamotrigine Combination

Lamotrigine is a novel antiepileptic agent acting through inhibition of voltage-sensitive channel sodium current and by inhibiting NMDAR, decreases the release of glutamate [186].

One of the first study was a research performed by Dursun and Deakin [186], who added lamotrigine or topiramate to 26 treatment-resistant schizophrenia patients in addition to their ongoing different antipsychotic medications. They found that patients receiving lamotrigine augmentation of clozapine had a significant decrease in BPRS scores after 2 weeks of treatment, but no significant improvement when lamotrigine was added to risperidone, haloperidol, olanzapine or flupenthixol. There was also no significant improvement observed with topiramate augmentation of clozapine, olanzapine, haloperidol and flupenthixol [186].

The therapeutic effects of lamotrigine augmentation were assessed by Tiihonen et al. in a randomized placebo-controlled cross-over 14-week study of 34 clozapine-resistant patients [187]. It was demonstrated that lamotrigine treatment significantly improved positive symptoms and general psychopathological symptoms, but had no effect on negative symptoms.

The efficacy of add-on lamotrigine up to 200 mg/day or placebo on clinical symptomatology and cognitive functioning of treatment-resistant schizophrenia patients receiving clozapine was examined in a 24-week double-blind, randomized, trial. The results demonstrated that addition of lamotrigine to a stable clozapine treatment led to a beneficial effect on the negative, positive and general psychopathological symptomatology. The findings provide evidence that lamotrigine augmentation of clozapine treatment is well tolerated and may be proposed as an effective therapeutic strategy to improve outcome in treatment-resistant schizophrenia [99].

Goff and coworkers tried to replicate previous lamotrigine trials [188]. They performed two multicenter, randomized, double-blind, 12-week, parallel-group trials in order to evaluate the potential role of lamotrigine augmentation in schizophrenia patients resistant to atypical antipsychotic medication. In these studies flexibly dosed lamotrigine (100–400 mg/day) were compared with placebo as add-on treatment in schizophrenia patients with stable, residual psychotic symptoms. These studies do not support the use of lamotrigine as an add-on to atypical antipsychotics in patients with refractory psychosis. In one trial, the researchers mention a positive effect of lamotrigine on cognition [188]. However, it is necessary to note that in these studies the majority of patients (85%) were treated with another antipsychotic medication than clozapine. Those patients did not receive greater benefit from lamotrigine compared with placebo, whereas 63 patients treated with clozapine showed from small to moderate effect sizes for the efficacy of lamotrigine.

Tiihonen and colleagues [97] performed a meta-analysis including 5 trials and total of 161 randomized clozapine patients aimed to study the efficacy of lamotrigine in treatment of clozapine-resistant schizophrenia. This meta-analysis suggests that lamotrigine augmentation may be an effective treatment for patients with clozapine-resistant schizophrenia. A substantial proportion of these most severely ill patients appeared to obtain clinically meaningful benefit from this combination [97]. To date it is the first evidence of efficacy for any pharmacological treatment in clozapine-resistant schizophrenia and it is noted by the authors that similar benefits may not be observed with lamotrigine and other antipsychotic agents apart from clozapine [189].

7.14.2 Clozapine-Topiramate Combination

Topiramate is a GABAergic anticonvulsant drug indicated as add-on pharmacotherapy for adults and children with primary generalized tonic–clonic and partial-onset seizures. It has been used for people with schizophrenia to correct a postulated glutamate deregulation due to NMDA receptor hypofunction [190, 191].

Afshar et al. conducted a 8 week randomized, double-blind trial, where maximum dose of 300 mg/day topirimate or placebo were added to schizophrenia patients with an incomplete clinical response to clozapine [192]. Clinical response (more than 20% reduction in PANSS) was significantly higher in the topirimate treatment than in the placebo group (50% vs. 12.5%). Similar significant decline patterns were found in all three subscales (negative, positive and psychopathology signs).

Side effects such as hypersalivation, psychomotor retardation, paresthesia, and weight loss were more prevalent in the topiramate group. The authors assume that topiramate can be an effective medication in controlling schizophrenic symptoms, considering its effect on negative symptoms and controlling antipsychotic-associated weight gain [192]. However, the authors did not assess a cognitive function. Cognitive impairment is one of the most important adverse effect of topiramate that is particularly relevant to people with schizophrenia [193–195].

Since cognitive impairment is a dose-dependent side effect of topiramate, another 24-week double-blind, randomized, placebo-controlled trial was performed in a sample of treatment-resistant schizophrenia patients treated with clozapine [18]. The authors reported about a significant reduction of bizarre behavior score emerged at the end of the trial in patients treated with clozapine-topiramate combination. However, in whole this trial showed that the addition of topiramate to clozapine does not appear to improve residual negative and positive symptoms in these patients despite an adequate trial of clozapine [18]. It is possible that negative results of this study were connected with a lower dose of topiramate (200 mg/day in comparison to 300 mg/day, which was used in the study by Afshar et al. [192]). From these studies it appears that relatively low doses of topiramate could preserve cognitive function, but they have a small benefit for clinical symptoms [189].

The third report: a 17-week, double-blind, placebo-controlled clinical trial was performed on 80 chronic schizophrenia patients resistant to at least two different antipsychotic therapy trials other than clozapine. All participants were treated with up to 300 mg/day of clozapine. In addition, participants randomly received either topiramate 200 mg/day (16 patients) or 300 mg/day (12 patients) or placebo. There were no statistically significant differences in PANSS score differences on any of the three subscales from baseline to endpoint between the clozapine and topiramate group compared to the clozapine and placebo group [196].

In a 12-week naturalistic, open study was examined the potential benefits of topiramate in clozapine-treated schizophrenia patients with a suboptimal clinical response. Augmentation with topiramate up to a maximum dose of 200 mg/day led to a 14% improvement in total BPRS scores and 2.5% decrease in body weight. This treatment was generally well tolerated. These findings support that topiramate may serve as a viable augmentation strategy in clozapine partial responders, with evidence of both clinical and metabolic benefits [86].

7.15 Clozapine-Lithium Combination

Lithium has not been shown to be an effective augmenting agent for schizophrenia in few trials, although some case studies have suggested its effectiveness [197]. The clozapine-lithium combination is considered as relatively contraindicated because of increased risks of seizures, neuroleptic malignant syndrome, and neurotoxic reactions. Other hazards of this combination may include masking of low leukocyte counts and other myeloid processes associated with agranulocytosis, increased body weight and blood sugar levels, ECG abnormalities, possible cardiomyopathy, EEG indications of reduced seizure threshold, and cognitive impairments. This combination is still a controversial issue, although the evidence base for this controversy remains weak and it has not been studied systematically [198].

Twenty hospitalized, treatment-resistant schizophrenia and schizoaffective patients treated with clozapine were included in a double-blind placebo-controlled study with repeated crossovers between lithium and placebo [199]. The patients received lithium citrate as a water solution with an initial dosage of 600 mg/day. Placebo consisted of the same-tasting liquor without lithium. Dosages were titrated to target plasma levels at least 0.5 mmol/l unless limited by side effects. There was improvement in CGI and PANSS total and negative symptom scales in schizoaffective patients, while schizophrenic patients were not improved [199].

Efficacy and safety of clozapine-lithium combination was also examined in retrospective study included 44 hospitalized schizophrenia resistant patients. Mean total duration of combined treatment was 23.5 months. The authors did not find additional risks are associated with a clozapine–lithium therapy that exceeds the risks reported for the respective monotherapies or the more common combination of lithium with other neuroleptics. The data also suggest somewhat enhanced efficacy of the combined therapy (e.g. when compared to the clozapine monotherapy). This combination was found to be effective in 84% patients concerning prophylaxis, treatment of affective symptoms or aggression/excitement, and augmentation of neuroleptic efficacy. At the same time adverse events were reported in 64% of the patients. Most adverse events were benign and transient. However, eight patients (18%) developed transient neurological adverse events that were genuinely novel in only three patients (7%). These side effects were observed in patients treated with high dosage of lithium and/or clozapine or with high plasma levels or serotonergic co-medication. The researchers conclude that combining clozapine with lithium treatment may be safe and effective, however it should be conducted under strict clinical guidelines (i.e. by administering at moderate doses with plasma-level monitoring) and by avoiding additional co-medication with serotonergic drugs or other substances that interfere clozapine metabolism and/or body clearance [198].

Ten men and one woman (aged 27–52 years) suffered from chronic schizophrenia or schizoaffective disorder benefited from a treatment with combination of lithium and clozapine. The clozapine-lithium treatment led to stabilization and improvement in all patients' mental condition [200].

Moldavsky and coworkers [201] found lithium-clozapine combination as effective in both the schizoaffective patients and the schizophrenic patients, reflected in the reduction of the BPRS, PANSS and CGI scores. The authors concluded that combined clozapine-lithium treatment may be effective in chronic schizophrenic or schizoaffective patients with notable affective or aggressive symptomatology, who are resistant to standard neuroleptics and to clozapine alone. There was no occurrence of agranulocytosis, neuroleptic malignant syndrome or other clinically significant adverse effects [201].

In one retrospective study was examined adjunct valproic acid (N = 15) or lithium (N = 9) in treatment-resistant schizophrenia patients added to clozapine and compared to clozapine monotherapy (N = 25). Six month total BPRS scores were similarly improved in all treatment groups, however significantly greater improvements were demonstrated in the first month in patients treated with valproic acid-clozapine or lithium-clozapine combinations vs. clozapine alone. Rates of sedation, tachycardia, orthostasis, gastrointestinal disturbances, confusion and dizziness were similar among all groups. The addition of valproic acid was significantly more effective in reducing global symptoms (driven by hostility and anxiety) in the first month of adjunct treatment as compared to clozapine monotherapy and to previous clozapine treatment [92].

7.16 Augmentation with NMDA Agonists and Antagonists

According to the glutamate hypothesis of schizophrenia, specifically N-Methyl-D-aspartate receptor (NMDAR) hypofunction, it was assumed that N-methyl-D-aspartate (NMDA)-enhancing agents might lead to beneficial effect in treatment resistant schizophrenia patients [202]. Antagonists of the NMDA subclass of glutamate receptors and agonists of the glycine-B co-agonist site of these receptors are important tools for characterizing the contributions of NMDAR pathophysiology to a large number of neuropsychiatric disturbances and for treating it.

Consistently with this hypothesis, glutamatergic agents such as glycine, D-serine, D-cycloserine, ampakine CX516, memantine, and N-methylglycine were investigated in several RCTs, which overall showed inconsistency or negative results.

Glycine is a full NMDA receptor agonist and D-cycloserine is a partial agonist. Results with these substances as augmenting agents in patients with schizophrenia were mixed. In two double blind placebo-controlled studies glycine plus clozapine was found effective [203, 204], while in the contrary, other two trials demonstrated it as not effective [83, 205].

The combinations clozapine with D-cycloserine [206, 207] and clozapine with D-serine [208] were not effective or even had deleterious effects, notably by worsening negative symptoms [206, 207]. Augmentation of clozapine with N-methylglycine for treatment resistant patients did not demonstrate any difference between placebo and treatment group [209]. Addition of AMPA-receptor-positive modulators (Ampakines) which facilitate learning and memory in animal models and in preliminary trials in human subjects also did not demonstrate its efficacy in two placebo-controlled studies [210, 211].

On the base of the membrane phospholipid hypothesis of schizophrenia [212], omega-3 fatty acid (ethyleicosapentaenoic acid) was added to clozapine as treatment of resistant schizophrenia patients. Two studies [213, 214], demonstrated a significant decrease in PANSS total score, while a third trial [215] failed to show any significant benefit. The most reported side effects over all studies were diarrhea and nausea.

7.16.1 Augmentation with Cognitive Enhancing Agents

Cognitive enhancing agents like memantine are drugs usually used as treatment of patients suffering from some kinds of dementia. To date there is only one double-blind trial where memantine (a weak, nonselective NMDA receptor antagonist) was added to 21 treatment resistant schizophrenia patients in order to examine an efficacy of this combination for negative symptoms [216]. Significant improvement was found in the active treatment group for the total BPRS score, and on the positive and negative symptom subscales. Additionally subjects from the memantine group showed a significant increase in mean score on the Mini-Mental State Examination (MMSE), although this test is not the most sensitive measure of cognitive functioning.

As a summary, we can notice that there is no definitive conclusion regarding these augmentations.

7.17 Augmentation with Antidepressants

Augmentation with selective serotonin reuptake inhibitors (SSRIs) is a strategy often employed when depressive or negative symptoms are prominent. Few studies have systematically examined the efficacy of antidepressants augmentation of clozapine. There is a variability of these trials results.

In two studies addition of fluvoxamine demonstrated beneficial effect on global symptomatology in refractory schizophrenia patients [217, 218]. However, this agent is a potent CYP1A2 inhibitor and substantially decreases clozapine metabolism, thus such interaction may increase the risk of side effects. An elevation of clozapine plasma levels might also explain the positive effects reported with fluvoxamine augmentation, at least partially. On the other hand, fluvoxamine decreases plasma levels of norclozapine (a toxic metabolite of clozapine), which has been reported to contribute to weight gain, hyperglycemia, and lipid abnormalities in clozapine treated patients [219]. Therefore, this strategy could be useful, but a close monitoring of drug doses and their serum concentrations are needed. The authors assume that the positive effect observed with fluvoxamine adjunction may be due to its peculiar pharmacological profile, in particular to its ability to block sigma receptors [220].

In contrast to fluvoxamine, fluoxetine augmentation does not have any clinical effect, although it also increases clozapine levels [221, 222]. It was suggested that agents with predominant serotoninergic effects such as fluoxetine are not effective in augmenting clozapine.

Two earlier reports concerning the mirtazapine augmentation to clozapine resistant patients [223, 224] found improvement negative symptoms and cognitive dysfunctions, but a recent double-blind placebo controlled trial [225] did not demonstrate any difference between addition of mirtazapine vs. placebo. The positive effect obtained adding mirtazapine may be explained by its peculiar pharmacological profile.

7.18 Clozapine—ECT Combination

An augmentation of clozapine by using ECT does not frequent use in clinical practice, since has been suggested that this combination could increase the risk of status epilepticus [226]. We found 14 reports describing 144 subjects concerning this strategy for schizophrenia treatment-resistant patients. Three were retrospective studies [85, 227, 228], two—open studies [229, 230] and nine case reports [91, 231–238]. Most researchers found this combination as safe and well tolerated. There is only one report of tardive grand mal seizures seemingly related to ECT in a patient previously treated with clozapine [237].

In general, researchers suppose that the augmentation of clozapine treatment with electroconvulsive therapy should be useful in treatment-resistant schizophrenia patients in cases when the clozapine monotherapy is ineffective or impossible to add another antipsychotic due to severe somatic diseases or side effects.

However, most studies were limited by small sample size, short follow-up period and an open trial design. Furthermore, data about clozapine and ECT dosages were not clearly reported, psychopathology measures are often lack, and clozapine serum levels are generally not reported. Thus, despite the fact that ECT plus clozapine could be effective for schizophrenia treatment-resistant patients, present literature data does not allow to jump into definitive conclusions.

7.19 Conclusions

Treatment with clozapine requires special knowledge and especially complex cases should preferably occur in specific clinics with sufficient knowledge and experienced with clozapine policy [239].

Although the assumed addition of an antipsychotic to facilitate dose reduction of clozapine is not supported by clinical data, but mainly based on clinical experience. However, one should keep in mind that most subjects receiving clozapine are complex patients that have already tried most evidence-based interventions and are often treated with high dosages and polypharmacy at the expense of dreadful side effects [68].

Some strategies of augmentation or combination used for clozapine treatment-resistant chronic schizophrenia patients, which we reviewed in this chapter, may be useful and relatively safe. Among antipsychotics, clozapine-amisulpride combination showed strong evidence-based support for these patients. Clozapine-aripiprazole maybe promising co-treatment. Augmentation of clozapine with lamotrigine among mood stabilizers and ECT among other strategies also seem to be promising attitude. However, further studies are needed to confirm the effectiveness and safety.

These data suggest that, at least, under certain circumstances, clozapine combinations may be superior to antipsychotic monotherapy regarding all-causes for discontinuation and general measures of efficacy.

References

1. Rossler W, Salize HJ, van Os J, Riecher-Rossler A (2005) Size of burden of schizophrenia and psychotic disorders. Eur Neuropsychopharmacol 15:399–409
2. Conley RR, Kelly DL (2001) Management of treatment resistance in schizophrenia. Biol Psychiatry 50:898–911
3. Lehman AF, Lieberman JA, Dixon LB, McGlashan TH, Miller AL, Perkins DO, Kreyenbuhl J (2004) Practice guideline for the treatment of patients with schizophrenia, second edition. Am J Psychiatry 161:1–56
4. Sheitman BB, Lieberman JA (1998) The natural history and pathophysiology of treatment resistant schizophrenia. J Psychiatr Res 32:143–150
5. McGlashan TH (1988) A selective review of recent North American long-term followup studies of schizophrenia. Schizophr Bull 14:515–542
6. Conley RR, Buchanan RW (1997) Evaluation of treatment-resistant schizophrenia. Schizophr Bull 23:663–674
7. Breier AF, Malhotra AK, Su TP, Pinals DA, Elman I, Adler CM, Lafargue RT, Clifton A, Pickar D (1999) Clozapine and risperidone in chronic schizophrenia: effects on symptoms, parkinsonian side effects, and neuroendocrine response. Am J Psychiatry 156:294–298
8. Loebel AD, Lieberman JA, Alvir JM, Mayerhoff DI, Geisler SH, Szymanski SR (1992) Duration of psychosis and outcome in first-episode schizophrenia. Am J Psychiatry 149:1183–1188
9. Kane J, Honigfeld G, Singer J, Meltzer H (1988) Clozapine for the treatment-resistant schizophrenic. A double-blind comparison with chlorpromazine. Arch Gen Psychiatry 45:789–796
10. Suzuki T, Remington G, Mulsant BH, Uchida H, Rajji TK, Graff-Guerrero A, Mimura M, Mamo DC (2012) Defining treatment-resistant schizophrenia and response to antipsychotics: a review and recommendation. Psychiatry Res 197(1):1–6
11. Suzuki T, Uchida H, Nomura K, Takeuchi H, Nakajima S, Tanabe A, Yagi G, Watanabe K, Kashima H (2008) Novel rating scales for schizophrenia—targeted inventory on problems in schizophrenia (TIP-Sz) and functional assessment for comprehensive treatment of schizophrenia (FACT-Sz). Schizophr Res 106:328–336
12. Meltzer HY (1997) Treatment-resistant schizophrenia—the role of clozapine. Curr Med Res Opin 14:1–20
13. Pantelis C, Lambert TJ (2003) Managing patients with "treatment-resistant" schizophrenia. Med J Aust 178(Suppl):S62–S66
14. Barnes TR, McEvedy CJ (1996) Pharmacological treatment strategies in the non-responsive schizophrenic patient. Int Clin Psychopharmacol 11(Suppl 2):67–71
15. Dixon LB, Lehman AF, Levine J (1995) Conventional antipsychotic medications for schizophrenia. Schizophr Bull 21:567–577
16. Carpenter WT Jr (2007) Schizophrenia: disease, syndrome, or dimensions? Fam Process 46:199–206
17. Kirkpatrick B, Buchanan RW, Ross DE, Carpenter WT Jr (2001) A separate disease within the syndrome of schizophrenia. Arch Gen Psychiatry 58:165–171
18. Muscatello MR, Bruno A, Pandolfo G, Mico U, Bellinghieri PM, Scimeca G, Cacciola M, Campolo D, Settineri S, Zoccali R (2011) Topiramate augmentation of clozapine in schizophrenia: a double-blind, placebo-controlled study. J Psychopharmacol 25:667–674
19. Jalenques I (1996) Drug-resistant schizophrenia. Treatment options. CNS Drugs 5:8–23
20. Dencker SJ, Kulhaet F (1988) Treatment resistance in schizophrenia. Springer, Braunschweig/Wiesbaden
21. Lawrie SM, Abukmeil SS, Chiswick A, Egan V, Santosh CG, Best JJ (1997) Qualitative cerebral morphology in schizophrenia: a magnetic resonance imaging study and systematic literature review. Schizophr Res 25:155–166
22. Ho BC, Andreasen NC, Nopoulos P, Arndt S, Magnotta V, Flaum M (2003) Progressive structural brain abnormalities and their relationship to clinical outcome: a longitudinal magnetic resonance imaging study early in schizophrenia. Arch Gen Psychiatry 60:585–594

23. Jarema M, Choma M, Kozlowski P, Poniatowska R, Krawczyk R (1997) Cortical atrophy in MRI, mental status and neuroleptic treatment effect in schizophrenia. Psychiatr Pol 31:547–557
24. Sheppard C, Collins L, Fiorentino D, Fracchia J, Merlis S (1969) Polypharmacy in psychiatric treatment. I. Incidence at a state hospital. Curr Ther Res Clin Exp 11:765–774
25. Barnes TR, Paton C (2011) Antipsychotic polypharmacy in schizophrenia: benefits and risks. CNS Drugs 25:383–399
26. Gaebel W, Weinmann S, Sartorius N, Rutz W, McIntyre JS (2005) Schizophrenia practice guidelines: international survey and comparison. Br J Psychiatry 187:248–255
27. Marder SR, Essock SM, Miller AL, Buchanan RW, Davis JM, Kane JM, Lieberman J, Schooler NR (2002) The Mount Sinai conference on the pharmacotherapy of schizophrenia. Schizophr Bull 28:5–16
28. National Institute for Health and Clinical Excellence (2010) Schizophrenia: core interventions in the treatment and management of schizophrenia in adults in primary and secondary care. Clinical guideline (updated 03 August, 2010). National Institute for Health and Clinical Excellence, London
29. Taylor D, Paton C, Kapur S (2009) The Maudsley prescribing guidelines, 10th edn. Informa Healthcare, London
30. Miller AL (2004) PORT treatment recommendations. Schizophr Bull 30:601–604
31. Stahl SM (1999) Selecting an atypical antipsychotic by combining clinical experience with guidelines from clinical trials. J Clin Psychiatry 60(Suppl 10):31–41
32. Biancosino B, Barbui C, Marmai L, Dona S, Grassi L (2005) Determinants of antipsychotic polypharmacy in psychiatric inpatients: a prospective study. Int Clin Psychopharmacol 20:305–309
33. Bret P, Bonnet F, Bret MC, Jaffre A (2002) Use of atypical antipsychotics in Charles perrens psychiatric hospital (Bordeaux) analysis of prescribing practices for amisulpride, clozapine, olanzapine and risperidone. Encéphale 28:329–342
34. Bret P, Bret MC, Queuille E (2009) Prescribing patterns of antipsychotics in 13 French psychiatric hospitals. Encéphale 35:129–138
35. Broekema WJ, de Groot IW, van Harten PN (2007) Simultaneous prescribing of atypical antipsychotics, conventional antipsychotics and anticholinergics—a European study. Pharm World Sci 29:126–130
36. De Hert M, Wampers M, Peuskens J (2006) Pharmacological treatment of hospitalised schizophrenic patients in Belgium. Int J Psychiatry Clin Pract 10:285–290
37. Florez Menendez G, Blanco Ramos M, Gomez-Reino Rodriguez I, Gayoso Diz P, Bobes Garcia J (2004) Polipharmacy in the antipsychotic prescribing in practices psychiatric outpatient clinic. Actas Esp Psiquiatr 32:333–339
38. Hamann J, Ruppert A, Auby P, Pugner K, Kissling W (2003) Antipsychotic prescribing patterns in Germany: a retrospective analysis using a large outpatient prescription database. Int Clin Psychopharmacol 18:237–242
39. Hemminki E (1977) Polypharmacy among psychiatric patients. Acta Psychiatr Scand 56:347–356
40. Heresco-Levy U, Brom D, Greenberg D (1993) Self-reported prescribing practices for schizophrenic patients among Israeli psychiatrists. Isr J Psychiatry Relat Sci 30:164–174
41. Paton C, Lelliott P, Harrington M, Okocha C, Sensky T, Duffett R (2003) Patterns of antipsychotic and anticholinergic prescribing for hospital inpatients. J Psychopharmacol 17:223–229
42. Tungaraza TE, Gupta S, Jones J, Poole R, Slegg G (2010) Polypharmacy and high-dose antipsychotic regimes in the community. The Psychiatrist 34:44–46
43. Yosselson-Superstine S, Sternik D, Liebenzon D (1979) Prescribing patterns in psychiatric hospitals in Israel. Acta Psychiatr Scand 60:477–482
44. Keks NA, Altson K, Hope J, Krapivensky N, Culhane C, Tanaghow A, Doherty P, Bootle A (1999) Use of antipsychosis and adjunctive medications by an inner urban community psychiatric service. Aust N Z J Psychiatry 33:896–901
45. Wheeler A, Humberstone V, Robinson G (2006) Trends in antipsychotic prescribing in schizophrenia in Auckland. Australas Psychiatry 14:169–174

46. Pai NB, Laidlaw M, Vella SC (2012) Augmentation of clozapine with another pharmacological agent: treatment for refractory schizophrenia in the 'real world'. Acta Psychiatr Scand 126(1):40–46
47. Procyshyn RM, Kennedy NB, Tse G, Thompson B (2001) Antipsychotic polypharmacy: a survey of discharge prescriptions from a tertiary care psychiatric institution. Can J Psychiatry 46:334–339
48. Chong SA, Sachdev P, Mahendran R, Chua HC (2000) Neuroleptic and anticholinergic drug use in Chinese patients with schizophrenia resident in a state psychiatric hospital in Singapore. Aust N Z J Psychiatry 34:988–991
49. Sim K, Su A, Fujii S, Yang SY, Chong MY, Ungvari GS, Si T, Chung EK, Tsang HY, Chan YH, Heckers S, Shinfuku N, Tan CH (2004) Antipsychotic polypharmacy in patients with schizophrenia: a multicentre comparative study in east Asia. Br J Clin Pharmacol 58:178–183
50. Ito C, Kubota Y, Sato M (1999) A prospective survey on drug choice for prescriptions for admitted patients with schizophrenia. Psychiatry Clin Neurosci 53(Suppl):S35–S40
51. Yoshimura R, Okamoto T, Nakamura J, Tateno M, Otsuka K, Takahashi H, Fujisawa D, Takamatsu T, Fujii S, Sato S, Inoue M, Sasaki H, Kuroki T, Shinfuku N (2006) Prescription pattern of antipsychotic drugs for schizophrenic inpatients in Japan: research on East Asia psychotropic prescription pattern-antipsychotics study. Psychiatry Clin Neurosci 60:778–779
52. Apiquian R, Fresan A, de la Fuente-Sandoval C, Ulloa RE, Nicolini H (2004) Survey on schizophrenia treatment in Mexico: perception and antipsychotic prescription patterns. BMC Psychiatry 4:12
53. Correll CU, Frederickson AM, Kane JM, Manu P (2007) Does antipsychotic polypharmacy increase the risk for metabolic syndrome? Schizophr Res 89:91–100
54. Faries D, Ascher-Svanum H, Zhu B, Correll C, Kane J (2005) Antipsychotic monotherapy and polypharmacy in the naturalistic treatment of schizophrenia with atypical antipsychotics. BMC Psychiatry 5:26
55. Ganguly R, Kotzan JA, Miller LS, Kennedy K, Martin BC (2004) Prevalence, trends, and factors associated with antipsychotic polypharmacy among Medicaid-eligible schizophrenia patients, 1998–2000. J Clin Psychiatry 65:1377–1388
56. Kreyenbuhl J, Valenstein M, McCarthy JF, Ganoczy D, Blow FC (2006) Long-term combination antipsychotic treatment in VA patients with schizophrenia. Schizophr Res 84:90–99
57. Lieberman JA, Stroup TS, McEvoy JP, Swartz MS, Rosenheck RA, Perkins DO, Keefe RS, Davis SM, Davis CE, Lebowitz BD, Severe J, Hsiao JK (2005) Effectiveness of antipsychotic drugs in patients with chronic schizophrenia. N Engl J Med 353:1209–1223
58. Tapp A, Wood AE, Secrest L, Erdmann J, Cubberley L, Kilzieh N (2003) Combination antipsychotic therapy in clinical practice. Psychiatr Serv 54:55–59
59. Chakos M, Lieberman J, Hoffman E, Bradford D, Sheitman B (2001) Effectiveness of second-generation antipsychotics in patients with treatment-resistant schizophrenia: a review and meta-analysis of randomized trials. Am J Psychiatry 158:518–526
60. Frogley C, Taylor D, Dickens G, Picchioni M (2012) A systematic review of the evidence of clozapine's anti-aggressive effects. Int J Neuropsychopharmacol 15(9):1351–1371
61. Munro J, O'Sullivan D, Andrews C, Arana A, Mortimer A, Kerwin R (1999) Active monitoring of 12,760 clozapine recipients in the UK and Ireland. Beyond pharmacovigilance. Br J Psychiatry 175:576–580
62. Bredbacka PE, Paukkala E, Kinnunen E, Koponen H (1993) Can severe cardiorespiratory dysregulation induced by clozapine monotherapy be predicted? Int Clin Psychopharmacol 8:205–206
63. Subramanian S, Völlm BA (2012) Clozapine dose for schizophrenia (Protocol). The Cochrane Library Issue 1 http://www.thecochranelibrary.com
64. Perry PJ, Miller DD, Arndt SV, Cadoret RJ (1991) Clozapine and norclozapine plasma concentrations and clinical response of treatment-refractory schizophrenic patients. Am J Psychiatry 148:231–235

65. Potkin SG, Bera R, Gulasekaram B, Costa J, Hayes S, Jin Y, Richmond G, Carreon D, Sitanggan K, Gerber B et al (1994) Plasma clozapine concentrations predict clinical response in treatment-resistant schizophrenia. J Clin Psychiatry 55(Suppl B):133–136
66. Porcelli S, Balzarro B, Serretti A (2011) Clozapine resistance: augmentation strategies. Eur Neuropsychopharmacol 22(3):165–182
67. Sernyak MJ, Rosenheck R (2004) Clinicians' reasons for antipsychotic coprescribing. J Clin Psychiatry 65:1597–1600
68. Nielsen J, Damkier P, Lublin H, Taylor D (2011) Optimizing clozapine treatment. Acta Psychiatr Scand 123:411–422
69. Miller AE (2005) Psychiatric management of treatment-resistant schizophrenia. In: The American Psychiatric Association, annual meeting, May 21–26, Atlanta, GA, Forum #4
70. Kane JM, Leucht S, Carpenter D, Docherty JP (2003) The expert consensus guideline series. Optimizing pharmacologic treatment of psychotic disorders. Introduction: methods, commentary, and summary. J Clin Psychiatry 64(Suppl 12):5–19
71. Cipriani A, Boso M, Barbui C (2009) Clozapine combined with different antipsychotic drugs for treatment resistant schizophrenia. Cochrane Database Syst Rev Jul 8;(3):CD006324
72. Correll CU, Rummel-Kluge C, Corves C, Kane JM, Leucht S (2009) Antipsychotic combinations vs monotherapy in schizophrenia: a meta-analysis of randomized controlled trials. Schizophr Bull 35:443–457
73. Taylor DM, Smith L (2009) Augmentation of clozapine with a second antipsychotic—a meta-analysis of randomized, placebo-controlled studies. Acta Psychiatr Scand 119:419–425
74. Muscatello MR, Bruno A, Pandolfo G, Mico U, Scimeca G, Di Nardo F, Santoro V, Spina E, Zoccali RA (2011) Effect of aripiprazole augmentation of clozapine in schizophrenia: a double-blind, placebo-controlled study. Schizophr Res 127:93–99
75. Weiner E, Conley RR, Ball MP, Feldman S, Gold JM, Kelly DL, Wonodi I, McMahon RP, Buchanan RW (2010) Adjunctive risperidone for partially responsive people with schizophrenia treated with clozapine. Neuropsychopharmacology 35:2274–2283
76. Ito H, Koyama A, Higuchi T (2005) Polypharmacy and excessive dosing: psychiatrists' perceptions of antipsychotic drug prescription. Br J Psychiatry 187:243–247
77. Mace S, Taylor D (2005) A prescription survey of antipsychotic use in England and Wales following the introduction of NICE guidance. Int J Psychiatry Clin Pract 9:124–129
78. Taylor D, Mir S, Mace S, Whiskey E (2002) Co-prescribing of atypical and typical antipsychotics—prescribing sequence and documented outcome. Psychiatr Bull 26:170–172
79. Buckley P, Miller A, Olsen J, Garver D, Miller DD, Csernansky J (2001) When symptoms persist: clozapine augmentation strategies. Schizophr Bull 27:615–628
80. Chen CK, Shiah IS, Yeh CB, Mao WC, Chang CC (2005) Combination treatment of clozapine and topiramate in resistant rapid-cycling bipolar disorder. Clin Neuropharmacol 28:136–138
81. Compton AD, Slemmer JE, Drew MR, Hyman JM, Golden KM, Balster RL, Wiley JL (2001) Combinations of clozapine and phencyclidine: effects on drug discrimination and behavioral inhibition in rats. Neuropharmacology 40:289–297
82. Dardennes RM, Al Anbar NN, Rouillon F (2010) Successful augmentation of clozapine-resistant treatment of schizophrenia with clonidine. Prog Neuropsychopharmacol Biol Psychiatry 34:724–725
83. Diaz P, Bhaskara S, Dursun SM, Deakin B (2005) Double-blind, placebo-controlled, cross-over trial of clozapine plus glycine in refractory schizophrenia negative results. J Clin Psychopharmacol 25:277–278
84. Doruk A, Uzun O, Ozsahin A (2008) A placebo-controlled study of extract of ginkgo biloba added to clozapine in patients with treatment-resistant schizophrenia. Int Clin Psychopharmacol 23:223–227
85. Gazdag G, Kocsis-Ficzere N, Tolna J (2006) The augmentation of clozapine treatment with electroconvulsive therapy. Ideggyogy Sz 59:261–267
86. Hahn MK, Remington G, Bois D, Cohn T (2010) Topiramate augmentation in clozapine-treated patients with schizophrenia: clinical and metabolic effects. J Clin Psychopharmacol 30:706–710

87. Havaki-Kontaxaki BJ, Ferentinos PP, Kontaxakis VP, Paplos KG, Soldatos CR (2006) Concurrent administration of clozapine and electroconvulsive therapy in clozapine-resistant schizophrenia. Clin Neuropharmacol 29:52–56
88. Hrdlicka M (2002) Combination of clozapine and maprotiline in refractory psychotic depression. Eur Psychiatry 17:484
89. Kalyoncu A, Mirsal H, Pektas O, Unsalan N, Tan D, Beyazyurek M (2005) Use of lamotrigine to augment clozapine in patients with resistant schizophrenia and comorbid alcohol dependence: a potent anti-craving effect? J Psychopharmacol 19:301–305
90. Kanaan RA, Kerwin RW (2006) Lithium and clozapine rechallenge: a retrospective case analysis. J Clin Psychiatry 67:756–760
91. Keller S, Drexler H, Lichtenberg P (2009) Very high-dose clozapine and electroconvulsive therapy combination treatment in a patient with schizophrenia. J ECT 25:280–281
92. Kelly DL, Conley RR, Feldman S, Yu Y, McMahon RP, Richardson CM (2006) Adjunct divalproex or lithium to clozapine in treatment-resistant schizophrenia. Psychiatr Q 77:81–95
93. Kreinin A, Miodownik C, Libov I, Shestakova D, Lerner V (2009) Moclobemide treatment of clozapine-induced hypersalivation: pilot open study. Clin Neuropharmacol 32:151–153
94. Pavlovic ZM (2008) Augmentation of clozapine's antiaggressive properties with lamotrigine in a patient with chronic disorganized schizophrenia. J Clin Psychopharmacol 28:119–120
95. Risch SC, Horner MD, McGurk SR, Palecko S, Markowitz JS, Nahas Z, DeVane CL (2007) Double-blind donepezil-placebo crossover augmentation study of atypical antipsychotics in chronic, stable schizophrenia: a pilot study. Schizophr Res 93:131–135
96. Stryjer R, Strous R, Bar F, Shaked G, Shiloh R, Rozencwaig S, Grupper D, Buchman N, Kotler M, Rabey JM, Weizman A (2004) Donepezil augmentation of clozapine monotherapy in schizophrenia patients: a double blind cross-over study. Hum Psychopharmacol 19:343–346
97. Tiihonen J, Wahlbeck K, Kiviniemi V (2009) The efficacy of lamotrigine in clozapine-resistant schizophrenia: a systematic review and meta-analysis. Schizophr Res 109:10–14
98. Zink M, Englisch S, Knopf U, Kuwilsky A, Dressing H (2007) Augmentation of clozapine with valproic acid for clozapine-induced obsessive-compulsive symptoms. Pharmacopsychiatry 40:202–203
99. Zoccali R, Muscatello MR, Bruno A, Cambria R, Mico U, Spina E, Meduri M (2007) The effect of lamotrigine augmentation of clozapine in a sample of treatment-resistant schizophrenic patients: a double-blind, placebo-controlled study. Schizophr Res 93:109–116
100. Potter WZ, Ko GN, Zhang LD, Yan WW (1989) Clozapine in China: a review and preview of US/PRC collaboration. Psychopharmacology (Berl) 99(Suppl):S87–S91
101. Mowerman S, Siris SG (1996) Adjunctive loxapine in a clozapine-resistant cohort of schizophrenic patients. Ann Clin Psychiatry 8:193–197
102. Friedman J, Ault K, Powchik P (1997) Pimozide augmentation for the treatment of schizophrenic patients who are partial responders to clozapine. Biol Psychiatry 42:522–523
103. Friedman JI, Lindenmayer JP, Alcantara F, Bowler S, Parak M, White L, Iskander A, Parrella M, Adler DN, Tsopelas ND, Tsai WY, Novakovick V, Harvey PD, Davis KL (2011) Pimozide augmentation of clozapine inpatients with schizophrenia and schizoaffective disorder unresponsive to clozapine monotherapy. Neuropsychopharmacology 36:1289–1295
104. Shiloh R, Zemishlany Z, Aizenberg D, Radwan M, Schwartz B, Dorfman-Etrog P, Modai I, Khaikin M, Weizman A (1997) Sulpiride augmentation in people with schizophrenia partially responsive to clozapine. A double-blind, placebo-controlled study. Br J Psychiatry 171:569–573
105. Shiloh R, Zemishlany Z, Aizenberg D, Weizman A (1997) Sulpiride adjunction to clozapine in treatment-resistant schizophrenic patients: a preliminary case series study. Eur Psychiatry 12:152–155
106. Stubbs JH, Haw CM, Staley CJ, Mountjoy CQ (2000) Augmentation with sulpiride for a schizophrenic patient partially responsive to clozapine. Acta Psychiatr Scand 102:390–393, discussion 393–4

107. Liu Q, Li X, Zhang Y (1996) A control study of clozapine in combination with sulpiride in alleviating the negative symptoms of schizophrenia. Chin J Psychiatry 29:87–90
108. Si S, Yuan C (1999) A comparative trial of the effects of sulpiride combined with clozapine in the treatment of schizophrenia. Shandong Arch Psychiatry 12:17–20
109. Wang C, Qin T, Lin Y, Zhao X (1994) A clinical effect and following-up study about sulpiride and clozapine for 105 cases of the schizophrenia type. Xinxiang Med Stud 11:148–151
110. Xao H (1999) A double-blind comparative study of the effects of sulpiride combined with clozapine in the treatment of schizophrenia. Sichuan Ment Health 12:250–251
111. Zhu Y, Zhang S, Zhang D (1999) A controlled trial comparing chlorimipramine and sulpiride as adjunct to clozapine in the treatment of negative symptoms of schizophrenia. J Clin Psychol Med 9:204–205
112. Zou G, Huang Y, Zou S, Yang Y (2003) A comparative trial of the beneficial effects of sulpiride combined with clozapine in the treatment of refractory schizophrenia. J Yichun Univ 25:94–96
113. Wang J, Omori IM, Fenton M, Soares B (2011) Sulpiride augmentation for schizophrenia. Cochrane Database Syst Rev 2010 Jan 20;(1):CD008125
114. Cubala WJ, Wichowicz HM, Landowski J (2007) Refractory schizophrenia treated with clozapine combined with zuclopenthixol. Prog Neuropsychopharmacol Biol Psychiatry 31: 781–783
115. Rajarethinam R, Gilani S, Tancer M, DeQuardo J (2003) Augmentation of clozapine partial responders with conventional antipsychotics. Schizophr Res 60:97–98
116. Mossaheb N, Sacher J, Wiesegger G, Klein N, Spindelegger CJ, Asenbaum S, Dudczak R, Kasper S (2006) Haloperidol in combination with clozapine in treatment-refractory patients with schizophrenia. Eur Neuropsychopharmacol 16(suppl 4):416
117. Jia Z, Zhang Z, Jin S (2000) A controlled trial for comparing clozapine combined with pipothiazine palmitate to clozapine alone in the treatment of negative symptoms in schizophrenic patients. Herald Med 19:142–143
118. Zhu H, Deng D (2002) A study of clozapine combined with or without pipotiazine palmitate in refractory schizophrenia. J Clin Psychol Med 12:15–17
119. Cooke C, de Leon J (1999) Adding other antipsychotics to clozapine. J Clin Psychiatry 60:710
120. Grohmann R, Ruther E, Sassim N, Schmidt LG (1989) Adverse effects of clozapine. Psychopharmacology (Berl) 99(Suppl):S101–S104
121. Peacock L, Gerlach J (1994) Clozapine treatment in Denmark: concomitant psychotropic medication and hematologic monitoring in a system with liberal usage practices. J Clin Psychiatry 55:44–49
122. Barbui C, Signoretti A, Mule S, Boso M, Cipriani A (2009) Does the addition of a second antipsychotic drug improve clozapine treatment? Schizophr Bull 35:458–468
123. Kontaxakis VP, Ferentinos PP, Havaki-Kontaxaki BJ, Roukas DK (2005) Randomized controlled augmentation trials in clozapine-resistant schizophrenic patients: a critical review. Eur Psychiatry 20:409–415
124. Taylor DM, Smith L, Gee SH, Jimmi N (2011) Augmentation of clozapine with a second antipsychotic—a meta-analysis. Acta Psychiatr Scand 125(1):15–24
125. Tamminga CA (2002) Partial dopamine agonists in the treatment of psychosis. J Neural Transm 109:411–420
126. Bolonna AA, Kerwin RW (2005) Partial agonism and schizophrenia. Br J Psychiatry 186:7–10
127. Rivas-Vasquez RA (2003) Aripiprazole: a novel antipsychotic with dopamine stabilising properties. Prof Psychol Res Pr 34:108–111
128. Clarke LA, Lindenmayer JP, Kaushik S (2006) Clozapine augmentation with aripiprazole for negative symptoms. J Clin Psychiatry 67:675–676
129. Lim S, Bowers MB (2007) Augmentation of clozapine treatment with aripiprazole. J Clin Psychiatry 68:798–799
130. Masopust J, Tuma I, Libiger J (2008) Adjunctive aripiprazole decreased metabolic side effects of clozapine treatment. Neuro Endocrinol Lett 29:435–437

131. Pigato G, Toffanin T, Perini GI (2009) Is a high dosage aripiprazole-clozapine combination an effective strategy for treatment-resistant schizophrenic patients? a case report. Prog Neuropsychopharmacol Biol Psychiatry 33:153–155
132. Rocha FL, Hara C (2006) Benefits of combining aripiprazole to clozapine: three case reports. Prog Neuropsychopharmacol Biol Psychiatry 30:1167–1169
133. Ziegenbein M, Sieberer M, Calliess IT, Kropp S (2005) Combination of clozapine and aripiprazole: a promising approach in treatment-resistant schizophrenia. Aust N Z J Psychiatry 39:840–841
134. Ziegenbein M, Wittmann G, Kropp S (2006) Aripiprazole augmentation of clozapine in treatment-resistant schizophrenia: a clinical observation. Clin Drug Investig 26:117–124
135. Mitsonis CI, Dimopoulos NP, Mitropoulos PA, Kararizou EG, Katsa AN, Tsakiris FE, Katsanou MN (2007) Aripiprazole augmentation in the management of residual symptoms in clozapine-treated outpatients with chronic schizophrenia: an open-label pilot study. Prog Neuropsychopharmacol Biol Psychiatry 31:373–377
136. Karunakaran K, Tungaraza TE, Harborne GC (2007) Is clozapine-aripiprazole combination a useful regime in the management of treatment-resistant schizophrenia? J Psychopharmacol 21:453–456
137. Benedetti A, Di Paolo A, Lastella M, Casamassima F, Candiracci C, Litta A, Ciofi L, Danesi R, Lattanzi L, Del Tacca M, Cassano GB (2010) Augmentation of clozapine with aripiprazole in severe psychotic bipolar and schizoaffective disorders: a pilot study. Clin Pract Epidemiol Ment Health 6:30–35
138. Millar H, Felter C, Landsberg W (2008) The effects of aripiprazole in combination with clozapine: patient functioning results from a double-blind, 16-week study in patients with schizophrenia. J Psychopharmacol 22:A17
139. Fleischhacker WW, Heikkinen ME, Olie JP, Landsberg W, Dewaele P, McQuade RD, Loze JY, Hennicken D, Kerselaers W (2010) Effects of adjunctive treatment with aripiprazole on body weight and clinical efficacy in schizophrenia patients treated with clozapine: a randomized, double-blind, placebo-controlled trial. Int J Neuropsychopharmacol 13:1115–1125
140. Barbui C, Accordini S, Nose M, Stroup S, Purgato M, Girlanda F, Esposito E, Veronese A, Tansella M, Cipriani A (2011) Aripiprazole versus haloperidol in combination with clozapine for treatment-resistant schizophrenia in routine clinical care: a randomized, controlled trial. J Clin Psychopharmacol 31:266–273
141. Chang JS, Ahn YM, Park HJ, Lee KY, Kim SH, Kang UG, Kim YS (2008) Aripiprazole augmentation in clozapine-treated patients with refractory schizophrenia: an 8-week, randomized, double-blind, placebo-controlled trial. J Clin Psychiatry 69:720–731
142. De Risio A, Pancheri A, Simonetti G, Giannarelli D, Stefanutto L, Gentile B (2011) Add-on of aripiprazole improves outcome in clozapine-resistant schizophrenia. Prog Neuropsychopharmacol Biol Psychiatry 35:1112–1116
143. Josiassen RC, Joseph A, Kohegyi E, Stokes S, Dadvand M, Paing WW, Shaughnessy RA (2005) Clozapine augmented with risperidone in the treatment of schizophrenia: a randomized, double-blind, placebo-controlled trial. Am J Psychiatry 162:130–136
144. Owens DG (1994) Extrapyramidal side effects and tolerability of risperidone: a review. J Clin Psychiatry 55(Suppl):29–35
145. Anil Yagcioglu AE, Kivircik Akdede BB, Turgut TI, Tumuklu M, Yazici MK, Alptekin K, Ertugrul A, Jayathilake K, Gogus A, Tunca Z, Meltzer HY (2005) A double-blind controlled study of adjunctive treatment with risperidone in schizophrenic patients partially responsive to clozapine: efficacy and safety. J Clin Psychiatry 66:63–72
146. Honer W, MacEwan GW, Williams R, Falkai P, McKenna PJ, Pomarol-Clotet E, Chen EY, Leung SP, Wong J, Stip E (2005) A randomized, placebo-controlled, double-blind trial of augmentation of clozapine with risperidone. Schizophr Bull 31:487
147. Honer WG, Thornton AE, Chen EY, Chan RC, Wong JO, Bergmann A, Falkai P, Pomarol-Clotet E, McKenna PJ, Stip E, Williams R, MacEwan GW, Wasan K, Procyshyn R (2006) Clozapine alone versus clozapine and risperidone with refractory schizophrenia. N Engl J Med 354:472–482

148. de Groot IW, Heck AH, van Harten PN (2001) Addition of risperidone to clozapine therapy in chronically psychotic inpatients. J Clin Psychiatry 62:129–130
149. Henderson DC, Goff DC (1996) Risperidone as an adjunct to clozapine therapy in chronic schizophrenics. J Clin Psychiatry 57:395–397
150. Taylor CG, Flynn SW, Altman S, Ehmann T, MacEwan GW, Honer WG (2001) An open trial of risperidone augmentation of partial response to clozapine. Schizophr Res 48:155–158
151. Adesanya A, Pantelis C (2000) Adjunctive risperidone treatment in patients with 'clozapine-resistant schizophrenia'. Aust N Z J Psychiatry 34:533–534
152. McCarthy RH, Terkelsen KG (1995) Risperidone augmentation of clozapine. Pharmacopsychiatry 28:61–63
153. Morera AL, Barreiro P, Cano-Munoz JL (1999) Risperidone and clozapine combination for the treatment of refractory schizophrenia. Acta Psychiatr Scand 99:305–306, discussion 306–7
154. Patel JK, Salzman C, Green AI, Tsuang MT (1997) Chronic schizophrenia: response to clozapine, risperidone, and paroxetine. Am J Psychiatry 154:543–546
155. Raskin S, Katz G, Zislin Z, Knobler HY, Durst R (2000) Clozapine and risperidone: combination/augmentation treatment of refractory schizophrenia: a preliminary observation. Acta Psychiatr Scand 101:334–336
156. Tyson SC, Devane CL, Risch SC (1995) Pharmacokinetic interaction between risperidone and clozapine. Am J Psychiatry 152:1401–1402
157. Beauchemin MA, Millaud F, Nguyen KA (2002) A case of neuroleptic malignant syndrome with clozapine and risperidone. Can J Psychiatry 47:886
158. Kontaxakis VP, Havaki-Kontaxaki BJ, Stamouli SS, Christodoulou GN (2002) Toxic interaction between risperidone and clozapine: a case report. Prog Neuropsychopharmacol Biol Psychiatry 26:407–409
159. Senechal A, Landry P, Deschamps R, Lessard M (2002) Neutropenia in a patient treated with clozapine in combination with other psychotropic drugs. Encéphale 28:567–569
160. Godleski LS, Sernyak MJ (1996) Agranulocytosis after addition of risperidone to clozapine treatment [letter]. Am J Psychiatry 153:735–736
161. Koreen AR, Lieberman JA, Kronig M, Cooper TB (1995) Cross-tapering clozapine and risperidone [letter]. Am J Psychiatry 152:1690
162. Chong SA, Tan CH, Lee HS (1996) Hoarding and clozapine-risperidone combination [letter]. Can J Psychiatry Revue Canadienne DePsychiatrie 41:315–316
163. Chong SA, Tan CH, Lee HS (1997) Atrial ectopics with clozapine-risperidone combination. J Clin Psychopharmacol 17:130–131
164. Agelink MW, Kavuk I, Ak I (2004) Clozapine with amisulpride for refractory schizophrenia. Am J Psychiatry 161:924–925
165. Allouche G, Joober R, Vanelle JM, Brochier T, Olie JP (1994) Sequence in prescribing neuroleptics: a therapeutic alternative in refractory schizophrenia? Encéphale 20:777–780
166. Assion HJ, Reinbold H, Lemanski S, Basilowski M, Juckel G (2008) Amisulpride augmentation in patients with schizophrenia partially responsive or unresponsive to clozapine. A randomized, double-blind, placebo-controlled trial. Pharmacopsychiatry 41:24–28
167. Cook B, Hoogenboom G (2004) Combined use of amisulpride and clozapine for patients with treatment-resistant schizophrenia. Australas Psychiatry 12:74–76
168. Croissant B, Hermann D, Olbrich R (2005) Reduction of side effects by combining clozapine with amisulpride: case report and short review of clozapine-induced hypersalivation—a case report. Pharmacopsychiatry 38:38–39
169. Genc Y, Taner E, Candansayar S (2007) Comparison of clozapine-amisulpride and clozapine-quetiapine combinations for patients with schizophrenia who are partially responsive to clozapine: a single-blind randomized study. Adv Ther 24:1–13
170. George S, Cowan C (2005) Effectiveness of amisulpride augmentation of clozapine in a non-responder to either drug alone: a case report. Acta Psychiatr Scand 111:163
171. Kampf P, Agelink MW, Naber D (2005) Augmentation of clozapine with amisulpride: a promising therapeutic approach to refractory schizophrenic symptoms. Pharmacopsychiatry 38:39–40

172. Kreinin A, Miodownik C, Sokolik S, Shestakova D, Libov I, Bergman J, Lerner V (2010) Amisulpride versus moclobemide in treatment of clozapine-induced hypersalivation. World J Biol Psychiatry 12(8):620–626
173. Kreinin A, Novitski D, Weizman A (2006) Amisulpride treatment of clozapine-induced hypersalivation in schizophrenia patients: a randomized, double-blind, placebo-controlled cross-over study. Int Clin Psychopharmacol 21:99–103
174. Lerner V, Bergman J, Borokhov A, Loewenthal U, Miodownik C (2005) Augmentation with amisulpride for schizophrenic patients nonresponsive to antipsychotic monotherapy. Clin Neuropharmacol 28:66–71
175. Munro J, Matthiasson P, Osborne S, Travis M, Purcell S, Cobb AM, Launer M, Beer MD, Kerwin R (2004) Amisulpride augmentation of clozapine: an open non-randomized study in patients with schizophrenia partially responsive to clozapine. Acta Psychiatr Scand 110:292–298
176. Zink M, Knopf U, Henn FA, Thome J (2004) Combination of clozapine and amisulpride in treatment-resistant schizophrenia—case reports and review of the literature. Pharmacopsychiatry 37:26–31
177. Gupta S, Sonnenberg SJ, Frank B (1998) Olanzapine augmentation of clozapine. Ann Clin Psychiatry 10:113–115
178. Rhoads E (2000) Polypharmacy of 2 atypical antipsychotics. J Clin Psychiatry 61:678–680
179. Nielsen J, Emborg C, Gydesen S, Dybbro J, Aagaard J, Haderup K, Glyngdal P, Fabricius S, Thode D, Lublin H, Andersen T, Damkier P, Taylor D (2012) Augmenting clozapine with sertindole: a double-blind, randomized, placebo-controlled study. J Clin Psychopharmacol 32:173–178
180. Nielsen RE, Levander S, Thode D, Nielsen J (2012) Effects of sertindole on cognition in clozapine-treated schizophrenia patients. Acta Psychiatr Scand 126(1):31–39
181. Kaye NS (2003) Ziprasidone augmentation of clozapine in 11 patients. J Clin Psychiatry 64:215–216
182. Ziegenbein M, Kropp S, Kuenzel HE (2005) Combination of clozapine and ziprasidone in treatment-resistant schizophrenia: an open clinical study. Clin Neuropharmacol 28:220–224
183. Zink M, Mase E, Dressing H (2004) Ziprasidone-augmentation of clozapine. Psychiatr Prax 31:259–261
184. Zink M, Mase E, Dressing H (2004) Combination of ziprasidone and clozapine in treatment-resistant schizophrenia. Hum Psychopharmacol 19:271–273
185. Coyle JT (2006) Glutamate and schizophrenia: beyond the dopamine hypothesis. Cell Mol Neurobiol 26:365–384
186. Dursun SM, Deakin JF (2001) Augmenting antipsychotic treatment with lamotrigine or topiramate in patients with treatment-resistant schizophrenia: a naturalistic case-series outcome study. J Psychopharmacol 15:297–301
187. Tiihonen J, Hallikainen T, Ryynanen OP, Repo-Tiihonen E, Kotilainen I, Eronen M, Toivonen P, Wahlbeck K, Putkonen A (2003) Lamotrigine in treatment-resistant schizophrenia: a randomized placebo-controlled crossover trial. Biol Psychiatry 54:1241–1248
188. Goff DC, Keefe R, Citrome L, Davy K, Krystal JH, Large C, Thompson TR, Volavka J, Webster EL (2007) Lamotrigine as add-on therapy in schizophrenia: results of 2 placebo-controlled trials. J Clin Psychopharmacol 27:582–589
189. McIlwain ME, Harrison J, Wheeler AJ, Russell BR (2011) Pharmacotherapy for treatment-resistant schizophrenia. Neuropsychiatr Dis Treat 7:135–149
190. Arnone D (2005) Review of the use of topiramate for treatment of psychiatric disorders. Ann Gen Psychiatry 4:5
191. Shank RP, Gardocki JF, Streeter AJ, Maryanoff BE (2000) An overview of the preclinical aspects of topiramate: pharmacology, pharmacokinetics, and mechanism of action. Epilepsia 41(Suppl 1):S3–S9
192. Afshar H, Roohafza H, Mousavi G, Golchin S, Toghianifar N, Sadeghi M, Talaei M (2009) Topiramate add-on treatment in schizophrenia: a randomised, double-blind, placebo-controlled clinical trial. J Psychopharmacol 23:157–162

193. Arif H, Buchsbaum R, Weintraub D, Pierro J, Resor SR Jr, Hirsch LJ (2009) Patient-reported cognitive side effects of antiepileptic drugs: predictors and comparison of all commonly used antiepileptic drugs. Epilepsy Behav 14:202–209
194. Lee S, Sziklas V, Andermann F, Farnham S, Risse G, Gustafson M, Gates J, Penovich P, Al-Asmi A, Dubeau F, Jones-Gotman M (2003) The effects of adjunctive topiramate on cognitive function in patients with epilepsy. Epilepsia 44:339–347
195. Thompson PJ, Baxendale SA, Duncan JS, Sander JW (2000) Effects of topiramate on cognitive function. J Neurol Neurosurg Psychiatry 69:636–641
196. Behdani F, Hebrani P, Rezaei Ardani A, Rafee E (2011) Effect of topiramate augmentation in chronic schizophrenia: a placebo-controlled trial. Arch Iran Med 14:270–275
197. Fayek M, Kingsbury SJ, Simpson G (2002) Treatment-resistant schizophrenia: making the determination. Psychiatric Times 19: http://www.psychiatrictimes.com/schizophrenia/content/article/10168/47931?pageNumber=1
198. Bender S, Linka T, Wolstein J, Gehendges S, Paulus HJ, Schall U, Gastpar M (2004) Safety and efficacy of combined clozapine-lithium pharmacotherapy. Int J Neuropsychopharmacol 7:59–63
199. Small JG, Klapper MH, Malloy FW, Steadman TM (2003) Tolerability and efficacy of clozapine combined with lithium in schizophrenia and schizoaffective disorder. J Clin Psychopharmacol 23:223–228
200. Bryois C, Ferrero F (1993) Clinical observation of 11 patients under clozapine-lithium association. Eur Psychiatry 8:213–218
201. Moldavsky M, Stein D, Benatov R, Sirota P, Elizur A, Matzner Y, Weizman A (1998) Combined clozapine-lithium treatment for schizophrenia and schizoaffective disorder. Eur Psychiatry 13:104–106
202. Olney JW, Newcomer JW, Farber NB (1999) NMDA receptor hypofunction model of schizophrenia. J Psychiatr Res 33:523–533
203. Evins AE, Fitzgerald SM, Wine L, Rosselli R, Goff DC (2000) Placebo-controlled trial of glycine added to clozapine in schizophrenia. Am J Psychiatry 157:826–828
204. Heresco-Levy U, Javitt DC, Ermilov M, Mordel C, Silipo G, Lichtenstein M (1999) Efficacy of high-dose glycine in the treatment of enduring negative symptoms of schizophrenia. Arch Gen Psychiatry 56:29–36
205. Potkin SG, Jin Y, Bunney BG, Costa J, Gulasekaram B (1999) Effect of clozapine and adjunctive high-dose glycine in treatment-resistant schizophrenia. Am J Psychiatry 156:145–147
206. Goff DC, Henderson DC, Evins AE, Amico E (1999) A placebo-controlled crossover trial of D-cycloserine added to clozapine in patients with schizophrenia. Biol Psychiatry 45:512–514
207. Goff DC, Tsai G, Manoach DS, Flood J, Darby DG, Coyle JT (1996) D-cycloserine added to clozapine for patients with schizophrenia. Am J Psychiatry 153:1628–1630
208. Tsai GE, Yang P, Chung LC, Tsai IC, Tsai CW, Coyle JT (1999) D-serine added to clozapine for the treatment of schizophrenia. Am J Psychiatry 156:1822–1825
209. Lane HY, Huang CL, Wu PL, Liu YC, Chang YC, Lin PY, Chen PW, Tsai G (2006) Glycine transporter I inhibitor, N-methylglycine (sarcosine), added to clozapine for the treatment of schizophrenia. Biol Psychiatry 60:645–649
210. Goff DC, Lamberti JS, Leon AC, Green MF, Miller AL, Patel J, Manschreck T, Freudenreich O, Johnson SA (2008) A placebo-controlled add-on trial of the ampakine, CX516, for cognitive deficits in schizophrenia. Neuropsychopharmacology 33:465–472
211. Goff DC, Leahy L, Berman I, Posever T, Herz L, Leon AC, Johnson SA, Lynch G (2001) A placebo-controlled pilot study of the ampakine CX516 added to clozapine in schizophrenia. J Clin Psychopharmacol 21:484–487
212. Horrobin DF (1998) The membrane phospholipid hypothesis as a biochemical basis for the neurodevelopmental concept of schizophrenia. Schizophr Res 30:193–208
213. Peet M, Horrobin DF (2002) A dose-ranging exploratory study of the effects of ethyl-eicosapentaenoate in patients with persistent schizophrenic symptoms. J Psychiatr Res 36:7–18

214. Emsley R, Myburgh C, Oosthuizen P, van Rensburg SJ (2002) Randomized, placebo-controlled study of ethyl-eicosapentaenoic acid as supplemental treatment in schizophrenia. Am J Psychiatry 159:1596–1598
215. Fenton WS, Dickerson F, Boronow J, Hibbeln JR, Knable M (2001) A placebo-controlled trial of omega-3 fatty acid (ethyl eicosapentaenoic acid) supplementation for residual symptoms and cognitive impairment in schizophrenia. Am J Psychiatry 158:2071–2074
216. de Lucena D, Fernandes BS, Berk M, Dodd S, Medeiros DW, Pedrini M, Kunz M, Gomes FA, Giglio LF, Lobato MI, Belmonte-de-Abreu PS, Gama CS (2009) Improvement of negative and positive symptoms in treatment-refractory schizophrenia: a double-blind, randomized, placebo-controlled trial with memantine as add-on therapy to clozapine. J Clin Psychiatry 70:1416–1423
217. Lu ML, Lane HY, Chen KP, Jann MW, Su MH, Chang WH (2000) Fluvoxamine reduces the clozapine dosage needed in refractory schizophrenic patients. J Clin Psychiatry 61:594–599
218. Silver H, Kushnir M, Kaplan A (1996) Fluvoxamine augmentation in clozapine-resistant schizophrenia: an open pilot study. Biol Psychiatry 40:671–674
219. Lu ML, Lane HY, Lin SK, Chen KP, Chang WH (2004) Adjunctive fluvoxamine inhibits clozapine-related weight gain and metabolic disturbances. J Clin Psychiatry 65:766–771
220. Hindmarch I, Hashimoto K (2010) Cognition and depression: the effects of fluvoxamine, a sigma-1 receptor agonist, reconsidered. Hum Psychopharmacol 25:193–200
221. Buchanan RW, Kirkpatrick B, Bryant N, Ball P, Breier A (1996) Fluoxetine augmentation of clozapine treatment in patients with schizophrenia. Am J Psychiatry 153:1625–1627
222. Spina E, Avenoso A, Facciola G, Fabrazzo M, Monteleone P, Maj M, Perucca E, Caputi AP (1998) Effect of fluoxetine on the plasma concentrations of clozapine and its major metabolites in patients with schizophrenia. Int Clin Psychopharmacol 13:141–145
223. Delle Chiaie R, Salviati M, Fiorentini S, Biondi M (2007) Add-on mirtazapine enhances effects on cognition in schizophrenic patients under stabilized treatment with clozapine. Exp Clin Psychopharmacol 15:563–568
224. Zoccali R, Muscatello MR, Cedro C, Neri P, La Torre D, Spina E, Di Rosa AE, Meduri M (2004) The effect of mirtazapine augmentation of clozapine in the treatment of negative symptoms of schizophrenia: a double-blind, placebo-controlled study. Int Clin Psychopharmacol 19:71–76
225. Berk M, Gama CS, Sundram S, Hustig H, Koopowitz L, D'Souza R, Malloy H, Rowland C, Monkhouse A, Monkhouse A, Bole F, Sathiyamoorthy S, Piskulic D, Dodd S (2009) Mirtazapine add-on therapy in the treatment of schizophrenia with atypical antipsychotics: a double-blind, randomised, placebo-controlled clinical trial. Hum Psychopharmacol 24:233–238
226. Bloch Y, Pollack M, Mor I (1996) Should the administration of ECT during clozapine therapy be contraindicated? Br J Psychiatry 169:253–254
227. Kupchik M, Spivak B, Mester R, Reznik I, Gonen N, Weizman A, Kotler M (2000) Combined electroconvulsive-clozapine therapy. Clin Neuropharmacol 23:14–16
228. Frankenburg FR, Suppes T, McLean PE (1993) Combined clozapine and electroconvulsive therapy. Convuls Ther 9:176–180
229. Kho KH, Blansjaar BA, de Vries S, Babuskova D, Zwinderman AH, Linszen DH (2004) Electroconvulsive therapy for the treatment of clozapine nonresponders suffering from schizophrenia—an open label study. Eur Arch Psychiatry Clin Neurosci 254:372–379
230. Masoudzadeh A, Khalilian AR (2007) Comparative study of clozapine, electroshock and the combination of ECT with clozapine in treatment-resistant schizophrenic patients. Pak J Biol Sci 10:4287–4290
231. Benatov R, Sirota P, Megged S (1996) Neuroleptic-resistant schizophrenia treated with clozapine and ECT. Convuls Ther 12:117–121
232. Bhatia SC, Bhatia SK, Gupta S (1998) Concurrent administration of clozapine and ECT: a successful therapeutic strategy for a patient with treatment-resistant schizophrenia. J ECT 14:280–283

233. Cardwell BA, Nakai B (1995) Seizure activity in combined clozapine and ECT: a retrospective view. Convuls Ther 11:110–113
234. Kales HC, Dequardo JR, Tandon R (1999) Combined electroconvulsive therapy and clozapine in treatment-resistant schizophrenia. Prog Neuropsychopharmacol Biol Psychiatry 23:547–556
235. Kumar S, Goswami U, Behera D, Khastgir U (2003) ECT and clozapine combination producing delirium: a case report. Indian J Psychiatry 45:193
236. Landy DA (1991) Combined use of clozapine and electroconvulsive therapy. Convuls Ther 7:218–221
237. Masiar SJ, Johns CA (1991) ECT following clozapine. Br J Psychiatry 158:135–136
238. Safferman AZ, Munne R (1992) Combining clozapine with ECT. Convuls Ther 8:141–143
239. McEvoy JP, Lieberman JA, Stroup TS, Davis SM, Meltzer HY, Rosenheck RA, Swartz MS, Perkins DO, Keefe RS, Davis CE, Severe J, Hsiao JK (2006) Effectiveness of clozapine versus olanzapine, quetiapine, and risperidone in patients with chronic schizophrenia who did not respond to prior atypical antipsychotic treatment. Am J Psychiatry 163:600–610

Chapter 8
Metabolic Syndrome and Antipsychotic Polypharmacy

Fuminari Misawa, Fujii Yasuo, Yasuyuki Okumura, and Hiroto Ito

Abstract Patients with schizophrenia are more likely than the general population to have metabolic syndrome and to live around 15 fewer years largely because of cardiovascular death. Recent studies have suggested that antipsychotic polypharmacy may be associated with metabolic disturbance including metabolic syndrome and the mortality related to it. Although antipsychotic polypharmacy is not recommended and there is limited evidence of its benefits, it is nevertheless becoming common in the treatment of schizophrenia. If it is indeed associated with a greater risk of metabolic syndrome, then more widespread use is a serious concern. In this chapter, we review the effects of antipsychotic polypharmacy on mortality, metabolic disturbance, and metabolic syndrome. The results of earlier studies indicate that antipsychotic polypharmacy might increase the risk of some metabolic disturbances and related mortality but not the risk of metabolic syndrome. The effects of antipsychotic polypharmacy on metabolic disturbance and metabolic syndrome may be unchanged in patients with schizophrenia even after changing unhealthy lifestyles. Further studies are still needed to clarify the association between antipsychotic polypharmacy and metabolic disturbance or metabolic syndrome. At present, in cases when antipsychotic polypharmacy is deemed necessary, it is recommended that testing for metabolic parameters should be undertaken more often in patients receiving polypharmacy than in those receiving monotherapy and stricter lifestyle interventions are needed.

F. Misawa (✉) • F. Yasuo
Yamanashi Prefectural KITA Hospital, Yamanashi, Japan
e-mail: misawa-ahme@ych.pref.yamanashi.jp

Y. Okumura • H. Ito
Department of Social Psychiatry, National Institute of Mental Health, Tokyo, Japan

M.S. Ritsner (ed.), *Polypharmacy in Psychiatry Practice, Volume II: Use of Polypharmacy in the "Real World"*, DOI 10.1007/978-94-007-5799-8_8,

Abbreviations

CI	Confidence interval
HDL	High-density lipoprotein
LDL	Low-density lipoprotein
OR	Odds ratio
RR	Rate ratio
TG/HDL	The triglycerides/high-density lipoprotein cholesterol ratio

8.1 Introduction

Metabolic syndrome is a cluster of metabolic dysfunctions that includes central obesity, hypertension, glucose, and lipid abnormalities. Individuals with metabolic syndrome have an increased incidence of diabetes mellitus and coronary heart disease, and increased mortality from cardiovascular disease [1].

Metabolic syndrome occurs more frequently in patients with schizophrenia than in the general population. A review by De Hert et al. [2] of 38 heterogeneous studies from around the world that were published between 2003 and 2008 revealed that the prevalence and incidence of metabolic syndrome were two to three times higher in patients with schizophrenia or schizoaffective disorder than in the general population. Moreover, individuals with schizophrenia are likely to live about 15 fewer years than those without schizophrenia largely because of cardiovascular deaths [3]. The risk to metabolic health in schizophrenia would reflect the combined effects of inherent biological risk, the contribution of lifestyle factors, and the metabolic impact of antipsychotic treatment [4].

Antipsychotic monotherapy is currently recommended in the treatment of patients with schizophrenia [5, 6]. However, antipsychotic polypharmacy is becoming more common in treatment; it has been reported to have been used in 13–90% of cases [7–11], despite there being limited evidence of its benefits to date. Antipsychotic polypharmacy has also been reported to be associated with, for example, extrapyramidal side effects [12–14], sedation [15], and hyperprolactinemia [16, 17]. In addition, recent data suggest that it may be associated with metabolic disturbance and the mortality related to it. It is therefore of serious concern that antipsychotic polypharmacy, which is not recommended for the treatment of schizophrenia, might promote premature death among such patients.

Given that antipsychotic polypharmacy seems to becoming increasingly widespread despite the recommendation to the opposite, it is a matter of urgency that we understand the association between it and metabolic disturbance. In this chapter, we begin by reviewing the literature on the association between antipsychotic polypharmacy and mortality. We then describe metabolic disturbance, focusing especially on metabolic syndrome. We conclude the chapter by discussing the effects of an unhealthy lifestyle on the association between antipsychotic polypharmacy and metabolic syndrome in schizophrenia.

8.2 Antipsychotic Polypharmacy and Mortality

Several studies have demonstrated a graded relationship between the number of antipsychotic drugs prescribed and mortality in patients with schizophrenia. Hollis et al. [18] explored the odds ratios (ORs) of death associated with antipsychotic medications dispensed to elderly subjects and found that the OR for mixed antipsychotics was 5.32 (95% confidence interval [CI] 3.49–8.10). Joukamaa et al. [19] found that a combination of antipsychotics seemed to increase the risk of mortality in individuals with schizophrenia. In their long-term study conducted over 17 years of follow-up, 39 of the 99 subjects died. When adjusted for potential confounders, the relative risk was 2.50 (95% CI 1.46–4.30) per increment of one antipsychotic. Waddington et al. [20] prospectively followed a cohort of 88 inpatients over a 10-year period with the aim of identifying predictors of survival among demographic, clinical, and treatment variables. Over the decade, 39 patients (44%) died, with no instances of suicide. Cox proportional hazards modeling showed that the greater the maximum number of antipsychotics given concurrently, the shorter patient survival was (relative risk 2.46, 95% CI 1.10–5.47).

Evidence to the contrary has been reported by Baandrup et al. [21] who conducted a population-based nested case control study using patient data obtained from central Danish registers. They found that antipsychotic polypharmacy did not contribute to excess mortality from natural causes. Specifically, risk of natural death did not increase with the number of concurrently used antipsychotic agents compared with antipsychotic monotherapy (no antipsychotics: adjusted odds ratio [AOR] 1.48, 95% CI 0.89–2.46; two antipsychotics: AOR 0.91, 95% CI 0.61–1.36; ≥3 antipsychotics: AOR 1.16, 95% CI 0.68–2.00).

Given that the case control study showed no risk of mortality in patients on antipsychotic polypharmacy, but the cohort studies did, we should take the view that antipsychotic polypharmacy could be a risk factor for death. Although the causality remains unclear, polypharmacy-induced metabolic disturbances could well carry some risk of death in light of the fact that the main cause of death for patients with schizophrenia is cardiovascular disease and that an association exists between antipsychotic polypharmacy and metabolic disturbance, as will be described next. In any case, it is a serious concern that antipsychotic polypharmacy, for which there is limited evidence of efficacy and a possible higher risk of death, is commonplace in the treatment of schizophrenia.

8.3 Antipsychotic Polypharmacy and Metabolic Disturbance

To date, it has been reported that antipsychotic polypharmacy could contribute to various metabolic disturbances. Nagamine [22] analyzed the results of laboratory parameters measured in 68 patients with schizophrenia during psychomotor excitation and approximately 1 month later during a medicated recovery phase. The polypharmacy group was found to have the second highest frequency of abnormal values after the olanzapine group. The frequency of abnormal values for parameters related to metabolic effects specifically during the recovery phase was increased in the polypharmacy group, and the incidence of metabolic abnormalities appeared to vary depending on the number of antipsychotic drugs being taken.

Kessing et al. [23] used data from linked registers of all prescribed antipsychotics, antidiabetics, and diagnoses of diabetes in Denmark to investigate and characterize the incidence of diabetes for people treated clinically with antipsychotic medications. In total, 345,937 patients who purchased antipsychotics and 1,426,488 unexposed individuals were included in the study. Compared with unexposed individuals, treatment with first-generation (rate ratio, RR 1.53, 95% CI 1.49–1.56) or second-generation (RR 1.32, 95% CI 1.22–1.42) antipsychotics was associated with increased risk of subsequent incident diabetes. The incidence of diabetes increased with the number of combined antipsychotic drugs taken (one antipsychotic: RR 1.48, 95% CI 1.44–1.51; two antipsychotics: RR 1.68, 95% CI 1.61–1.76; three antipsychotics: RR 1.96, 95% CI 1.82–1.56; four antipsychotics: RR 2.38, 95% CI 2.13–2.65; ≥5 antipsychotics: RR 3.41, 95% CI 3.03–3.83. On the basis of these results, Kessing et al. suggested that the development of diabetes was related to the antipsychotic drugs per se rather than to the psychiatric illnesses, although an effect of illness could not be excluded.

Looking now at the association between antipsychotic polypharmacy and metabolic disturbance, few well-designed prospective studies appear to have been conducted. There have been some randomized controlled studies investigating the efficacy of antipsychotic combination therapy, and the data on metabolic parameters from double-blind controlled studies of antipsychotic polypharmacy are summarized in Table 8.1. Anil Yagcioglu et al. [15] carried out a placebo-controlled trial of the efficacy, safety, and tolerability of adjunctive treatment with risperidone in patients with schizophrenia who were partially responsive to clozapine. The mean ± standard deviation (SD) increase in weight was 0.5 ± 2.4 kg in the placebo group and 0.9 ± 2.2 kg in the risperidone group. Using the mixed model approach, only the treatment-group effect was significant for weight. However, the authors speculated that it reflected the small variance in weight gain more than it reflected a large effect of risperidone.

Honer et al. [24] investigated whether augmentation with risperidone would alleviate psychotic symptoms in patients with an incomplete response to treatment with clozapine. No significant differences were seen in weight, waist circumference, or body mass index (BMI) between the risperidone and placebo groups. There were also no significant differences in fasting glucose between the two groups, in mean value at baseline or at 8-week follow-up. However, fasting blood glucose was increased more in the risperidone group than in the placebo group at 8 weeks (16.2 vs. 1.8 mg/dl, $p = 0.04$). The level of total cholesterol, triglycerides, low-density lipoprotein (LDL) cholesterol, and high-density lipoprotein (HDL) cholesterol did not differ significantly between the two groups at baseline or at 8 weeks, and there were no significant differences between the two groups in the changes in these measurements between baseline and 8 weeks.

Table 8.1 Double-blind controlled studies of antipsychotic polypharmacy

First author (ref.)	Combination of antipsychotics	Metabolic disturbance
Anil Yagcioglu [15]	CLZ + RIS	Weight gain: CLZ + RIS > or CLZ Vital signs: CLZ + RIS ≅ CLZ
Honer [24]	CLZ + RIS	Weight gain, waist circumference, BMI, cholesterol, triglycerides: CLZ + RIS ≅ CLZ Fasting glucose: CLZ + RIS > CLZ
Weiner [25]	CLZ + RIS	Fasting glucose, weight gain, vital signs: CLZ + RIS ≅ CLZ
Fleischhacker [26]	CLZ + APZ	Weight gain, BMI, waist circumference, total and LDL cholesterol: CLZ + APZ < CLZ HDL cholesterol, triglycerides, fasting glucose: CLZ + APZ ≅ CLZ
Muscatello [27]	CLZ + APZ	Blood pressure, weight gain: CLZ + APZ ≅ CLZ
Kane [28]	RIS or QTP + APZ	Fasting glucose, cholesterol, triglycerides, weight gain: RIS or QTP + APZ ≅ RIS or QTP

CLZ clozapine, *RIS* risperidone, *APZ* aripiprazole, *QTP* quetiapine

Weiner et al. [25] examined the efficacy and safety of adjunctive risperidone in a treatment-resistant population optimally treated with clozapine. There were no significant differences between the risperidone and placebo groups in mean value for fasting glucose, weight gain, or vital signs at baseline or at 16 weeks, and there were also no significant differences between the two groups in the changes in these measurements between baseline and 16 weeks.

Fleischhacker et al. [26] conducted a randomized, double-blind, placebo-controlled trial to provide a robust evaluation of the effects of adjunctive therapy with aripiprazole + clozapine versus clozapine monotherapy on body weight and clinical efficacy in patients with schizophrenia. The participants were not optimally controlled while on a stable dose of clozapine for >3 months and had experienced weight gain of ≥2.5 kg while taking clozapine. At week 16, the mean decrease in body weight was significantly greater with adjunctive aripiprazole than with adjunctive placebo (−2.53 vs.−0.38 kg, respectively, $p<0.001$). Patients receiving adjunctive aripiprazole had adjusted median reductions in BMI and waist circumference of 0.8 kg/m^2 and 2.0 cm, compared with no change in the adjunctive placebo group ($p<0.001$, $p=0.001$, respectively). Compared to the adjunctive placebo, adjunctive aripiprazole was associated with a significant decrease in total and LDL cholesterol from baseline. There were no significant differences in HDL cholesterol, triglycerides, or fasting glucose between the groups.

In a 24-week double-blind, randomized, placebo-controlled trial of adjunctive aripiprazole to clozapine therapy conducted by Muscatello et al. [27], the combination was generally well tolerated. There were no clinically significant changes in blood pressure or body weight. Kane et al. [28] performed a 16-week multicenter, randomized, double-blind, placebo-controlled study to investigate the efficacy of aripiprazole adjunctive to risperidone or quetiapine for treating schizophrenia and schizoaffective disorder. There were no significant differences in median changes from baseline to week 16 in fasting glucose, total cholesterol, fasting triglycerides, LDL cholesterol, or HDL cholesterol between the aripiprazole and placebo groups. Most patients experienced no change in metabolic parameters during the 16 weeks of treatment. Mean weight change was similar between subjects receiving adjunctive aripiprazole and adjunctive placebo. Clinically relevant weight gain was observed in 13.4% of patients in the adjunctive aripiprazole group and in 9.9% of patients in the adjunctive placebo group ($p = 0.445$).

In most of these studies, an antipsychotic was added to clozapine in patients with treatment-resistant schizophrenia. Therefore, the effects of antipsychotic polypharmacy on metabolic disturbances may have been underestimated because of the ceiling effect of clozapine. On the other hand, adding aripiprazole, which has a mostly weight-neutral profile [29], to second-generation antipsychotics might not worsen metabolic side effects and in fact might reduce them. This is a very interesting speculation and requires further study.

It remains unclear why antipsychotic polypharmacy is correlated with metabolic disturbance. Olanzapine and clozapine, which have the greatest effects on metabolic disturbance, have high affinity for the 5-HT_{2C} and histamine H_1 receptors, which implicate these receptors in antipsychotic-induced weight gain, while peripheral M_3 muscarinic receptor antagonism as well as central 5-HT_{2C} effects may contribute to obesity-independent diabetes. Other receptor mechanisms may have additive or synergistic effects; dopamine D_2 receptor antagonism can enhance 5-HT_{2C}-mediated effects on food intake, as well as influence lipid and glucose metabolism via disinhibition of prolactin secretion [30]. Given the above, several processes in the pharmacological mechanisms contributing to metabolic disturbance must be considered. We speculate that the complex receptor binding profiles of antipsychotic polypharmacy might be one of the causes of metabolic disturbance.

8.4 The Association Between Antipsychotic Polypharmacy and Metabolic Syndrome

Although many studies have investigated the association between metabolic syndrome and schizophrenia or antipsychotics, few have examined the association between it and antipsychotic polypharmacy. According to the findings of studies in which the main outcome was not the association between metabolic syndrome and antipsychotic polypharmacy, the prevalence of metabolic syndrome could be higher with antipsychotic polypharmacy. However, this speculation remains to be confirmed as there is insufficient data at present.

Of the studies that have examined the association between metabolic syndrome and antipsychotic polypharmacy, Krane-Gartiser et al. [31] conducted a cross-sectional, observational study to assess the prevalence of metabolic syndrome among Danish psychiatric outpatients and compare it with that in the general population.

They found that 48.2% of patients taking antipsychotics fulfilled the International Diabetes Federation criteria for metabolic syndrome, compared with 29.6% of the general population. Of the 170 patients involved, 107 patients (62.9%) prescribed one antipsychotic drug and 63 (37.1%) were prescribed two or three different antipsychotics. The rates of metabolic syndrome in these two patient groups were not statistically significant however, at 44.9 and 54.0%, respectively.

Huang et al. [32] recruited 650 patients with schizophrenia or schizoaffective disorder and assessed the prevalence of metabolic syndrome. Overall prevalence was 34.9 and was 38.9% in female patients and 31.5% in male patients. Of the 115 (20.2%) patients on antipsychotic polypharmacy, 51 (44.3%) had metabolic syndrome. Logistic regression analysis using status of metabolic syndrome as a dependent variable, and sex, age, strata, BMI (Body Mass Index), type of antipsychotic, and number of antipsychotics as independent variables showed a marginally significant association between polypharmacy and prevalence of metabolic syndrome (OR 1.6, 95% CI 1.0–2.6).

Early on, when there was very little evidence of any association between metabolic syndrome and antipsychotic polypharmacy, Correll et al. [33] were the first to conduct research to examine the relationship between antipsychotic polypharmacy and rates of metabolic syndrome and insulin resistance. They assessed antipsychotic polypharmacy and the presence of metabolic syndrome in 364 newly admitted adults being treated with second-generation antipsychotics, using the triglycerides/high-density lipoprotein cholesterol ratio (TG/HDL) as a sensitive marker of insulin resistance. The correlates of antipsychotic polypharmacy and associations with metabolic syndrome and TG/HDL were determined by univariate comparisons and multiple logistic regression analyses. Compared with antipsychotic monotherapy, polypharmacy was associated with elevated rates of metabolic syndrome (50.0 vs. 34.3%, $p=0.015$) and TG/HDL (50.7 vs. 35.0%, $p=0.016$) in univariate comparisons. They then conducted stepwise multiple regression analyses in which they entered into the model antipsychotic polypharmacy, sex, age, race as well as all of the variables that univariate analyses had identified to be significantly different between patients on antipsychotic monotherapy or polypharmacy at a level of $p\leq 0.1$ (i.e., body mass index (BMI), diagnosis of schizophrenia, bipolar disorder and depressive disorder, treatment with olanzapine, quetiapine, risperidone, aripiprazole, ziprasidone, clozapine or a first-generation antipsychotic, and cotreatment with antidepressant or anticholinergic drugs). Metabolic syndrome was shown to be significantly associated with higher BMI, older age, a diagnosis of bipolar disorder or schizophrenia, and cotreatment with a first-generation antipsychotic (r^2 0.25, $p<0.0001$). The TG/HDL marker of insulin resistance was associated with higher BMI, male sex, Caucasian race, and absence of aripiprazole treatment (r^2 0.14, $p<0.0001$). Antipsychotic polypharmacy dropped out of both multivariate models. On the basis of these results, Correll et al. suggested that patients receiving antipsychotic polypharmacy represent a subgroup that is more obese and inactive and thus is more prone to metabolic risks than patients receiving antipsychotic monotherapy. In short, they concluded that antipsychotic polypharmacy is not independently associated with the prevalence of metabolic abnormalities.

8.5 Antipsychotic Polypharmacy, Lifestyle, and Metabolic Syndrome

There is no doubt that an unhealthy lifestyle contributes to metabolic disturbance included metabolic syndrome in patients with schizophrenia. Patients living in the community make significantly poorer dietary choices, take less exercise, and smoke more heavily than the general population [34]. However, little information is available on the association between metabolic syndrome and antipsychotic polypharmacy in conjunction with patients' lifestyle. Against this background, in a cross-sectional study we investigated the degree that antipsychotic polypharmacy contributed to metabolic syndrome in 334 outpatients with schizophrenia, after adjustment for the effects of lifestyle [35]. We measured the components comprising metabolic syndrome and interviewed the participants about their lifestyle. In addition, psychiatrists in charge of the participants assessed them using the Global Assessment of Functioning (GAF) Scale. We classified metabolic syndrome into the following four groups according to severity of metabolic disturbance: metabolic syndrome, pre-metabolic syndrome, visceral fat obesity, and normal groups. We used multinomial logistic regression models to assess the association of metabolic syndrome with antipsychotic polypharmacy, adjusting for lifestyle. Seventy-four (22.2%) patients were classified into the metabolic syndrome group, 61 (18.3%) into the premetabolic syndrome group, and 41 (12.3%) into the visceral fat obesity group. A total of 167 (50.0%) patients were receiving antipsychotic polypharmacy. Multinomial logistic regression analyses revealed that the metabolic syndrome group was associated with being male, longer duration of psychiatric treatment, and heavier smoking habit. The pre-metabolic syndrome group was associated with being male and antipsychotic polypharmacy. The visceral fat obesity group was associated with being male and higher antipsychotic total daily dose. Antipsychotic polypharmacy was significantly associated with the pre-metabolic syndrome group (AOR 2.348; 95% CI 1.181–4.668), but not with the metabolic syndrome group (AOR 1.269; 95% CI 0.679–2.371). Thus, overall, antipsychotic polypharmacy was not related to the severity of symptoms in the metabolic syndrome group but was related to it in the pre-metabolic syndrome group. The association between metabolic syndrome and antipsychotic polypharmacy cannot be said to be a definitive one, however, because of the effect of antipsychotic polypharmacy on lowering blood pressure. It was reported by Silver et al. [36] that polypharmacy was associated with a significantly higher drop in systolic pressure than monotherapy. This might be due to the effects of a higher dose than that received during monotherapy or a drug interaction that led to dopaminergic and noradrenergic deficiency, such as in Shy-Drager syndrome. In our study, patients receiving antipsychotic polypharmacy were less likely to fulfill the criterion of elevated blood pressure for metabolic syndrome. Consequently, because antipsychotic polypharmacy tended not to be associated with elevated blood pressure, which is one of the three criteria for metabolic syndrome, this is why it may not have been correlated with metabolic syndrome, which requires two or more of the three criteria to be fulfilled. Instead it was associated with pre-metabolic syndrome, which requires one or more of the criteria to be fulfilled. We speculate that antipsychotic polypharmacy is in fact directly associated with metabolic disturbance and increases the risk for metabolic syndrome, but its effect that lowers blood pressure masks the diagnosis of metabolic syndrome.

Another reason for our finding that polypharmacy contributes in some way to metabolic syndrome is that psychiatrists might be reluctant to prescribe additional antipsychotics for patients with metabolic syndrome to avoid worsening their metabolic profiles; however, for patients with pre-metabolic syndrome, they might not hesitate to prescribe an additional antipsychotic.

8.6 Conclusions and Future Directions

Antipsychotic polypharmacy seems not to increase the risk of metabolic syndrome directly, but it could be associated with some metabolic disturbances regardless of patients' unhealthy lifestyles. Moreover, antipsychotic polypharmacy may increase the risk of cardiovascular death associated with metabolic disturbance. However, at present there is insufficient data to judge to what degree antipsychotic polypharmacy contributes to metabolic disturbance or metabolic syndrome. Further studies to clarify the association are warranted.

According to the evidence available to date, we recommend that the number of antipsychotics be minimized for patients with schizophrenia, and when antipsychotic polypharmacy is deemed necessary, that testing for metabolic parameters be undertaken more often than for patients receiving monotherapy. In addition, stricter lifestyle interventions are needed with patients on antipsychotic polypharmacy.

References

1. Lakka HM, Laaksonen DE, Lakka TA et al (2002) The metabolic syndrome and total and cardiovascular disease mortality in middle-aged men. JAMA 288(21):2709–2716
2. De Hert M, van Winkel R, Van Eyck D et al (2006) Prevalence of diabetes, metabolic syndrome and metabolic abnormalities in schizophrenia over the course of the illness: a cross-sectional study. Clin Pract Epidemiol Ment Health 2:14
3. Hennekens CH, Hennekens AR, Hollar D et al (2005) Schizophrenia and increased risks of cardiovascular disease. Am Heart J 150(6):1115–1121
4. Meyer JM, Stahl SM (2009) The metabolic syndrome and schizophrenia. Acta Psychiatr Scand 119(1):4–14
5. Lehman AF, Lieberman JA, Dixon LB et al (2004) Practice guideline for the treatment of patients with schizophrenia, second edition. Am J Psychiatry 161(2 Suppl):1–56
6. Miller AL, Hall CS, Buchanan RW et al (2004) The Texas medication algorithm project antipsychotic algorithm for schizophrenia: 2003 update. J Clin Psychiatry 65(4):500–508
7. Miller AL, Craig CS (2002) Combination antipsychotics: pros, cons, and questions. Schizophr Bull 28(1):105–109

8. Schumacher JE, Makela EH, Griffin HR (2003) Multiple antipsychotic medication prescribing patterns. Ann Pharmacother 37(7–8):951–955
9. Tapp A, Wood AE, Secrest L et al (2003) Combination antipsychotic therapy in clinical practice. Psychiatr Serv 54(1):55–59
10. Rittmannsberger H, Meise U, Schauflinger K et al (1999) Polypharmacy in psychiatric treatment. Patterns of psychotropic drug use in Austrian psychiatric clinics. Eur Psychiatry 14(1):33–40
11. Williams CL, Johnstone BM, Kesterson JG et al (1999) Evaluation of antipsychotic and concomitant medication use patterns in patients with schizophrenia. Med Care 37(4 Suppl Lilly):AS81–AS86
12. Procyshyn RM, Kennedy NB, Tse G et al (2001) Antipsychotic polypharmacy: a survey of discharge prescriptions from a tertiary care psychiatric institution. Can J Psychiatry 46(4):334–339
13. Sim K, Su A, Fujii S et al (2004) Antipsychotic polypharmacy in patients with schizophrenia: a multicentre comparative study in East Asia. Br J Clin Pharmacol 58(2):178–183
14. Hida H, Faber M, Alberto-Gondouin MC et al (1997) Analysis of prescriptions for psychotropic drugs in a psychiatric hospital. Therapie 52(6):573–578
15. Anil Yagcioglu AE, Kivircik Akdede BB, Turgut TI et al (2005) A double-blind controlled study of adjunctive treatment with risperidone in schizophrenic patients partially responsive to clozapine: efficacy and safety. J Clin Psychiatry 66(1):63–72
16. Shiloh R, Zemishlany Z, Aizenberg D et al (1997) Sulpiride adjunction to clozapine in treatment-resistant schizophrenic patients: a preliminary case series study. Eur Psychiatry 12(3):152–155
17. Montgomery J, Winterbottom E, Jessani M et al (2004) Prevalence of hyperprolactinemia in schizophrenia: association with typical and atypical antipsychotic treatment. J Clin Psychiatry 65(11):1491–1498
18. Hollis J, Touyz S, Grayson D et al (2006) Antipsychotic medication dispensing and associated odds ratios of death in elderly veterans and war widows, 2001. Aust N Z J Psychiatry 40(11–12):981–986
19. Joukamaa M, Heliovaara M, Knekt P et al (2006) Schizophrenia, neuroleptic medication and mortality. Br J Psychiatry 188:122–127
20. Waddington JL, Youssef HA, Kinsella A (1998) Mortality in schizophrenia. Antipsychotic polypharmacy and absence of adjunctive anticholinergics over the course of a 10-year prospective study. Br J Psychiatry 173:325–329
21. Baandrup L, Gasse C, Jensen VD et al (2010) Antipsychotic polypharmacy and risk of death from natural causes in patients with schizophrenia: a population-based nested case–control study. J Clin Psychiatry 71(2):103–108
22. Nagamine T (2010) Abnormal laboratory values during the acute and recovery phases in schizophrenic patients: a retrospective study. Neuropsychiatr Dis Treat 6:281–288
23. Kessing LV, Thomsen AF, Mogensen UB et al (2010) Treatment with antipsychotics and the risk of diabetes in clinical practice. Br J Psychiatry 197(4):266–271
24. Honer WG, Thornton AE, Chen EY et al (2006) Clozapine alone versus clozapine and risperidone with refractory schizophrenia. N Engl J Med 354(5):472–482
25. Weiner E, Conley RR, Ball MP et al (2010) Adjunctive risperidone for partially responsive people with schizophrenia treated with clozapine. Neuropsychopharmacology 35(11):2274–2283
26. Fleischhacker WW, Heikkinen ME, Olie JP et al (2010) Effects of adjunctive treatment with aripiprazole on body weight and clinical efficacy in schizophrenia patients treated with clozapine: a randomized, double-blind, placebo-controlled trial. Int J Neuropsychopharmacol 13(8):1115–1125
27. Muscatello MR, Bruno A, Pandolfo G et al (2011) Effect of aripiprazole augmentation of clozapine in schizophrenia: a double-blind, placebo-controlled study. Schizophr Res 127(1–3):93–99
28. Kane JM, Correll CU, Goff DC et al (2009) A multicenter, randomized, double-blind, placebo-controlled, 16-week study of adjunctive aripiprazole for schizophrenia or schizoaffective

disorder inadequately treated with quetiapine or risperidone monotherapy. J Clin Psychiatry 70(10):1348–1357
29. Goodwin G, Fleischhacker W, Arango C et al (2009) Advantages and disadvantages of combination treatment with antipsychotics ECNP consensus meeting, March 2008, Nice. Eur Neuropsychopharmacol 19(7):520–532
30. Riordan H, Antonini P, Murphy M (2011) Atypical antipsychotics and metabolic syndrome in patients with schizophrenia: risk factors, monitoring, and health care implications. Am Health Drug Benefits 4(5):292–302
31. Krane-Gartiser K, Breum L, Glumrr C et al (2011) Prevalence of the metabolic syndrome in Danish psychiatric outpatients treated with antipsychotics. Nord J Psychiatry 65(5):345–352
32. Huang MC, Lu ML, Tsai CJ et al (2009) Prevalence of metabolic syndrome among patients with schizophrenia or schizoaffective disorder in Taiwan. Acta Psychiatr Scand 120(4):274–280
33. Correll CU, Frederickson AM, Kane JM et al (2007) Does antipsychotic polypharmacy increase the risk for metabolic syndrome? Schizophr Res 89(1–3):91–100
34. Connolly M, Kelly C (2005) Life style and physical health in schizophrenia. Adv Psychiatry Treat 11:125–132
35. Misawa F, Shimizu K, Fujii Y et al (2011) Is antipsychotic polypharmacy associated with metabolic syndrome even after adjustment for lifestyle effects?: a cross-sectional study. BMC Psychiatry 11:118
36. Silver H, Kogan H, Zlotogorski D (1990) Postural hypotension in chronically medicated schizophrenics. J Clin Psychiatry 51(11):459–462

Part II
Polypharmacy for Other Psychiatric Conditions

Chapter 9
Evidence Based Combination Therapy for Bipolar Disorder

Stamatia Magiria, Melina Siamouli, Xenia Gonda, Apostolos Iacovides, and Konstantinos N. Fountoulakis

Abstract The treatment of bipolar illness is complex and full of caveats for the clinician, and it seems that at least some aspects of the disorder are rather refractory to treatment. While some agents are efficacious as monotherapy, the overall outcome is unsatisfactory. However, only specific combinations have solid evidence supporting their efficacy. Antidepressants should only be used in combination with an antimanic agent, because they can induce switching to mania/hypomania/mixed states/or rapid cycling when utilized as monotherapy however only fluoxetine in combination with olanzapine has data supporting its usefulness for the treatment of bipolar depression. Adding an antipsychotic to acutely manic patients who are partial responders to lithium/valproate/carbamazepine is a reasonable choice. The combination with best data in acute bipolar depression is lithium plus lamotrigine. Patients stabilized on combination treatment might do worse if shifted to monotherapy during maintenance, and patients refractory to monotherapy could benefit with add on treatment with olanzapine, valproate, an antidepressant or lamotrigine, depending on the index acute phase. Combination therapy may improve treatment outcome but it also carries more side-effect burden. Further research is necessary as well as the development of better guidelines and algorithms for the step-by-step rational treatment.

S. Magiria • M. Siamouli • A. Iacovides • K.N. Fountoulakis, M.D., Ph.D. (✉)
3rd Department of Psychiatry, School of Medicine, Aristotle University of Thessaloniki, Thessaloniki, Greece
e-mail: kostas_fountoulakis@yahoo.com

X. Gonda
Department of Clinical and Theoretical Mental Health, Faculty of Medicine, Semmelweis University, Budapest, Hungary

M.S. Ritsner (ed.), *Polypharmacy in Psychiatry Practice, Volume II: Use of Polypharmacy in the "Real World"*, DOI 10.1007/978-94-007-5799-8_9,

Abbreviations

BD	Bipolar Disorder
ECT	Electroconvulsive Therapy
HDRS-21	Hamilton Depression Rating Scale-21
Li	Lithium
MADRS	Montgomery-Asberg Depression Rating Scale
OFC	Olanzapine-fluoxetine combination
RCT	Randomised Controlled Studies
YMRS	Young Mania Rating Scale

9.1 Introduction

There have been made many important developments in the understanding of bipolar disorder (BD) and its treatment, during the recent years. The first to describe manic-depressive illness as an illness of the mind were Hippocrates (460–357 BC), Galen (131–201 AD) and Areteus from Kappadokia (second century AD) who is also considered to be the one who saw the strong connection between mania and melancholy and his description of manic episodes was very close to modern theories, including, seasonality and psychotic features. Eventually, it was Emil Kraepelin (1856–1926) who separated manic-depressive illness from schizophrenia and established it as a nosological entity on the basis of longitudinal follow-up, heredity and a relatively favourable outcome. Lately, BD-I and II subtypes were defined and described, and some more subtypes such as BD-III and IV have been suggested to further improve the nosology [1–3].

BD (previously described as manic-depressive psychosis) according to the formal contemporary classification consists of a depressive episode and at least one manic (BD-I), hypomanic (BD-II), or mixed episode. Symptoms as mood alterations are described for several other DSM disorders which have a bipolar character [4]. The definition 'rapid cycling' refers to patients who are suffering from at least four mood episodes in a year. Females are more often rapid-cyclers and also higher social class subjects. In bipolar patients is common to meet psychotic features including hallucinations or delusions of any type and those features can either be congruent or non-congruent and both could occur in the context of any type of episode. Substance and alcohol abuse seem to be very common problems among patients with BD [5]. Recent studies report that there is an important degree of psychosocial impairment even during the euthymic period and suggest that only a minority of them achieves a complete functional recovery [6–12].

Although BD was considered, according to traditional understanding, as an episodic illness with a return to premorbid level of functioning between the episodes and a favourable outcome compared to schizophrenia [13], today we know that this is not always the case [14] and the Kraepelinian concept largely corresponds to BD-I.

Earlier studies suggested that the classic manic-depressive psychosis had a lifetime prevalence of around 1% (0.4–1.6%). However, the prevalence seems to depend on the definition, with the wider spectrum of bipolarity ('the bipolar spectrum') having an overall rate of 3–6.5% [15–19].

All the above put further more weight on the fact that the treatment approach to BD till now was too simplistic and unsatisfactory. Nowadays, the suboptimal outcome of mood disorders is better documented, and is related more to younger age of onset and to substance and alcohol abuse. Another important issue is that 75% of patients who commit suicide were found to suffer from some type of mood disorder. The World Health Organization has recently ranked bipolar disorder amongst the ten most disabling medical conditions world-wide [20].

The treatment of bipolar illness still is complex and full of caveats for the clinicians [21–23], and it seems that at least some aspects of the disorder are rather refractory to treatment.

9.2 Combination Treatment of Acute Mania

Acute mania is the best-studied phase with a significant number of monotherapy treatment strategies existing and with solid evidence support.

Concerning combination treatment, the data are few. An older study on the combination of haloperidol plus lithium failed to increase response rates compared to haloperidol alone [24]. On the contrary a more recent study combining valproate or lithium with 2–12 mg haloperidol or 1–6 mg risperidone suggested that the combination was more efficacious against acute mania than adding placebo (response rate 50% vs. 53% vs. 35% respectively for the combined lithium-valproate sample) [25]. Another study reports that the combination of lithium with haloperidol at low dose (5 mg/daily) but not at high dosage (25 mg/daily) increases the efficacy against acute mania. Lorazepam was found to be of no effect neither on the low nor on the high dosage [26]. Adding haloperidol on lithium was reported to be similar to adding lorazepam [27], but this was not a placebo controlled study. Lithium plus carbamazepine was equal to lithium plus haloperidol [28], and haloperidol plus carbamazepine was superior to haloperidol plus lithium [29] especially in improving agitation in manic patients. Olanzapine plus carbamazepine was not better than carbamazepine alone [30] and lithium plus tamoxifen was superior to lithium alone [31]. An add-on study of gabapentin was negative [32] while another one of phenytoin was positive but the sample size was small [33].

There are also a few add-on RCTs (Randomised Controlled Studies) on the treatment of acute mania in patients previously considered to be partial responders to lithium or valproate.

In partial responders under lithium, carbamazepine or valproate at therapeutic levels adding 1–6 mg risperidone proved to be superior to lithium, valproate or carbamazeprine alone (response rate: 48% vs. 31% at week 1; 61% vs. 43% at week 3) [34]. An 8-week trial on 52 incomplete responders to lithium utilized adding carbamazepine or oxcarbazepine (600–1,200 mg daily) during maintenance treatment. Although this trial was designed on patients in the 'maintenance' phase the design and the results are more relevant to the acute manic phase. The study sample constituted of manic, mixed and depressed patients. Both groups improved with the addition of either of the two drugs, but those receiving oxcarbazepine improved significantly more, also their YMRS score [35] did. In partially responsive manic patients already receiving valproate or lithium, adding olanzapine 5–20 mg daily improves the outcome after 6 weeks (response rate 67.7% vs 44.7% with placebo) with a robust effect on mixed-depressive symptoms [36] and on suicidality [37]. In a 3-weeks combination treatment study, patients under lithium (0.7–1.0 mEq/L) or valproate (50–100 μg/mL) were randomized to receive quetiapine (up to 800 mg daily) or placebo and the response rate was higher for the quetiapine group (54.3% vs. 32.6%) [38]. Adding up to 800 mg of quetiapine daily on lithium or valproate in partial responders, improved the response rate at week 3 (55.7% vs. 41.6% with placebo) [39]. However a more recent 6-week RCT does not support adding quetiapine to lithium or valproate in partial responders [40]. Adding aripiprazole on lithium (0.6–1.0 mmol/liter) or valproate (50–125 μg/ml) in partial responders produced higher response rate at week 6 (62.8% vs. 48.5% concerning both lithium and valproate groups) [41]. One study reported that adding valproate to neuroleptics improves the outcome (70% vs. 46%) [42].

Two unpublished studies of add on ziprasidone exist and are both negative concerning the primary outcome. The first utilized 80–120 mg ziprasidone daily vs placebo on top of lithium [43] while the second concerned a comparison of ziprasidone (40–80 or 80–160 mg daily) vs. placebo on top of lithium or divalproex [44]. Data as an adjunctive therapy are negative for topiramate [45]. There is also one negative study for paliperidone 3–12 mg daily as adjunctive therapy to lithium or valproate [46].

The results of a 12-week placebo controlled study on the safety and efficacy of asenapine when added to lithium or valproate was positive. Recent trials with licarbazepine reported negative results.

A recent placebo-controlled 4-week RCT supported the efficacy and safety of the purinergic agents allopurinol and dipyridamole adjunctive to lithium in acute bipolar mania [47]. Also another placebo controlled RCT supported the usefulness of celecoxib as an adjunct in the treatment of mixed episodes with a rapid action [48]. Folic acid was also found to be useful as an adjunct to valproate [49]. A small pilot study suggested that adding valnoctamide 600–1,200 mg/day (which is an anticonvulsant analog of valproate that does not undergo biotransformation to the corresponding free acid and in mice has been shown to be distinctly less teratogenic than valproate) on risperidone was more efficacious against acute mania in comparison to risperidone plus placebo [50]. A pilot study on the usefulness of adjunctive ramelteon was positive [51].

The grading of efficacy data for the acute mania/mixed treatment phase (up to 12 weeks) is shown in Table 9.1.

In conclusion, combination and add-on studies suggest that in acutely manic patients partial responders to lithium, valproate or carbamazepine, a good strategy

Table 9.1 Grading of efficacy data for the acute mania/mixed treatment phase (up to 12 weeks)

Agent/modality (alphabetical order)	Combination with:				
	Mood stabilizer	Carbamazepine	Lamotrigine	Lithium	Valproate
Aripiprazole	–	–	–	Good[a]	Good
Asenapine	–	–	–	Good	Good
Haloperidol	–	Fair[b]	–	Good	Good
Lithium	–	Fair	–	–	–
Olanzapine	–	Negative data	–	Good	Good
Oxcarbazepine	–	–	–	+	–
Paliperidone	–	–	–	Negative data	Negative data
Quetiapine	–	–	–	Good	Good
Risperidone, oral	–	Good	–	Good	Good
Topiramate	Negative data	–	–	–	–
Valproate	–	–	–	–	–
Ziprasidone	–	–	–	Negative data	–

[a] Good research-based evidence, supported by at least one placebo controlled study of sufficient magnitude. If there are non-placebo trials controlled with a comparator and with different results, the placebo controlled is the only taken into consideration

[b] Fair research-based evidence, from at least one randomised, double-blind controlled trial which, however, fail to fulfil all the criteria above (e.g., very small sample size or no placebo control)

would be to add haloperidol, risperidone, olanzapine, quetiapine or aripiprazole. Adding oxcarbazepine to lithium is also a choice. The clinician could also choose to add alternative agents for whose usefulness data are available (purinergic agents, celecoxib, folic acid).

9.3 Combination Treatment of Acute Bipolar Depression

Acute bipolar depression is not well studied, only a limited number of RCTs exist and the common practice to carry the clinical data and wisdom from the treatment of unipolar to bipolar depression is proven to be wrong. Quetiapine is the only monotherapy with proven efficacy.

As for combination treatment, the first add on studies used imipramine as adjunctive therapy on lithium in bipolar depression and were negative [52–54]. More recently one study used imipramine or paroxetine vs placebo as add on to lithium and reported that antidepressants were beneficial for patients with low but not for high levels of lithium [55]. Desipramine was reported to be equal to bupropion when added on a mood stabilizer [56]. Another study reported that adding venlafaxine, sertraline or bupropion on a mood stabilizer increases the response rate [57–59]. Similar findings were reported for citalopram [60] and paroxetine and amitriptyline [61].

RCTs fulfilling the modern quality standards suggest that the Olanzapine-Fluoxetine combination (OFC) is efficacious against bipolar I depression with remission rates 24.5% for placebo 32.8% for olanzapine and 48.8% for the OFC. However, the study sample was small concerning the OFC arm (N=86) [62]. Another study suggested that the OFC is somewhat superior to lamotrigine although the response rates did not differ between groups. (OFC: 68.8% vs. lamotrigine 59.7%). Thus one could interpret this study as somewhat negative for the OFC since lamotrigine is proven to be non-effective. Secondary indices showed that the time to response was significantly shorter for the OFC-treated patients (OFC 17 days vs. lamotrigine 23 days) and there were lesser 'suicidal and self-injurious behavior' among OFC treated patients (OFC, 0.5% vs. lamotrigine 3.4%) [63].

In a recent double-blind, placebo-controlled study, adding an antidepressant (including paroxetine) on a mood stabilizer in 179 bipolar depressed patients was not significant better than placebo after 26 weeks of treatment and the recovery rates (23.5% in the antidepressant group vs. 27.3% in the placebo group) and switch rates were similar. Thus this study does not support the usefulness of adjunctive antidepressant therapy [64], while on the contrary another earlier one supported the usefulness of paroxetine as add on therapy [65]. Adding L-sulpiride was similar to adding amitriptyline on lithium but the study was not controlled [66]. A more recent trial reported that the combination of risperidone plus paroxetine was not more efficacious than either agent alone [67]. However these data should be read with caution because paroxetine played a significant role in the design since these trials predated the negative trial of paroxetine vs. quetiapine [68]. A more recent study reported that adding lamotrigine to lithium was better than placebo in patients with bipolar depression at week 8, [69] however it is doubtful that the effect persists beyond week 12 [70, 71]. Another recent 8-week trial on 52 incomplete responders utilized adding carbamazepine or oxcarbazepine (600–1,200 mg daily) during maintenance treatment with lithium. Although this trial was on patients in 'maintenance' phase the design and the results are more relevant to the acute depressive phase since the study sample included depressed patients. Both groups improved with the addition of either drug but those receiving oxcarbazepine improved significantly more concerning their Montgomery-Asberg Depression Rating Scale (MADRS) and Hamilton Depression Rating Scale (HDRS-21) scores [35]. A small placebo-controlled adjunctive study of aripiprazole on lithium and citalopram was negative [72].

Recently one study with ziprasidone was negative [73]. The small add on study of leviracetam was negative [74]. A placebo controlled study suggested that in patients with treatment-resistant bipolar depression under lithium or valproate, robust and rapid antidepressant effects resulted from a single intravenous dose of ketamine hydrochloride (an N-methyl-D-aspartate antagonist) [75].

The grading of efficacy data for the acute depressive treatment phase (up to 12 weeks) is shown in Table 9.2.

Treatment algorithms with adding agents on a step-by-step basis are yet to be researched adequately [71].

Table 9.2 Grading of efficacy data for the acute depressive treatment phase (up to 12 weeks)

Agent/modality (alphabetical order)	Combination with:				
	Mood stabilizer	Carbamazepine	Lamotrigine	Lithium	Valproate
Aripiprazole	–	–	–	Negative data	–
Bupropion	–	Negative data	–	Negative data	Negative data
Lamotrigine	–	–	–	Good[a]	–
Lithium	–	–	Good	–	–
Oxcarbazepine	–	–	–	Fair[b]	–
Paroxetine	Negative data	Negative data	–	Negative data	Negative data
Ziprasidone	Negative data	–	–	–	–

[a]Good research-based evidence, supported by at least one placebo controlled study of sufficient magnitude. If there are non-placebo trials controlled with a comparator and with different results, the placebo controlled is the only taken into consideration
[b]Fair research-based evidence, from at least one randomised, double-blind controlled trial which, however, fail to fulfil all the criteria above (e.g., very small sample size or no placebo control)

9.4 Combination Treatment During the Maintenance Phase

Three combination studies with lithium plus imipramine, carbamazepine or perphenazine and carbamazepine or valproate plus perphenazine were negative. In the first one, 22 bipolar II patients in remission for at least 6 months and randomly assigned them to lithium, imipramine, lithium plus imipramine, or placebo. No effect or interaction of imipramine was found in either group [54]. In the second study, the combination of lithium plus carbamazepine did not produce further improvement for patients although rapid cycling patients do better under combination than under monotherapy (28.0% responded to lithium; 19.0% responded to carbamazepine and 56.3% to their combination) [76]. In the third study, which was a 6-months maintenance study with a placebo-controlled double blind design of perphenazine plus lithium, carbamazepine, or valproate or a mood stabilizer plus placebo in patients just remitted from an acute manic episode, the results suggested that patients receiving perphenazine had not a better course in comparison to those receiving placebo, but on the contrary they had a shorter time to depressive relapse, more drop-outs, and have increased rates of dysphoria and depressive symptoms [77].

The olanzapine-fluoxetine combination (OFC) data have already been reported above [78].

On the contrary, a recent placebo-controlled combination trial of quetiapine plus mood stabilizer during maintenance treatment, suggests that quetiapine is superior to placebo in the prevention of manic and depressive recurrences in either manic, depressive, or mixed index episode over a period of 2-years [79, 80]. This combination study appears to be the first to report prevention on both depression and mania regardless of the type of index episode.

One small study of add-on gabapentin to ongoing treatment was positive however the sample size was too small ($N=25$) [81]. The same holds true for phenytoin [82], while a small pilot study on oxcarabazepine plus lithium was negative [83].

One placebo controlled 18-month discontinuation study on olanzapine as add on lithium or valproate during the 6-weeks acute phase suggested that patients which responded to the combination during the acute phase did not do longitudinally better under the combination than under monotherapy with lithium or valproate [84]. Another discontinuation 6 month RCT of the combination of mood stabilizer plus ziprasidone (80–160 mg/day) vs mood stabilizer alone was in favour of the combination (relapse rate 19.7% vs 32.4%; longer median time to intervention for the combination: 43.0 days vs. 26.5 days) [85, 86]. Refractory patients to lithium or valproate during the acute phase are reported to benefit from continuation treatment with adjunctive aripiprazole [87].

The recently published BALANCE could neither reliably confirm nor refute a benefit of combination therapy compared with lithium monotherapy [88] at least partially because of methodological flaws [89].

Add on studies suggest that at least some strategies could be useful in patients with inadequate response to monotherapy.

One randomized add-on study suggested clozapine is superior to treatment as usual in the prevention of mania in refractory patients [90]. Adding olanzapine to lithium or valproate improves outcome [84] and may reduce suicidality [37]. Another study reported that valproate was more efficacious than lithium when added on antidepressants for the prevention of bipolar depression [91], and a recent double blind study suggested that adding an antidepressant (bupropion, sertraline or venlafaxine) on a mood stabilizer improved both the acute phase outcome and after 1 year follow up without inducing mania [59]. One study reports that adding lamotrigine to lithium was better than placebo in patients with bipolar depression [69] and its extension with the addition of paroxetine gave some additional positive results [70]. There is also one positive add on study on long acting injectable risperidone [92].

A 40-week placebo controlled study of the safety and efficacy of Asenapine when added to lithium or valproate and a 40 week extension study of asenapine vs. olanzapine (Ares 7501007) are expected to be announced.

The efficacy data for the maintenance treatment phase is shown in Table 9.3.

Overall, there is no compelling data that combination treatment does better than monotherapy. However patients stabilized on combination treatment might do worse if shifted to monotherapy, and patients refractory to monotherapy could benefit with add on treatment with olanzapine, valproate, an antidepressant or lamotrigine, depending on the index acute phase.

9.5 Combination Treatment of Mixed Episodes

Most studies include mixed patients; however they include mixed episodes together with manic/hypomanic episodes. Mixed depressive cases are not usually reported in depressive RCTs. Thus there are not much data available specifically for

Table 9.3 Efficacy data for the maintenance treatment phase

Agent/modality (alphabetical order)	Index episode	Enriched sample	Combination with: Treatment as usual	Mood stabilizer	Lamotrigine	Lithium	Valproate
Aripiprazole	m	Yes	–	–	–	m	m
Lamotrigine	m/d	Yes	–	–	–	d	–
Lithium	m/d	No	–	–	d	–	–
Olanzapine	m	Yes	–	m/d	–	m/d	m/d
Perphenazine	m	Yes	–	neg	–	–	–
Quetiapine	m/d	Yes	–	m/d	–	m/d	m/d
Long-acting injectable risperidone	m	Yes	m	–	–	–	–
Valproate	m	Yes	–	–	–	–	–
Ziprasidone	m	Yes	–	m	–	m	m
Cognitive-behavioral therapy	d	No	d	–	–	–	–
Psychoeducation	m/d	No	m/d	–	–	–	–

m mania/mixed, *d* depression, *m/d* both mania and depression

mixed patients. Some studies report separately the outcome for mixed patients; however there is a significant question concerning methodology that is most studies report the response only of the manic component of the mixed episode.

Adding risperidone or haloperidol on valproate or lithium significantly improves the manic component but there was no report on the depressive one [25]. Adding olanzapine on valproate or lithium improved both components [36].

The efficacy of olanzapine versus placebo as augmentation strategy to ongoing valproate treatment was also assessed in mixed patients during a more recent 6-week, placebo-controlled RCT. This study is the only existing RCT examining treatment effects on mixed bipolar patients. It included 202 mixed bipolar patients refractory to divalproex, who were administered adjunctive olanzapine or placebo. Adjunctive olanzapine was superior to placebo in improving both manic and depressive symptoms. The manic component responded from day 2 and the depressive from day 14 [93]. A secondary analysis of this study suggested early response of a component (at day 2) predicted full remission of the specific component [94].

The meta-analysis of the olanzapine-fluoxetine RCT against acute bipolar depression [62] separated patients suffering from non-mixed versus mixed depression [95] and reported that the response rates in patients with non-mixed versus those with mixed depression were similar in the OFC arm (48.9% vs. 43.2%; *odds ratio* = 1.24), but somewhat differed in the olanzapine arm (39.9% vs. 26.6%; *odds ratio* = 1.84) and in the placebo arm (27.5% vs. 16.3%; *OR* = 1.94). OFC response was independent of the number of manic/hypomanic symptoms, whereas a higher number of baseline concurrent manic/hypomanic symptoms predicted a lower response rate in the olanzapine and placebo arms [95].

Concerning the maintenance phase, combination of quetiapine with lithium or valproate protected from any mood episode in patients with an index mixed episode [79].

9.6 Combination Treatment of Rapid Cycling

There are no studies investigating the efficacy of treatment modalities in rapid cycling patients. All the data we have comes from post-hoc and meta-analytic studies and are poor concerning the overall response of the disorder.

Combination of lithium plus carbamazepine is better for rapid cycling patients do better under combination than under monotherapy (28.0% responded to lithium; 19.0% responded to carbamazepine and 56.3% to their combination) but not for non-rapid cyclers [76]. A 6-months study comparing lithium monotherapy vs. lithium plus valproate in rapid cycling patients with comorbid substance abuse reported that both options are equal, however the dropout rate was extremely high [96].

A 12-week study of adjunct lamotrigine vs. placebo on lithium or valproate in rapid cycling depressive bipolar patients was positive [97]. Also negative was a 6-month add-on study with lamotrigine vs. or placebo monotherapy on 182 patients with rapid-cycling bipolar disorder (DSM-IV criteria) although it showed some benefits for lamotrigine [98].

From 1,742 bipolar I and II patients in the STEP-BD at entry, 32% met the DSM-IV criteria for rapid cycling in the pre-study year. Of the 1,742 patients, 551 (32%) did not complete 1 year of treatment. Rapid cyclers were more likely to have further recurrences, although not necessarily more than four episodes per year. At the end of 12 months, only 5% of the patients could be classified as rapid cyclers. Antidepressant use during follow-up was associated with more frequent mood episodes [99].

9.7 Treatment of Comorbid Conditions

Comorbidity is a significant issue in bipolar patients and often needs specific therapeutic intervention. Often it requires to combine the standard anti-bipolar therapy with another treatment modality.

Lithium can be used for the treatment of concomitants substance abuse [100, 101], quetiapine for alcohol abuse [102] and anxiety symptoms [103], while risperidone can reduce drug craving [104] and anxiety [105]. Benzodiazepines can be used as adjunctive medication for sedation or for the treatment of anxiety, although abuse, tolerance and dependence constitute important problems. Pregabaline might be a useful agent for the treatment of anxiety disorders that commonly accompany bipolar illness and could substitute bendodiazepines. A significant advantage is that it is not metabolized in the liver. Topiramate is unique because of its ability to cause weight loss at dosages of 50–200 mg daily. It is reported that more than 70% of patients taking topiramate for a mean duration of 5 months lost a mean of 5–6 kilograms. Thus topiramate could be useful to treat weight gain which is a common problem in bipolar patients [106]. Naltrexone could be useful in outpatients with bipolar disorder and alcohol dependence [107].

9.8 Combination Treatment with Other Agents and Therapeutic Modalities

A variety of agents and treatment modalities are useful in the treatment of bipolar illness. Benzodiazepines can be used as adjunctive medication for sedation or for the treatment of anxiety, although abuse, tolerance and dependence constitute important problems. Dopaminergic agents and especially pramipexole could be useful in the treatment of bipolar depression either as monotherapy or as add on therapy [108]. In refractory depressive patients, inositol [109] and N-acetyl cysteine for maintenance [110, 111] could also be used as augmenting agents. Recently a placebo-controlled study of adjunctive modafinil has been shown to improve the outcome of bipolar depression without switching to mania or hypomania [112], however subclinical switches could be present [113]. The proof of concept study for adjunct armodafinil (the longer lasting isomer of modafinil) on lithium, valproate or olanzapine was positive [114]. Celecoxib was proved efficient an adjunct in the treatment of depressive or mixed with rapid onset of the effect [48]. Electroconvulsive therapy (ECT) could be a valuable option in mania [115, 116] and in treatment resistant bipolar depression [116, 117]. Transcranial Magnetic Stimulation especially when combined with brain navigation could be efficient and well tolerated against refractory bipolar depression [118]. Sleep deprivation and other noninvasive circadian-related interventions could be useful add-on treatment in order to accelerate and sustain antidepressant response [119]. Some data are in support of the usefulness of omega-3 fatty acids as adjunctive therapy in bipolar depression but not mania [120–125].

Naltrexone could be useful in outpatients with bipolar disorder and alcohol dependence [107].

A list of agents studied for augmentation strategies is shown in Table 9.4.

9.9 Conclusions and Future Directions

Historically, the modern approach in the treatment of bipolar illness starts with lithium when Frederik Lange in the late 19th century [126], and latter John Cade in 1949 [127–129] used it for the treatment of affective patients. However, Mogens Schou established the effectiveness of Li for the treatment of Bipolar Disorder [130, 131]

Table 9.4 List of agents studied for augmentation strategies

Agent/modality	Indication for augmentation
Celecoxib	Mania/mixed
Dopaminergic agents (pramipexole)	Bipolar depression
Electroconvulsive therapy	Bipolar depression or mania/mixed
Folic acid	Mania/mixed
Inositol	Bipolar depression
Modafinil/armodafinil	Bipolar depression
N-acetyl cysteine	Bipolar depression
Purinergic agents	Mania/mixed
Sleep deprivation	Bipolar depression
Transcranial magnetic stimulation	Bipolar depression or mania/mixed

together with Poul Christian Baastrup [132–134] by performing among other things a placebo-control discontinuation study of prophylaxis [135].

Our knowledge concerning the treatment of BD has changed radically during the last couple of decades. Earlier studies report a global and high effectiveness for older agents on all facets of bipolar disorder and a high prevalence of switching with antidepressants, which were not confirmed by newer studies. However the suboptimal outcome is well established and the need to go beyond the first line monotherapy treatment is pressing.

Concerning the treatment of acute mania some studies suggest that combination therapies give equivocal results and do not support combination treatment as first line treatment for all patients [24–30]. On the contrary, many combination and add-on studies report that in acutely manic patients the combination of Li or valproate with aripiprazole, olanzapine, risperidone, and maybe quetiapine or asenapine is recommended. Adding oxcarbazepine to lithium is also a choice. Anecdotal data suggest the use of ECT or higher dosages of neuroleptics, but the data are insufficient.

Unfortunately, there are few data to support a valid strategy about combination therapy in bipolar depressive cases. Quetiapine and the OFC are the only treatment options with proven efficacy against this condition. Some data on the combination of lithium plus lamotrigine also exist.

About the maintenance phase, favorable data exist concerning the OFC, quetiapine olanzapine or ziprasidone plus a mood stabilizer, specific antidepressants plus a mood stabilizer and lithium plus lamotrigine.

The paucity of data leaves the clinician with the heavy burden to decide on the basis of clinical experience and wisdom. In this frame, existing treatment guidelines cannot be considered to rely on hard data after their first step recommendations. Future research is essential and necessary to test possible treatment approaches for refractory patients of all kinds. Add-on studies or combination studies might give some kind of information; however the interpretation is complex and so far failed to provide reliable ground for decision-making.

References

1. Ng B, Camacho A, Lara DR et al (2007) A case series on the hypothesized connection between dementia and bipolar spectrum disorders: bipolar type VI? J Affect Disord 107:307–315
2. Akiskal HS (1996) The prevalent clinical spectrum of bipolar disorders: beyond DSM-IV. J Clin Psychopharmacol 16(2 Suppl 1):4S–14S
3. Akiskal HS, Pinto O (1999) The evolving bipolar spectrum prototypes I, II, III, and IV. Psychiatr Clin North Am 22(3):517–534, vii
4. Akiskal HS, Benazzi F (2004) Validating Kraepelin's two types of depressive mixed states: "depression with flight of ideas" and "excited depression". World J Biol Psychiatry 5(2):107–113
5. Winokur G, Turvey C, Akiskal H et al (1998) Alcoholism and drug abuse in three groups—bipolar I, unipolars and their acquaintances. J Affect Disord 50(2–3):81–89
6. Goldberg JF, Harrow M, Grossman LS (1995) Course and outcome in bipolar affective disorder: a longitudinal follow-up study. Am J Psychiatry 152(3):379–384
7. Goldberg JF, Harrow M, Grossman LS (1995) Recurrent affective syndromes in bipolar and unipolar mood disorders at follow-up. Br J Psychiatry 166(3):382–385
8. Keck PE Jr, McElroy SL, Strakowski SM et al (1998) 12-month outcome of patients with bipolar disorder following hospitalization for a manic or mixed episode. Am J Psychiatry 155(5):646–652
9. Strakowski SM, Keck PE Jr, McElroy SL et al (1998) Twelve-month outcome after a first hospitalization for affective psychosis. Arch Gen Psychiatry 55(1):49–55
10. Martinez-Aran A, Vieta E, Torrent C et al (2007) Functional outcome in bipolar disorder: the role of clinical and cognitive factors. Bipolar Disord 9(1–2):103–113
11. Mur M, Portella MJ, Martinez-Aran A et al (2007) Persistent neuropsychological deficit in euthymic bipolar patients: executive function as a core deficit. J Clin Psychiatry 68(7):1078–1086
12. Daban C, Martinez-Aran A, Torrent C et al (2006) Specificity of cognitive deficits in bipolar disorder versus schizophrenia a systematic review. Psychother Psychosom 75(2):72–84
13. Kraepelin E (1921) Manic-depressive insanity and paranoia. Robertson GM, Barclay RM (translator, ed), Livingstone, Edinburgh
14. Tohen M, Waternaux CM, Tsuang MT (1990) Outcome in mania. A 4-year prospective follow-up of 75 patients utilizing survival analysis. Arch Gen Psychiatry 47(12):1106–1111
15. Angst J (1998) The emerging epidemiology of hypomania and bipolar II disorder. J Affect Disord 50:143–151
16. Judd LL, Akiskal HS (2003) The prevalence and disability of bipolar spectrum disorders in the US population: re-analysis of the ECA database taking into account subthreshold cases. J Affect Disord 73(1–2):123–131
17. Acorn S (1993) Mental and physical health of homeless persons who use emergency shelters in Vancouver. Hosp Community Psychiatry 44(9):854–857
18. Angst J, Azorin JM, Bowden CL et al (2011) Prevalence and characteristics of undiagnosed bipolar disorders in patients with a major depressive episode: the BRIDGE study. Arch Gen Psychiatry 68(8):791–798
19. Angst J, Gamma A, Bowden CL et al (2011) Diagnostic criteria for bipolarity based on an international sample of 5,635 patients with DSM-IV major depressive episodes. Eur Arch Psychiatry Clin Neurosci
20. World Health Organization (2003) The world health report 2003—shaping the future. WHO, Geneva
21. Fountoulakis KN, Grunze H, Panagiotidis P et al (2008) Treatment of bipolar depression: an update. J Affect Disord 109(1–2):21–34
22. Fountoulakis KN, Vieta E, Sanchez-Moreno J et al (2005) Treatment guidelines for bipolar disorder: a critical review. J Affect Disord 86(1):1–10

23. Fountoulakis KN, Vieta E, Siamouli M et al (2007) Treatment of bipolar disorder: a complex treatment for a multi-faceted disorder. Ann Gen Psychiatry 6:27
24. Garfinkel PE, Stancer HC, Persad E (1980) A comparison of haloperidol, lithium carbonate and their combination in the treatment of mania. J Affect Disord 2(4):279–288
25. Sachs GS, Grossman F, Ghaemi SN et al (2002) Combination of a mood stabilizer with risperidone or haloperidol for treatment of acute mania: a double-blind, placebo-controlled comparison of efficacy and safety. Am J Psychiatry 159(7):1146–1154
26. Chou JC, Czobor P, Charles O et al (1999) Acute mania: haloperidol dose and augmentation with lithium or lorazepam. J Clin Psychopharmacol 19(6):500–505
27. Lenox RH, Newhouse PA, Creelman WL et al (1992) Adjunctive treatment of manic agitation with lorazepam versus haloperidol: a double-blind study. J Clin Psychiatry 53(2):47–52
28. Small JG, Klapper MH, Marhenke JD et al (1995) Lithium combined with carbamazepine or haloperidol in the treatment of mania. Psychopharmacol Bull 31(2):265–272
29. Klein E, Bental E, Lerer B et al (1984) Carbamazepine and haloperidol v placebo and haloperidol in excited psychoses a controlled study. Arch Gen Psychiatry 41(2):165–170
30. Tohen M, Bowden CL, Smulevich AB et al (2008) Olanzapine plus carbamazepine v. carbamazepine alone in treating manic episodes. Br J Psychiatry 192(2):135–143
31. Amrollahi Z, Rezaei F, Salehi B, et al (2010) Double-blind, randomized, placebo-controlled 6-week study on the efficacy and safety of the tamoxifen adjunctive to lithium in acute bipolar mania. J Affect Disord (in press)
32. Pande AC, Crockatt JG, Janney CA et al (2000) Gabapentin in bipolar disorder: a placebo-controlled trial of adjunctive therapy gabapentin bipolar disorder study group. Bipolar Disord 2(3 Pt 2):249–255
33. Mishory A, Yaroslavsky Y, Bersudsky Y et al (2000) Phenytoin as an antimanic anticonvulsant: a controlled study. Am J Psychiatry 157(3):463–465
34. Yatham LN, Grossman F, Augustyns I et al (2003) Mood stabilisers plus risperidone or placebo in the treatment of acute mania. International, double-blind, randomised controlled trial. Br J Psychiatry 182:141–147
35. Juruena MF, Ottoni GL, Machado-Vieira R et al (2009) Bipolar I and II disorder residual symptoms: oxcarbazepine and carbamazepine as add-on treatment to lithium in a double-blind, randomized trial. Prog Neuropsychopharmacol Biol Psychiatry 33(1):94–99
36. Tohen M, Chengappa KN, Suppes T et al (2002) Efficacy of olanzapine in combination with valproate or lithium in the treatment of mania in patients partially nonresponsive to valproate or lithium monotherapy. Arch Gen Psychiatry 59(1):62–69
37. Houston JP, Ahl J, Meyers AL et al (2006) Reduced suicidal ideation in bipolar I disorder mixed-episode patients in a placebo-controlled trial of olanzapine combined with lithium or divalproex. J Clin Psychiatry 67(8):1246–1252
38. Sachs G, Chengappa KN, Suppes T et al (2004) Quetiapine with lithium or divalproex for the treatment of bipolar mania: a randomized, double-blind, placebo-controlled study. Bipolar Disord 6(3):213–223
39. Yatham LN, Paulsson B, Mullen J et al (2004) Quetiapine versus placebo in combination with lithium or divalproex for the treatment of bipolar mania. J Clin Psychopharmacol 24(6):599–606
40. Yatham LN, Vieta E, Young AH et al (2007) A double blind, randomized, placebo-controlled trial of quetiapine as an add-on therapy to lithium or divalproex for the treatment of bipolar mania. Int Clin Psychopharmacol 22(4):212–220
41. Vieta E, T'Joen C, McQuade RD et al (2008) Efficacy of adjunctive aripiprazole to either valproate or lithium in bipolar mania patients partially nonresponsive to valproate/lithium monotherapy: a placebo-controlled study. Am J Psychiatry 165(10):1316–1325
42. Muller-Oerlinghausen B, Retzow A, Henn FA et al (2000) Valproate as an adjunct to neuroleptic medication for the treatment of acute episodes of mania: a prospective, randomized, double-blind, placebo-controlled, multicenter study European Valproate Mania Study Group. J Clin Psychopharmacol 20(2):195–203

43. Weisler R, Dunn J, English P (2003) Adjunctive Ziprasidone for acute bipolar mania: randomized, placebo-controlled trial. 4th international forum on mood and anxiety disorders, November 19–21, Monte Carlo, Monaco 2003
44. unpublished A three-week, double-blind, multicenter, placebo-controlled study evaluating the efficacy and safety of add-on oral ziprasidone in subjects with acute mania treated with lithium or divalproex 2011 [September 5th, 2011]. Available from: http://www.clinicalstudyresults.org/documents/company-study_9884_0.pdf
45. Roy Chengappa KN, Schwarzman LK, Hulihan JF et al (2006) Adjunctive topiramate therapy in patients receiving a mood stabilizer for bipolar I disorder: a randomized, placebo-controlled trial. J Clin Psychiatry 67(11):1698–1706
46. Berwaerts J, Lane R, Nuamah IF, et al (2010) Paliperidone extended-release as adjunctive therapy to lithium or valproate in the treatment of acute mania: a randomized, placebo-controlled study. J Affect Disord (in press)
47. Machado-Vieira R, Soares JC, Lara DR et al (2008) A double-blind, randomized, placebo-controlled 4-week study on the efficacy and safety of the purinergic agents allopurinol and dipyridamole adjunctive to lithium in acute bipolar mania. J Clin Psychiatry 69(8):1237–1245
48. Nery FG, Monkul ES, Hatch JP et al (2008) Celecoxib as an adjunct in the treatment of depressive or mixed episodes of bipolar disorder: a double-blind, randomized, placebo-controlled study. Hum Psychopharmacol 23(2):87–94
49. Behzadi AH, Omrani Z, Chalian M et al (2009) Folic acid efficacy as an alternative drug added to sodium valproate in the treatment of acute phase of mania in bipolar disorder: a double-blind randomized controlled trial. Acta Psychiatr Scand 120(6):441–445
50. Bersudsky Y, Applebaum J, Gaiduk Y et al (2010) Valnoctamide as a valproate substitute with low teratogenic potential in mania: a double-blind, controlled, add-on clinical trial. Bipolar Disord 12(4):376–382
51. McElroy SL, Winstanley EL, Martens B et al (2010) A randomized, placebo-controlled study of adjunctive ramelteon in ambulatory bipolar I disorder with manic symptoms and sleep disturbance. Int Clin Psychopharmacol 26(1):48–53
52. Prien RF, Kupfer DJ, Mansky PA et al (1984) Drug therapy in the prevention of recurrences in unipolar and bipolar affective disorders. Report of the NIMH Collaborative Study Group comparing lithium carbonate, imipramine, and a lithium carbonate-imipramine combination. Arch Gen Psychiatry 41(11):1096–1104
53. Prien RF, Klett CJ, Caffey EM Jr (1973) Lithium carbonate and imipramine in prevention of affective episodes. A comparison in recurrent affective illness. Arch Gen Psychiatry 29(3):420–425
54. Kane JM, Quitkin FM, Rifkin A et al (1982) Lithium carbonate and imipramine in the prophylaxis of unipolar and bipolar II illness: a prospective, placebo-controlled comparison. Arch Gen Psychiatry 39(9):1065–1069
55. Nemeroff CB, Evans DL, Gyulai L et al (2001) Double-blind, placebo-controlled comparison of imipramine and paroxetine in the treatment of bipolar depression. Am J Psychiatry 158(6):906–912
56. Sachs GS, Lafer B, Stoll AL et al (1994) A double-blind trial of bupropion versus desipramine for bipolar depression. J Clin Psychiatry 55(9):391–393
57. Post RM, Altshuler LL, Frye MA et al (2001) Rate of switch in bipolar patients prospectively treated with second-generation antidepressants as augmentation to mood stabilizers. Bipolar Disord 3(5):259–265
58. Post RM, Altshuler LL, Leverich GS et al (2006) Mood switch in bipolar depression: comparison of adjunctive venlafaxine, bupropion and sertraline. Br J Psychiatry 189:124–131
59. Altshuler LL, Post RM, Hellemann G et al (2009) Impact of antidepressant continuation after acute positive or partial treatment response for bipolar depression: a blinded, randomized study. J Clin Psychiatry 70(4):450–457
60. Schaffer A, Zuker P, Levitt A (2006) Randomized, double-blind pilot trial comparing lamotrigine versus citalopram for the treatment of bipolar depression. J Affect Disord 96(1–2):95–99

61. Pilhatsch M, Wolf R, Winter C et al (2010) Comparison of paroxetine and amitriptyline as adjunct to lithium maintenance therapy in bipolar depression: a reanalysis of a randomized, double-blind study. J Affect Disord 126(3):453–457
62. Tohen M, Vieta E, Calabrese J et al (2003) Efficacy of olanzapine and olanzapine-fluoxetine combination in the treatment of bipolar I depression. Arch Gen Psychiatry 60(11):1079–1088
63. Brown EB, McElroy SL, Keck PE Jr et al (2006) A 7-week, randomized, double-blind trial of olanzapine/fluoxetine combination versus lamotrigine in the treatment of bipolar I depression. J Clin Psychiatry 67(7):1025–1033
64. Sachs GS, Nierenberg AA, Calabrese JR et al (2007) Effectiveness of adjunctive antidepressant treatment for bipolar depression. N Engl J Med 356(17):1711–1722
65. Young LT, Joffe RT, Robb JC et al (2000) Double-blind comparison of addition of a second mood stabilizer versus an antidepressant to an initial mood stabilizer for treatment of patients with bipolar depression. Am J Psychiatry 157(1):124–126
66. Bocchetta A, Bernardi F, Burrai C et al (1993) A double-blind study of L-sulpiride versus amitriptyline in lithium-maintained bipolar depressives. Acta Psychiatr Scand 88(6):434–439
67. Shelton RC, Stahl SM (2004) Risperidone and paroxetine given singly and in combination for bipolar depression. J Clin Psychiatry 65(12):1715–1719
68. McElroy SL, Weisler RH, Chang W et al (2010) A double-blind, placebo-controlled study of quetiapine and paroxetine as monotherapy in adults with bipolar depression (EMBOLDEN II). J Clin Psychiatry 71(2):163–174
69. van der Loos ML, Mulder PG, Hartong EG et al (2009) Efficacy and safety of lamotrigine as add-on treatment to lithium in bipolar depression: a multicenter, double-blind, placebo-controlled trial. J Clin Psychiatry 70(2):223–231
70. van der Loos ML, Mulder P, Hartong EG et al (2011) Long-term outcome of bipolar depressed patients receiving lamotrigine as add-on to lithium with the possibility of the addition of paroxetine in nonresponders: a randomized, placebo-controlled trial with a novel design. Bipolar Disord 13(1):111–117
71. van der Loos ML, Mulder P, Hartong EG et al (2010) Efficacy and safety of two treatment algorithms in bipolar depression consisting of a combination of lithium, lamotrigine or placebo and paroxetine. Acta Psychiatr Scand 122(3):246–254
72. Quante A, Zeugmann S, Luborzewski A et al (2010) Aripiprazole as adjunct to a mood stabilizer and citalopram in bipolar depression: a randomized placebo-controlled pilot study. Hum Psychopharmacol 25(2):126–132
73. Sachs GS, Ice KS, Chappell PB et al (2011) Efficacy and safety of adjunctive oral ziprasidone for acute treatment of depression in patients with bipolar I disorder: a randomized, double-blind, placebo-controlled trial. J Clin Psychiatry 72:1413
74. Saricicek A, Maloney K, Muralidharan A et al (2010) Lvetiracetam in the management of bipolar depression: a randomized, double-blind, placebo-controlled trial. J Clin Psychiatry 72:744–750
75. Diazgranados N, Ibrahim L, Brutsche NE et al (2010) A randomized add-on trial of an N-methyl-D-aspartate antagonist in treatment-resistant bipolar depression. Arch Gen Psychiatry 67(8):793–802
76. Denicoff KD, Smith-Jackson EE, Disney ER et al (1997) Comparative prophylactic efficacy of lithium, carbamazepine, and the combination in bipolar disorder. J Clin Psychiatry 58(11):470–478
77. Zarate CA Jr, Tohen M (2004) Double-blind comparison of the continued use of antipsychotic treatment versus its discontinuation in remitted manic patients. Am J Psychiatry 161(1):169–171
78. Brown E, Dunner DL, McElroy SL et al (2009) Olanzapine/fluoxetine combination vs. lamotrigine in the 6-month treatment of bipolar I depression. Int J Neuropsychopharmacol 12(6):773–782
79. Vieta E, Suppes T, Eggens I et al (2008) Efficacy and safety of quetiapine in combination with lithium or divalproex for maintenance of patients with bipolar I disorder (international trial 126). J Affect Disord 109(3):251–263

80. Suppes T, Vieta E, Liu S et al (2009) Maintenance treatment for patients with bipolar I disorder: results from a north american study of quetiapine in combination with lithium or divalproex (trial 127). Am J Psychiatry 166(4):476–488
81. Vieta E, Manuel Goikolea J, Martinez-Aran A et al (2006) A double-blind, randomized, placebo-controlled, prophylaxis study of adjunctive gabapentin for bipolar disorder. J Clin Psychiatry 67(3):473–477
82. Mishory A, Winokur M, Bersudsky Y (2003) Prophylactic effect of phenytoin in bipolar disorder: a controlled study. Bipolar Disord 5(6):464–467
83. Vieta E, Cruz N, Garcia-Campayo J et al (2008) A double-blind, randomized, placebo-controlled prophylaxis trial of oxcarbazepine as adjunctive treatment to lithium in the long-term treatment of bipolar I and II disorder. Int J Neuropsychopharmacol 11(4):445–452
84. Tohen M, Chengappa KN, Suppes T et al (2004) Relapse prevention in bipolar I disorder: 18-month comparison of olanzapine plus mood stabiliser v. mood stabiliser alone. Br J Psychiatry 184:337–345
85. Bowden CL, Vieta E, Ice KS et al (2010) Ziprasidone plus a mood stabilizer in subjects with bipolar I disorder: a 6-month, randomized, placebo-controlled, double-blind trial. J Clin Psychiatry 71(2):130–137
86. Citrome L (2010) Ziprasidone HCl capsules for the adjunctive maintenance treatment of bipolar disorder in adults. Expert Rev Neurother 10(7):1031–1037
87. Marcus R, Khan A, Rollin L et al (2011) Efficacy of aripiprazole adjunctive to lithium or valproate in the long-term treatment of patients with bipolar I disorder with an inadequate response to lithium or valproate monotherapy: a multicenter, double-blind, randomized study. Bipolar Disord 13(2):133–144
88. Geddes JR, Goodwin GM, Rendell J et al (2010) Lithium plus valproate combination therapy versus monotherapy for relapse prevention in bipolar I disorder (BALANCE): a randomised open-label trial. Lancet 375(9712):385–395
89. Fountoulakis KN (2010) The BALANCE trial. Lancet 375(9723):1343–1344, author reply 1344
90. Suppes T, Webb A, Paul B et al (1999) Clinical outcome in a randomized 1-year trial of clozapine versus treatment as usual for patients with treatment-resistant illness and a history of mania. Am J Psychiatry 156(8):1164–1169
91. Gyulai L, Bowden CL, McElroy SL et al (2003) Maintenance efficacy of divalproex in the prevention of bipolar depression. Neuropsychopharmacology 28(7):1374–1382
92. Macfadden W, Alphs L, Haskins JT et al (2009) A randomized, double-blind, placebo-controlled study of maintenance treatment with adjunctive risperidone long-acting therapy in patients with bipolar I disorder who relapse frequently. Bipolar Disord 11(8):827–839
93. Houston JP, Tohen M, Degenhardt EK et al (2009) Olanzapine-divalproex combination versus divalproex monotherapy in the treatment of bipolar mixed episodes: a double-blind, placebo-controlled study. J Clin Psychiatry 70(11):1540–1547
94. Houston JP, Ketter TA, Case M et al (2011) Early symptom change and prediction of subsequent remission with olanzapine augmentation in divalproex-resistant bipolar mixed episodes. J Psychiatr Res 45(2):169–173
95. Benazzi F, Berk M, Frye MA et al (2009) Olanzapine/fluoxetine combination for the treatment of mixed depression in bipolar I disorder: a post hoc analysis. J Clin Psychiatry 70(10):1424–1431
96. Kemp DE, Gao K, Ganocy SJ et al (2009) A 6-month, double-blind, maintenance trial of lithium monotherapy versus the combination of lithium and divalproex for rapid-cycling bipolar disorder and co-occurring substance abuse or dependence. J Clin Psychiatry 70(1):113–121
97. Wang Z, Gao K, Kemp DE et al (2010) Lamotrigine adjunctive therapy to lithium and divalproex in depressed patients with rapid cycling bipolar disorder and a recent substance use disorder: a 12-week, double-blind, placebo-controlled pilot study. Psychopharmacol Bull 43(4):5–21

98. Calabrese JR, Suppes T, Bowden CL et al (2000) A double-blind, placebo-controlled, prophylaxis study of lamotrigine in rapid-cycling bipolar disorder. Lamictal 614 study group. J Clin Psychiatry 61(11):841–850
99. Schneck CD, Miklowitz DJ, Miyahara S et al (2008) The prospective course of rapid-cycling bipolar disorder: findings from the STEP-BD. Am J Psychiatry 165:370–377
100. Geller B, Cooper TB, Sun K et al (1998) Double-blind and placebo-controlled study of lithium for adolescent bipolar disorders with secondary substance dependency. J Am Acad Child Adolesc Psychiatry 37(2):171–178
101. Geller B, Cooper TB, Watts HE et al (1992) Early findings from a pharmacokinetically designed double-blind and placebo-controlled study of lithium for adolescents comorbid with bipolar and substance dependency disorders. Prog Neuropsychopharmacol Biol Psychiatry 16(3):281–299
102. Brown ES, Garza M, Carmody TJ (2008) A randomized, double-blind, placebo-controlled add-on trial of quetiapine in outpatients with bipolar disorder and alcohol use disorders. J Clin Psychiatry 69(5):701–705
103. Lydiard RB, Culpepper L, Schioler H et al (2009) Quetiapine monotherapy as treatment for anxiety symptoms in patients with bipolar depression: a pooled analysis of results from 2 double-blind, randomized, placebo-controlled studies. Prim Care Companion J Clin Psychiatry 11(5):215–225
104. Nejtek VA, Avila M, Chen LA et al (2008) Do atypical antipsychotics effectively treat co-occurring bipolar disorder and stimulant dependence? A randomized, double-blind trial. J Clin Psychiatry 69(8):1257–1266
105. Sheehan DV, McElroy SL, Harnett-Sheehan K et al (2009) Randomized, placebo-controlled trial of risperidone for acute treatment of bipolar anxiety. J Affect Disord 115(3):376–385
106. Arnone D (2005) Review of the use of Topiramate for treatment of psychiatric disorders. Ann Gen Psychiatry 4(1):5
107. Sherwood Brown E, Carmody TJ, Schmitz JM et al (2009) A randomized, double-blind, placebo-controlled pilot study of naltrexone in outpatients with bipolar disorder and alcohol dependence. Alcohol Clin Exp Res 33(11):1863–1869
108. Zarate CA Jr, Payne JL, Singh J et al (2004) Pramipexole for bipolar II depression: a placebo-controlled proof of concept study. Biol Psychiatry 56(1):54–60
109. Eden Evins A, Demopulos C, Yovel I et al (2006) Inositol augmentation of lithium or valproate for bipolar depression. Bipolar Disord 8(2):168–174
110. Berk M, Copolov DL, Dean O et al (2008) N-acetyl cysteine for depressive symptoms in bipolar disorder—a double-blind randomized placebo-controlled trial. Biol Psychiatry 64(6):468–475
111. Magalhaes PV, Dean OM, Bush AI et al (2011) N-acetyl cysteine add-on treatment for bipolar II disorder: a subgroup analysis of a randomized placebo-controlled trial. J Affect Disord 129(1–3):317–320
112. Frye MA, Grunze H, Suppes T et al (2007) A placebo-controlled evaluation of adjunctive modafinil in the treatment of bipolar depression. Am J Psychiatry 164(8):1242–1249
113. Fountoulakis KN, Siamouli M, Panagiotidis P et al (2008) Ultra short manic-like episodes after antidepressant augmentation with modafinil. Prog Neuropsychopharmacol Biol Psychiatry 32(3):891–892
114. Calabrese JR, Ketter TA, Youakim JM et al (2010) Adjunctive armodafinil for major depressive episodes associated with bipolar I disorder: a randomized, multicenter, double-blind, placebo-controlled, proof-of-concept study. J Clin Psychiatry 71(10):1363–1370
115. Hiremani RM, Thirthalli J, Tharayil BS et al (2008) Double-blind randomized controlled study comparing short-term efficacy of bifrontal and bitemporal electroconvulsive therapy in acute mania. Bipolar Disord 10(6):701–707
116. Loo C, Katalinic N, Mitchell PB et al (2010) Physical treatments for bipolar disorder: a review of electroconvulsive therapy, stereotactic surgery and other brain stimulation techniques. J Affect Disord 132:1–13

117. Kessler U, Vaaler AE, Schoyen H et al (2010) The study protocol of the Norwegian randomized controlled trial of electroconvulsive therapy in treatment resistant depression in bipolar disorder. BMC Psychiatry 10(1):16
118. Dell'Osso B, Mundo E, D'Urso N et al (2009) Augmentative repetitive navigated transcranial magnetic stimulation (rTMS) in drug-resistant bipolar depression. Bipolar Disord 11(1):76–81
119. Wu JC, Kelsoe JR, Schachat C et al (2009) Rapid and sustained antidepressant response with sleep deprivation and chronotherapy in bipolar disorder. Biol Psychiatry 66(3):298–301
120. Sarris J, Mischoulon D, Schweitzer I (2011) Omega-3 for bipolar disorder: meta-analyses of use in mania and bipolar depression. J Clin Psychiatry 73:81–86
121. Frangou S, Lewis M, McCrone P (2006) Efficacy of ethyl-eicosapentaenoic acid in bipolar depression: randomised double-blind placebo-controlled study. Br J Psychiatry 188:46–50
122. Frangou S, Lewis M, Wollard J et al (2007) Preliminary in vivo evidence of increased N-acetyl-aspartate following eicosapentanoic acid treatment in patients with bipolar disorder. J Psychopharmacol 21(4):435–439
123. Keck PE Jr, Mintz J, McElroy SL et al (2006) Double-blind, randomized, placebo-controlled trials of ethyl-eicosapentanoate in the treatment of bipolar depression and rapid cycling bipolar disorder. Biol Psychiatry 60(9):1020–1022
124. Chiu CC, Huang SY, Chen CC et al (2005) Omega-3 fatty acids are more beneficial in the depressive phase than in the manic phase in patients with bipolar I disorder. J Clin Psychiatry 66(12):1613–1614
125. Stoll AL, Severus WE, Freeman MP et al (1999) Omega 3 fatty acids in bipolar disorder: a preliminary double-blind, placebo-controlled trial. Arch Gen Psychiatry 56(5):407–412
126. Lange F (1894) De vigtigste sindssygdomme (The most important pychiatric disorders). Gyldendal, Copenhagen
127. Cade J (1949) Lithium salts in the treatment of psychotic excitement. Med J Aust 36:349–352
128. Cade J (1970) The story of lithium. In: Ayd F, Blackwell B (eds) Discoveries in biological psychiatry. Lippincott, Philadelphia
129. Bech P (2006) The full story of lithium. A tribute to Mogens Schou (1918–2005). Psychother Psychosom 75(5):265–269
130. Schou M, Juel-Nielsen N, Stromgren E et al (1954) The treatment of manic psychosis by the administration of lithium salts. J Neurol Neurosurg Psychiatry 17:250–260
131. Schou M (1997) Forty years of lithium treatment. Arch Gen Psychiatry 54:9
132. Baastrup P (1964) The use of lithium in manic-depressive psychosis. Compr Psychiatry 5:396–408
133. Baastrup PC, Schou M (1967) Lithium as a prophylactic agents its effect against recurrent depressions and manic-depressive psychosis. Arch Gen Psychiatry 16(2):162–172
134. Schou M, Baastrup PC (1967) Lithium treatment of manic-depressive disorder dosage and control. JAMA 201(9):696–698
135. Baastrup PC, Poulsen JC, Schou M et al (1970) Prophylactic lithium: double blind discontinuation in manic-depressive and recurrent-depressive disorders. Lancet 2(7668):326–330

Chapter 10
Antidepressant Combination Strategies for Major Depressive Disorder

André F. Carvalho, Danielle S. Macêdo, Thomas N. Hyphantis, and Roger S. McIntyre

Abstract The majority of patients with major depressive disorder (MDD) fail to remit after initial antidepressant (AD) treatment trials. The results of the Treatment Alternatives to Relieve Depression (STAR*D) trial suggest that most MDD patients require a 'next-step' treatment, which include AD combination therapies, as well as various AD augmentation strategies. Antidepressant combination strategies are widely used by clinicians for the management of treatment-resistant depression (TRD). The aim of this chapter was to review current evidence on antidepressant combination strategies for TRD. There are limited evidences to guide even the most widely used combination strategies for TRD. This stands in marked contrast to several augmentation strategies for AD non-responders, including adjunctive lithium, thyroid hormone or atypical antipsychotics, for which there are stronger evidences from well designed randomized controlled trials to support efficacy. Recently, a few randomized trials have investigated the efficacy of different antidepressant combination strategies for MDD from treatment initiation. These trials provided discrepant results thus far. Potential clinical advantages of various combination

A.F. Carvalho, M.D., Ph.D. (✉)
Department of Clinical Medicine and Psychiatry Research Group,
Faculty of Medicine, Federal University of Ceará, Fortaleza, CE, Brazil
e-mail: andrefc7@terra.com.br

D.S. Macêdo, Ph.D.
Department of Physiology and Pharmacology, Faculty of Medicine,
Federal University of Ceará, Fortaleza, CE, Brazil

T.N. Hyphantis, M.D., Ph.D.
Department of Psychiatry, Medical School, University of Ioaninna, Ioaninna, Greece

R.S. McIntyre, M.D., FRCPC
Department of Psychiatry, University of Toronto, Toronto, ON, Canada

Mood Disorders Psychopharmacology Unit, University Health Network,
Toronto, ON, Canada

M.S. Ritsner (ed.), *Polypharmacy in Psychiatry Practice, Volume II: Use of Polypharmacy in the "Real World"*, DOI 10.1007/978-94-007-5799-8_10,

strategies are also discussed (for example, avoidance of discontinuation-emergent symptoms). This chapter deals with pharmacological aspects of TRD and will not cover evidence-based psychotherapeutic and neuromodulatory (for example, electroconvulsive therapy) approaches for TRD. This chapter underscores the need for the design of adequately powered randomized controlled trials to provide a clearer evidence base for this widely employed clinical practice.

Abbreviations

5-HT	Serotonin
AD	Antidepressant
ADHD	Attention deficit hyperactivity disorder
EBM	Evidence-based medicine
ECT	Electroconvulsive therapy
HDRS	Hamilton depression rating scale
MADRS	Montgomery-Asberg Depression Rating Scale
MAOI	Monoamine oxidase inhibitor
MDD	Major depressive disorder
NRI	Norepinephrine reuptake inhibitor
RCT	Randomized controlled trial
SNRI	Serotonin and norepinephrine reuptake inhibitor
SNRI	Serotonin norepinephrine reuptake inhibitor
SSRI	Selective serotonin reuptake inhibitors
STAR*D	Sequenced Treatment Alternatives to Relieve Depression
TCA	Tricyclic antidepressant
TRT	Treatment-resistant depression

10.1 Introduction

The pharmacotherapy of major depressive disorder (MDD) has evolved through the introduction of more selective antidepressants in clinical practice. Newer antidepressant (AD) drugs, including selective serotonin reuptake inhibitors (SSRIs) and dual serotonin and norepinephrine reuptake inhibitors (SNRIs), have gained wide acceptance, primarily because of their relative favorable tolerability and safety profiles; however, response rates for this drugs typically are in the range of 60–70% in RCTs [1, 2]. Patients who met the traditional definition of response (typically a 50% improvement on a depression scale) could still have significant functional impairment [3]. The treatment of MDD is now directed to symptomatic remission (e.g., a score $\leq$7 on the 17-item HDRS) [4]. However, far fewer patients achieve full remission.

For those patients who fail to achieve remission on a given AD trial, several so-called second-step strategies have been proposed, such as: (i) increasing the dose of the antidepressant; (ii) switching to another antidepressant (either from the same

Table 10.1 Phase and rush staging method for treatment-resistant depression

Stage I: Failure of at least one adequate trial of one major class of antidepressant
Stage II: Stage I resistance *plus* failure of adequate trial of an antidepressant in a distinctly different class from that used in Stage I
Stage III: Stage II resistance *plus* failure of an adequate trial of tricyclic antidepressant (TCA) agent
Stage IV: Stage III resistance *plus* failure of an adequate trial of a monoamine oxidase inhibitor (MAOI)
Stage V: Stage IV resistance *plus* failure of a course of bilateral electroconvulsive therapy (ECT)

class or from a different class); (iv) augmentation therapies and (v) combining two antidepressants [5]. There are several definitions for treatment-resistant depression (TRD). However, Thase and Rush [5] introduced a 5-stage model for TRD that yields a categorical assignment of degree of resistance (Table 10.1). This model has heuristic value as it might provide useful information for the clinician.

Augmentation and combination therapies are commonly employed by clinicians treating patients with various levels of TRD [6, 7]. Augmentation refers to the addition of a drug that is not a standard AD to ongoing AD treatment [1, 2]. Several augmentation strategies have been tested for the management of TRD. However, there is a dearth of well designed RCTs to guide current practice. Augmentation strategies with lithium [1, 2], T3 thyroid hormone [1, 2] and atypical antipsychotics [8] have a stronger level of evidence thus far.

The rationale behind either augmentation or combination strategies for TRD is to add novel pharmacological mechanisms to ongoing AD treatment [9].Theoretically, these procedures would lead to remission in patients with either non-response or partial response to ADs. Furthermore, these strategies have been tested to improve specific residual symptoms of MDD patients (e.g., insomnia and fatigue) [10]. Combination protocols may offer several advantages for the management of TRD, namely: (i) avoidance of discontinuation-emergent symptoms and cross-titration schedules; (ii) the second AD should be as effective in combination as it would be in monotherapy following a switch and (iii) the probability of complementary neuropharmacological mechanisms that may enhance efficacy or improve tolerability [9–11]. Recently, some investigators had also suggested that the combination of ADs at the onset of treatment would enhance the likelihood of achieving remission [9, 10].

This chapter provides a critical review of the existing literature on AD combination treatment strategies for MDD.

10.2 Antidepressant Combination Strategies for MDD

The introduction of SSRIs changed the therapeutics of MDD in many ways and, for the most part, these changes have been beneficial to our patients. Indeed the SSRIs became so widely prescribed that—by mid-1990—they had supplanted the tricyclic antidepressants (TCAs) as first line treatment for outpatients with MDD. The popularity of SSRIs directly led to a new unmet need: the identification of effective strategies for those patients who would not achieve remission with SSRIs. The perceived magnitude of this need may have been a direct result of the high selectivity of the SSRIs, compared with the TCAs, were arguably at the expense of a somewhat reduced efficacy, especially for patients with severe forms of depression. Although this assumption is still controversial even two decades later, it was initially supported by the results of several early inpatient trials that compared clomipramine with the SSRIs citalopram [12] and paroxetine [13], and further supported by the results of a meta-analysis of 25 inpatient RCTs [14]. Regarding the relevance of selectivity, it is noteworthy that Anderson and coworkers found no clear difference in efficacy in the studies that contrasted the SSRIs with the more noradrenergically selective, secondary amine TCAs (e.g., desipramine and nortriptyline) and their tetracyclic congener, maprotyline [14]. It was thus hypothesized that the apparently greater efficacy of tertiary amine TCAs, such as amitryptiline and clomipramine, was attributable to their broader actions, including direct actions on 5-HT and noradrenergic neurotransmission. One immediate therapeutic consequence for this hypothesis was the possibility that the effectiveness of SSRIs could be subsequently enhanced by adding a noradrenergically active TCA. A meta-analysis by Papakostas and colleagues [15] suggest that treatment of MDD patients with SNRIs is associated with higher response rates when compared to SSRIs. Although the clinical significance of their results (Number Needed to Treat=24) are questionable, they give support to the notion that ADs with broader actions might offer greater clinical efficacy.

As clinical experience with SSRIs plus TCAs combinations expanded in psychiatric practice, it became apparent that the SSRIs were safer to use in tandem with TCAs than were monoamine oxidase inhibitors (MAOIs), and aside for some concerns, pertaining to drug-drug interactions, these combinations were generally well tolerated. Such positive clinical experiences led to the rapidly expansion of AD combination strategies to include combinations with other newer generation ADs (e.g., bupropion, mirtazapine and the SNRI venlafaxine) [16].

Despite the fact that clinical experience provides important input for the management of MDD, the various combination strategies for the treatment of MDD should be empirically validated by the standard procedures of evidence-based medicine (EBM). Thus, the current state of the evidence of each AD combination strategy is critically reviewed below.

10.2.1 TCA Plus SSRI Combinations

An early study using a historical control has suggested that a combination of TCA plus SSRI may produce a more rapid onset of action [17]. A more recent, prospective randomized trial found remission rates were significantly higher with desipramine *plus* fluoxetine than with either drug alone [18]. The results are consistent with uncontrolled observations that desipramine and other TCAs are effective in combination with SSRIs in small cohorts of TRD patients [10, 19]. The efficacy of

TCAs combined with SSRIs has been challenged by two studies that found that adding low-dose desipramine to fluoxetine was less effective than increasing the dose of fluoxetine in patients unresponsive to 8 weeks of treatment with fluoxetine 20 mg/day [20, 21].

A third study by Nelson et al. [18], which was not limited to patients with TRD, evaluated the combination of fluoxetine and higher doses of desipramine. In this trial, 39 inpatients were randomly assigned to 6 weeks of double-blind treatment with fluoxetine or desipramine, singly or in combination. The fluoxetine dosage was fixed at 20 mg daily; and desipramine dosages were adjusted by an unblended monitor to ensure adequate plasma levels. Average dosages of desipramine were 98 mg daily in the combined therapy group and 294 mg daily in the monotherapy group. In contrast to the findings of Fava et al [21], the previous study found evidence of an additive effect with a significant difference in remission rates favoring the group in combined therapy (54%), compared to the groups that received either fluoxetine (7%) or desipramine (0%) monotherapy. These findings are consistent with the meta-analysis of Anderson [14], namely, that for inpatients, AD strategies that target both norepinephrine and 5-HT are superior to more highly selective ADs. Further research should investigate whether these findings would apply to outpatients with less severe MDD.

Since TCAs are substrates of the cytochrome P450 2D6 isoenzyme, TCA serum levels may rise when co-administered with some SSRIs that inhibit this metabolic pathway, with the potential for cardiac toxicity, anticholinergic side effects and orthostatic hypotension. Therefore, low doses of TCAs (25–75 mg/day) are typically used and monitoring of TCA blood levels is necessary.

10.2.2 SSRIs Plus Bupropion

In the United States, bupropion had largely replaced the TCAs as the drug of choice for combining with SSRIs by the mid-1990's [11]. When compared with TCAs, important perceived advantages included:

- Bupropion has a more favourable side effect and tolerability profile than TCAs;
- Bupropion may help to counteract the adverse effects of SSRIs over sexual function.

Early anecdotal case series had suggested that this combination strategy was both well tolerated and effective (see [16] for a review). The state of the evidence did not change much during the past decade. Two open-label active comparator studies have been published, and when considered together, these trials provide only limited support for the strong clinical enthusiasm for this combination [22, 23]. In a small (n = 61), non-randomized, open label trial, the combination of bupropion-SR and citalopram was more effective than switching to the other medication in patients who had not responded to either one of these two medications [22].

10.2.3 SSRIs and (or) SNRIs Plus Mirtazapine and (or) Mianserin

Mirtazapine and mianserin are closely related drugs that are mechanistically distinct from other ADs as they have no appreciable effects on monoamine uptake transporters. However, these drugs do modulate norepinephrine and 5-HT neurotransmission via complex mechanisms that include antagonism of alfa-2 autoreceptors and heteroreceptors, as well as, blockade of 5-HT_2, 5-HT_3 and histamine receptors. There several potential advantages of combining these drugs with SSRIs and SNRIs, namely: (i) 'boosting' monoaminergic neurotransmission; (ii) broadening symptomatic coverage for insomnia and diminished appetite and (iii) counteracting troublesome gastrointestinal side effects of SSRIs and SNRIs [11].

The efficacy of mianserin combination for TRD has been evaluated by at least two RCTs [16]. Both studies of mianserin augmentation of SSRI non-responders yielded some evidence in favour of the combination, compared to fluoxetine alone. Anecdotal evidences have shown that combining mianserin was an effective strategy for patients unresponsive to TCAs alone [24]. A previous trial has reported that fluoxetine nonresponders showed greater improvement when mianserin was added than when placebo was added [25]. A third, more recent, RCT has shown that adding mianserin to sertraline nonresponders offered no advantage over adding placebo [25]. However, the initial trial with sertraline monotherapy was too brief and a dose increase of sertraline was carried out 2 weeks prior to randomization, thereby confounding the results. Overall, these studies do suggest that the addition of mianserin might increase response/remission rates in MDD patients unresponsive to TCAs or SSRIs.

Mirtazapine (15–30 mg q.h.s) has been found to be effective in combination with SSRIs in open label studies and case series of patients nonresponsive to SSRIs [26]. Mirtazapine was found to be effective in a subsequent small (n=20), double-blind study of SSRI-resistant participants, although sedation and weight gain emerged as significant adverse effects among mirtazapine-treated patients [27].

10.2.4 Reboxetine/Atomoxetine Plus SSRIs

Reboxetine and atomoxetine are norepinephrine reuptake inhibitors (NRIs). Reboxetine is available in Europe for the treatment of depression; atomoxetine is marketed in the US for the treatment of ADHD. Three open-label trials, using doses of reboxetine up to 8 mg/day, have suggested the usefulness of combining this drug with SSRIs in TRD, as reviewed elsewhere [10]. In the US, a number of clinicians have been using atomoxetine in combination with SSRIs. An open trial suggests its efficacy in antidepressant non-responders [28]. Clearly, RCTs are needed to evaluate this off-label use of atomoxetine.

10.2.5 *Nefazodone/Trazodone Plus SSRIs*

Anecdotal reports or case series suggest efficacy of combining SSRIs with trazodone [29] or nefazodone [30], which are antidepressants with significant serotonin 5-HT_2 antagonism. Furthermore, a study on patients with residual with residual symptoms of insomnia while taking fluoxetine or bupropion has found greater efficacy for trazodone over placebo in treating these symptoms [31]. However, the combination of nefazodone with SSRIs has been linked to fatal cases of hepatotoxicity and to serotonin syndrome [10]. Combining trazodone to SSRIs, on the other hand, may lead to sedation or orthostatic hypotension.

10.3 The STAR*D Trial

The results of the STAR*D study-the largest depression clinical trial ever done outside the pharmaceutical industry-have been recently published (see Sinyor et al. [32]. for a review). This study was a practical clinical trial with broad inclusion criteria, resulting in a highly representative sample of the US population. Undertaken in both psychiatric and primary care settings, STAR*D used up to four successive treatment steps, including switch, combination and augmentation strategies (see Fig. 10.1 for details). The study lacked a placebo group and was not a purely randomized trial (both patients and doctors had a degree of choice throughout trial levels). Furthermore, the trial was predominantly unblinded (both patients and doctors were informed about what arm they have been randomized) [33]. The ultimate goal of the trial was full remission. Despite these limitations, the STAR*D trial provided important insights regarding the remission rates of several depression treatments in a 'real world scenario'. Thus, remission rates in step one to four were disappointing at 36.8%, 30.6%, 13.7%, and 13.0%, respectively, with a cumulative remission rate of 67% after all four steps.

Importantly, two antidepressant combination strategies were tested in the STAR*D trial. Among more than 2,700 patients that received citalopram therapy, about 1,200 did not remit and participated in a second treatment trial [34, 35]. An unanticipated consequence of the randomization was that few patients were at equipoise about the decision to switch, compared to augment/combine, and it was not possible to conduct a planned comparison of the group that received citalopram *plus* bupropion, compared to the groups that received the most relevant switch strategies. Therefore, the only relevant contrast possible was the one comparing citalopram *plus* bupropion with citalopram plus the nonbenzodiazepine anxiolytic buspirone [34, 35]. A total of 565 patients were randomized to these two arms. There were no differences in remission rates between the two treatments in the primary outcome measure (HDRS score; both groups had a remission of ~ 30%) [34, 35].

A total of 109 patients who had not responded to three sequential STAR*D treatment trials were randomly assigned to treatment with either the AD combination (mirtazapine, mean dosage 36 mg daily; venlafaxine extended release: 210 mg

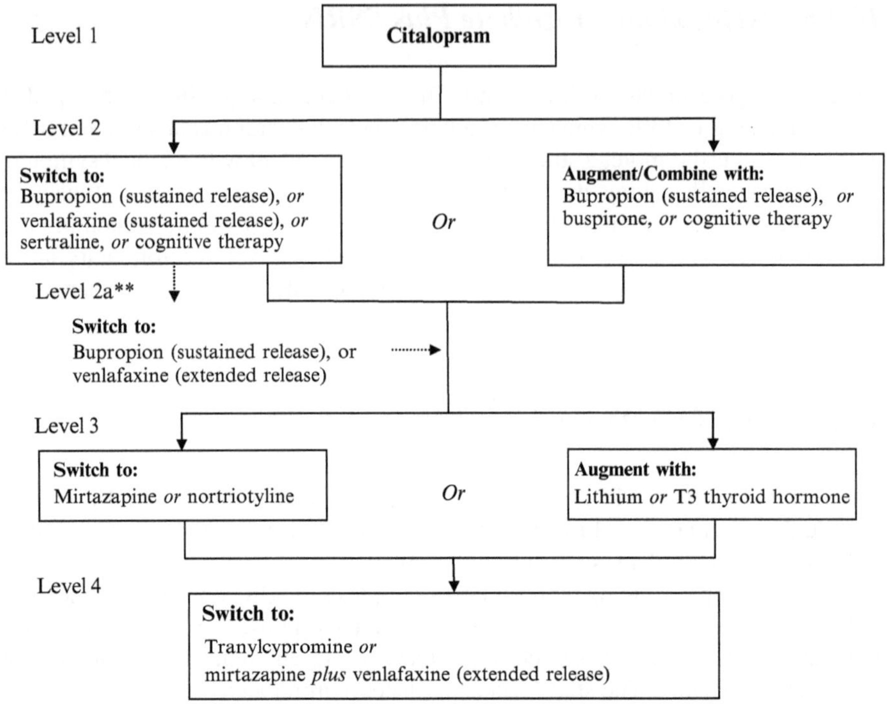

Fig. 10.1 Overview of the steps of the sequenced treatment alternatives to relieve depression (STAR*D) trial. **Only for those who were randomized to cognitive therapy

daily) or the MAOI tranylcypromine (mean dosage, 37 mg daily) [36]. Neither treatment was particularly effective, with final remission rates of 7% and 14% for the tranylcypromine and AD therapy combination groups, respectively. Nevertheless, the combination strategy was associated with significantly greater reduction of depressive symptoms and lower attrition, owing to side effects [36].

10.4 Combination of Antidepressants from the Inception of Treatment

Some researchers have conducted open-label studies using two AD drugs from treatment initiation in an attempt to obtain either a more rapid onset of therapeutic action or a greater efficacy. Nelson et al. performed the first randomized, controlled trial of AD combination from treatment initiation [18]. These authors had found that the combination of fluoxetine plus desipramine was more effective than either drug alone in a sample 39 inpatients with nonpsychotic MDD. In a small (n = 60) 6-week, randomized, double-blind, trial, improvement on the MADRS was 10 points greater in patients receiving combination therapy with the SSRI paroxetine and mirtazapine than in participants treated with each drug alone [37]. The same research group performed a larger trial (n = 105), in which MDD patients were randomly assigned to receive fluoxetine (20 mg/Kg), fluoxetine (20 mg/day) *plus* mirtazapine (30 mg/day), venlafaxine (225 mg/day titrated in 14 days) *plus* mirtazapine (30 mg/day), or bupropion (150 mg/day) *plus* mirtazepine (30 mg/day) for 6 weeks [38]. Participants allocated to AD combination groups were twice as likely to achieve remission (HDRS score < 7; remission rates: 52% for fluoxetine *plus* mirtazapine, 46% for mirtazapine *plus* bupropion and 58% for venlafaxine *plus* mirtazapine) than patients on monotherapy groups (remission rate: 25% for fluoxetine). An important limitation of this study is that patients allocated to the fluoxetine monotherapy group received a fixed dose of 20 mg/day (some patients may respond to higher fluoxetine doses), thereby underestimating the efficacy of AD monotherapy.

The *Combining Medications to Enhance Depression Outcomes* (CO-MED) study is a large (n = 665) that recruited MDD outpatients from both primary care and psychiatric services who were randomly allocated at the onset of treatment to one of the following groups: escitalopram (up to 20 mg/day) *plus* placebo, sustained-release bupropion (up to 400 mg/day) *plus* escitalopram (up to 20 mg/day), or extended-release venlafaxine (up to 300 mg/day) plus mirtazapine (up to 45 mg/day) [39]. At 7 months, of response/remission rates. By the end of the trial (7 months) remission rates (41.8–46.6%) were not significantly different across groups. Furthermore, the mean number of worsening adverse events was higher for the venlafaxine-mirtazapine than for escitalopram-placebo. A secondary analysis has shown that there were no differences in response/remission rates as a function of melancholic features in each of the four treatment groups of the CO-MED trial [40].

10.5 Conclusions and Future Perspectives

The present review indicates that although there are some evidences that antidepressant combination strategies are probably effective and there is substantial clinical experience that many of the newer antidepressants can be safely combined, there remains an absolute problem, namely, there is a dearth of clinical trials on the efficacy of combined antidepressant treatment. Given the high prevalence of major depressive disorder and that non-response to a first antidepressant trial is a common occurrence in major depressive disorder treatment, the design of adequately powered clinical trials testing both absolute (compared with placebo) and relative (compared with other standard strategies) of combined antidepressant treatment are needed. According to current evidence-based medicine guidelines, at least two well-designed (i.e., adequately powered) RCT trials with positive outcomes are needed to provide consistent evidence of efficacy to a given treatment modality. This criterion has not been met thus far in the case of AD combination therapies for MDD. There is an urgent need for industry-academy-federal collaborations to provide empirical validation for the inclusion of AD combination strategies in the sequential algorithm-based treatment of MDD.

The role of AD combination strategies for MDD at the beginning of treatment is another topic that merits further research. At least three RCT do support the use of AD combination therapies at the inception of depression treatment. However, these trials were small (i.e., <30 patients per treatment arm). The CO-MED trial (i.e., the largest trial to date testing this treatment aspect) failed to demonstrate significant benefits of AD combination therapies when compared with standard AD monotherapy at the beginning of MDD treatment.

Furthermore, long-term antidepressant combination trials should indicate for how long antidepressant combination therapies should be maintained once remission has been achieved. In conclusion, until we have robust evidences to guide the choice and determine the efficiency of the various antidepressant combination strategies, clinicians should rely on their clinical judgment and on the limited available evidence to combine antidepressants for the management of major depressive disorder.

References

1. Carvalho AF, Cavalcante JL, Castelo MS, Lima MC (2007) Augmentation strategies for treatment-resistant depression: a literature review. J Clin Pharm Ther 32:415–428
2. Carvalho AF, Machado JR, Cavalcante JL (2009) Augmentation strategies for treatment-resistant depression. Curr Opin Psychiatry 22:7–12
3. Miller IW, Keitner GI, Schatzberg AF et al (1998) The treatment of chronic depression, part 3: psychosocial functioning before and after treatment with Sertraline or imipramine. Curr Opin Psychiatry 59:608–619
4. Thase ME (2003) Evaluating antidepressant therapies: remission as the optimal outcome. Curr Opin Psychiatry 64(Suppl 13):18–25
5. Thase ME, Rush AJ (1997) When at first you don't succeed: sequential strategies for antidepressant nonresponders. Curr Opin Psychiatry 58(Suppl 13):23–29
6. Mischoulon D, Nierenberg AA, Kizilbash L, Rosenbaum JF, Fava M (2000) Strategies for managing depression refractory to selective serotonin reuptake inhibitor treatment: a survey of clinicians. Can J Psychiatry 45:476–481
7. Horgan D, Dodd S, Berk M (2007) A survey of combination antidepressant use in Australia. Australas Psychiatry 15:26–29
8. Nelson JC, Papakostas GI (2009) Atypical antipsychotic augmentation in major depressive disorder: a meta-analysis of placebo-controlled randomized trials. Am J Psychiatry 166:980–991
9. Stahl SM (2010) Enhancing outcomes from major depression: using antidepressant combination therapies with multifunctional pharmacologic mechanisms from the initiation of treatment. CNS Spectr 15:79–94
10. Fava M, Rush AJ (2006) Current status of augmentation and combination treatments for major depressive disorder: a literature review and a proposal for a novel approach to improve practice. Psychother Psychosom 75:139–153
11. Thase ME (2011) Antidepressant combinations: widely used, but far from empirically validated. Can J Psychiatry 56:317–323
12. Danish University Antidepressant Group (1986) Citalopram: clinical effect profile in comparison with clomipramine. A controlled multicenter study. Psychopharmacology (Berl) 90:131–138
13. Danish University Antidepressant Group (1990) Paroxetine: a selective serotonin reuptake inhibitor showing better tolerance, but weaker antidepressant effect than clomipramine in a controlled multicenter study. J Affect Disord 18:289–299

14. Anderson IM (1998) SSRIS versus tricyclic antidepressants in depressed inpatients: a meta-analysis of efficacy and tolerability. Depress Anxiety 7(Suppl 1):11–17
15. Papakostas GI, Thase ME, Fava M, Nelson JC, Shelton RC (2007) Are antidepressant drugs that combine serotonergic and noradrenergic mechanisms of action more effective than the selective serotonin reuptake inhibitors in treating major depressive disorder? A meta-analysis of studies of newer agents. Biol Psychiatry 62:1217–1227
16. Lam RW, Wan DD, Cohen NL, Kennedy SH (2002) Combining antidepressants for treatment-resistant depression: a review. J Clin Psychiatry 63:685–693
17. Nelson JC, Mazure CM, Bowers MB Jr, Jatlow PI (1991) A preliminary, open study of the combination of fluoxetine and desipramine for rapid treatment of major depression. Arch Gen Psychiatry 48:303–307
18. Nelson JC, Mazure CM, Jatlow PI, Bowers MB Jr, Price LH (2004) Combining norepinephrine and serotonin reuptake inhibition mechanisms for treatment of depression: a double-blind, randomized study. Biol Psychiatry 55:296–300
19. Zajecka JM, Jeffries H, Fawcett J (1995) The efficacy of fluoxetine combined with a heterocyclic antidepressant in treatment-resistant depression: a retrospective analysis. J Clin Psychiatry 56:338–343
20. Fava M, Rosenbaum JF, McGrath PJ, Stewart JW, Amsterdam JD, Quitkin FM (1994) Lithium and tricyclic augmentation of fluoxetine treatment for resistant major depression: a double-blind, controlled study. Am J Psychiatry 151:1372–1374
21. Fava M, Alpert J, Nierenberg A, Lagomasino I, Sonawalla S, Tedlow J et al (2002) Double-blind study of high-dose fluoxetine versus lithium or desipramine augmentation of fluoxetine in partial responders and nonresponders to fluoxetine. J Clin Psychopharmacol 22:379–387
22. Lam RW, Hossie H, Solomons K, Yatham LN (2004) Citalopram and bupropion-SR: combining versus switching in patients with treatment-resistant depression. J Clin Psychiatry 65:337–340
23. Leuchter AF, Lesser IM, Trivedi MH et al (2008) An open pilot study of the combination of escitalopram and bupropion-SR for outpatients with major depressive disorder. J Psychiatr Pract 14:271–280
24. Medhus A, HesKestad S, Thue JF (1994) Mianserin added to tricyclic antidepressants in depressed patients not responding to a tricyclic antidepressant alone. Nord J Psychiatry 48:355–358
25. Licht RW, Qvitzau S (2002) Treatment strategies in patients with major depression not responding to first-line sertraline treatment. A randomised study of extended duration of treatment, dose increase or mianserin augmentation. Psychopharmacology (Berl) 161:143–151
26. Carpenter LL, Jocic Z, Hall JM, Rasmussen SA, Price LH (1999) Mirtazapine augmentation in the treatment of refractory depression. J Clin Psychiatry 60:45–49
27. Carpenter LL, Yasmin S, Price LH (2002) A double-blind, placebo-controlled study of antidepressant augmentation with mirtazapine. Biol Psychiatry 51:183–188
28. Carpenter LL, Milosavljevic N, Schecter JM, Tyrka AR, Price LH (2005) Augmentation with open-label atomoxetine for partial or nonresponse to antidepressants. J Clin Psychiatry 66:1234–1238
29. Nierenberg AA, Cole JO, Glass L (1992) Possible trazodone potentiation of fluoxetine: a case series. J Clin Psychiatry 53:83–85
30. Taylor FB, Prather MR (2003) The efficacy of nefazodone augmentation for treatment-resistant depression with anxiety symptoms or anxiety disorder. Depress Anxiety 18:83–88
31. Nierenberg AA, Adler LA, Peselow E et al (1994) Trazodone for antidepressant-associated insomnia. Am J Psychiatry 151:1069–1072
32. Sinyor M, Schaffer A, Levitt A (2010) The sequenced treatment alternatives to relieve depression (STAR*D) trial: a review. Can J Psychiatry 55:126–135
33. Deakin J, O'Loughlin C (2009) STAR*D: a summary and UK perspective. J Psychopharmacol 23:605–612
34. Rush AJ, Trivedi MH, Wisniewski SR et al (2006) Bupropion-SR, sertraline, or venlafaxine-XR after failure of SSRIs for depression. N Engl J Med 354:1231–1242
35. Trivedi MH, Fava M, Wisniewski SR et al (2006) Medication augmentation after the failure of SSRIs for depression. N Engl J Med 354:1243–1252

36. McGrath PJ, Stewart JW, Fava M et al (2006) Tranylcypromine versus venlafaxine plus mirtazapine following three failed antidepressant medication trials for depression: a STAR*D report. Am J Psychiatry 163:1531–1541
37. Blier P, Gobbi G, Turcotte JE et al (2009) Mirtazapine and paroxetine in major depression: a comparison of monotherapy versus their combination from treatment initiation. Eur Neuropsychopharmacol 19:457–465
38. Blier P, Ward HE, Tremblay P et al (2010) Combination of antidepressant medications from treatment initiation for major depressive disorder: a double-blind randomized study. Am J Psychiatry 167:281–288
39. Rush AJ, Trivedi MH, Stewart JW et al (2011) Combining medications to enhance depression outcomes (CO-MED): acute and long-term outcomes of a single-blind randomized study. Am J Psychiatry 168:689–701
40. Bobo WV, Chen H, Trivedi MH et al (2011) Randomized comparison of selective serotonin reuptake inhibitor (escitalopram) monotherapy and antidepressant combination pharmacotherapy for major depressive disorder with melancholic features: a CO-MED report. J Affect Disord 133:467–476

Chapter 11
Herbal Remedies and Nutraceuticals as Augmentation or Adjunct for Mood and Anxiety Disorders: Evidence for Benefit and Risk

Arun V. Ravindran and Tricia L. da Silva

Abstract Background: Complementary and alternative medicine (CAM) therapies have considerable patient appeal. Perceived as better, safer and more economical than conventional treatments, such as pharmacotherapy and psychotherapy, they are often used by patients to self-treat symptoms of depression and anxiety, usually in combination with existing medications and without medical supervision. CAM therapies include physical therapies (e.g. exercise), herbal remedies (e.g. St. John's wort) and nutraceuticals/dietary supplements (e.g. omega-3 fatty acids). This chapter will review the published evidence for the use of herbal and dietary supplements as augmenting or adjunctive agents in depressive and anxiety disorders.

Methods: A PubMed search was conducted for all randomized controlled trials, open trials and case reports available and published up to May 2012 on the use of herbal remedies and dietary supplements, as augmentation or combination, particularly to medications, in the treatment of unipolar depression, bipolar disorder and anxiety conditions.

Results: Overall, the published literature is sparse. Among available data in depressive disorders, there is a moderate level of evidence to support adjunctive use of Free and Easy Wanderer Plus (FEWP) and folate in unipolar depression, and FEWP and omega-3 fatty acids in bipolar depression. Several other herbal remedies and

A.V. Ravindran, M.B.B.S. M.Sc., Ph.D., FRCPC, FRCPsych (✉)
Departments of Psychiatry, Psychology and Institute of Medical Sciences, University of Toronto, Toronto, ON, Canada

Mood and Anxiety Disorders Program, Centre for Addiction and Mental Health, Toronto, ON, Canada
e-mail: arun.ravindran@camh.ca

T.L. da Silva, M.A.
Mood and Anxiety Disorders Program, Centre for Addiction and Mental Health, Toronto, ON, Canada
e-mail: tricia.dasilva@camh.ca

M.S. Ritsner (ed.), *Polypharmacy in Psychiatry Practice, Volume II: Use of Polypharmacy in the "Real World"*, DOI 10.1007/978-94-007-5799-8_11,

nutraceuticals have preliminary evidence of benefit as augmentation to pharmacotherapy, including S-adenosylmethionine (SAM-e), dehydroepiandrosterone (DHEA), folate, and zinc, in unipolar depression; magnesium in mania; N-acetylcysteine (NAC) in bipolar depression; and E. M. Power Plus (EMP+) in bipolar disorder. Surprisingly, there is no published evidence to support the benefit of St. John's wort as adjunct to antidepressants. Similarly, evidence of benefits for other herbal and dietary supplements remains limited. In anxiety disorders, there is, as yet, little evidence that herbal and dietary supplements are useful as augmenting agents.

Limitations: The overall evidence base remains limited and studies often had methodological problems, including small samples, variability in dose, short duration of treatment, and unknown quality of the agent. Though the supplements were generally well tolerated in reported studies, there is limited long-term safety and tolerability data, and drug-drug interaction information.

Conclusions: While several herbal and dietary supplements have evidence of benefit as add-on agents in depressive disorders, none can currently be recommended for anxiety conditions, and safety issues should be carefully considered prior to use in clinical practice. Larger well-designed studies are needed to provide a broad and reliable base of data for further evaluations.

Abbreviations

5-HTP	5-hydroxy tryptophan
CAM	Complementary and alternative medicine
CBZ	Carbamazepine
DBRCT	Double-blind randomized controlled trial
DHA	Docosahexaenoic acid
DHEA	Dehydroepiandrosterone
DNA	Dioxyribonucleic acid
EMP	E. M. Power Plus
EPA	Eicosapentanoic acid
FEWP	Free and Easy Wanderer Plus
GABA	Gamma-aminobutyric acid
GAD	Generalized anxiety disorder
HPA	Hypothalamic-pituitary adrenocortical
HRT	Hormone replacement therapy
MDD	Major depressive disorder
NAC	N-acetylcysteine
NMDA	N-methyl-D-aspartic acid
OCD	Obsessive-compulsive disorder
PD	Panic disorder
PTSD	Post-traumatic stress disorder
RCT	Randomized controlled trial

RNA	Ribonucleic acid
SAD	Social anxiety disorder
SAM-e	S-adenosylmethionine
STEP-BD	Systematic Treatment Enhancement Program for Bipolar Disorder
SSRI	Selective serotonin reuptake inhibitor
TCA	Tricyclic antidepressant
TRD	Treatment-resistant depression

11.1 Introduction

Depressive and anxiety disorders are the most common psychiatric conditions found in the general population. Depressive disorders, which encompass unipolar depression and bipolar disorder, have an estimated 12-month prevalence of up to 11%, while anxiety conditions, which include generalized anxiety disorder (GAD), panic disorder (PD), obsessive-compulsive disorder (OCD), social anxiety disorder (SAD) and post-traumatic stress disorder (PTSD), have a 1 year prevalence of up to 18% [1, 2].

Despite the wide range of pharmacological and psychological interventions available for depressive and anxiety conditions, up to a quarter of patients show partial or no response even with adequate treatment, and for many, a chronic course of illness is common [3–5]. Side effects (with medications), time and accessibility (with psychotherapy), and cost factors can be further obstacles to patient compliance and full recovery [6, 7]. These limitations are frequently cited among the reasons that many patients turn to complementary and alternative medication (CAM) therapies for symptom relief, under the perception that these 'natural' therapies are more effective, affordable and tolerable [8–10]. It is quite common for patients to use CAM therapies without medical supervision, and while also receiving conventional treatments [11, 12].

CAMs fall into three main categories: physical therapies (e.g. exercise, acupuncture), nutraceuticals (i.e. dietary and nutritional supplements such as vitamins and minerals) and herbal remedies (i.e. plants and plant extracts) [9]. Although the data on the utility of such treatments is not as extensive as that for more conventional treatments, the field of research is growing in response to patient interest and use. Published data suggests that several CAMs have shown some benefits in depression and anxiety, both as monotherapy and as adjunctive treatments to pharmacotherapy. As the benefits and risks of physical therapies have been reviewed extensively and recently elsewhere [e.g. 13–15], this chapter will focus on the data relating to nutraceuticals and herbal remedies as augmentation or combination with conventional treatments for mood and anxiety disorders.

A search of the psychiatric literature, using PubMed, was conducted for all articles relating to the use of herbal and dietary supplements as augmenting agents in mood and anxiety disorders and published in English up to May 2012. The range of disorders covered in this review include: Major depressive disorder (MDD), dysthymia, psychotic depression, treatment resistant depression (TRD), chronic depression, bipolar disorder, generalized anxiety disorder (GAD), panic disorder (PD), social anxiety disorder (SAD), obsessive-compulsive disorder (OCD), and post-traumatic stress disorder (PTSD). Information was summarized on the design, methods and outcomes of these studies. Study results were evaluated using the standard methodology for considering the strength of evidence for efficacy and tolerability.

The data reviewed below on herbal and dietary supplements used as augmenting or combination agents in depressive and anxiety disorders is also summarized in Tables 11.1, 11.2, 11.3 and 11.4. In published literature, "augmentation" refers to the addition of an agent to an existing treatment regime, usually antidepressants [65]. "Combination" refers to the concurrent use of two or more agents, who individually have antidepressant/anti-anxiety effects on their own, as treatment. "Add-on" refers to either strategy. The studies described below used one or other of these strategies.

11.2 Supplements

11.2.1 Herbal Remedies

Herbal remedies are non-prescription, natural health products derived from plants and plant extracts, such as leaves, flowers, roots, bark and berries. They are frequently used individually or in combination to support general wellness or resolve symptoms of physical or mental stress. A literature search on the use of herbs as augmenting or combination agents found research evidence relating to St. John's wort, lavender, and kava kava, as well as specific Chinese and Japanese herbal compounds.

Several other herbs that have been evaluated only as monotherapy in depressive and anxiety disorders, and are therefore not reviewed in this chapter. These include saffron (*Crocus sativus*), roseroot (*Rhodiola rosea*), borage (*Echium amoenum*), gingko biloba, passionflower (*Passiflora incarnate*) and valerian (*Valeriana officinalis*) see reviews [9, 66, 67].

11.2.1.1 St. John's Wort

St. John's wort (*Hypericum perforatum*) is a flowering plant whose extracts, which include hypericin and hyperforin, are candidates for its active ingredients [68]. Though St. John's wort has shown some efficacy in depressive and anxiety conditions, its mechanism of action is not fully elucidated. It is proposed that such action may be mediated by its effect on monoaminergic systems and modulation of hypothalamic-pituitary adrenocortical (HPA) axis activity [66, 68].

Table 11.1 Evidence for CAM therapies as augmentation in depression and co-morbid anxiety

Refs.	Study	Type	N	Duration	Agent	Comparator	Efficacy results[a]
St. John's wort							
[16]	Sarris et al. (2009)	DBRCT, cross-over design	MDD with co-morbid GAD/SAD/PD = 28	8 weeks	St. John's wort (1,800 mg) + kava kava (2,660 mg)	Placebo	Combination > placebo for depression in first phase ($p = 0.003$), but combination = placebo after cross-over. No treatment effects on anxiety.
[17]	Muller et al. (2003)	Open trial, random-ized	MDD with GAD = 2,462	6 weeks	St. John's wort (600 mg) + valerian (500 mg) St. John's wort (600 mg) + Valerian (1,000 mg)	None	Both groups improved similarly, but p values not reported.
Kava Kava							
[16]	Sarris et al. (2009)	DBRCT, cross-over design	MDD with co-morbid GAD/SAD/PD = 28	8 weeks	St. John's wort (1,800 mg) + kava kava (2,660 mg)	Placebo	Combination > placebo for depression in first phase ($p = 0.003$), but no group differences after cross-over. No treatment effects on anxiety.
[18]	Cagnacci et al. (2003)	Open trial, random-ized	Subsyndromal depression with moderate anxiety (self-reported) = 68	3 months	Calcium (1,000 mg) + kava kava (100 mg) Calcium (1,000 mg) + kava kava (200 mg)	Calcium (1,000 mg)	Calcium + kava groups similar and > calcium alone for anxiety ($p < 0.001$). All groups improved depression comparably ($p < 0.002$).

[a] Results statistically significant at $p < 0.05$

Table 11.2 Evidence for CAM therapies as augmentation in unipolar depression

Refs.	Study	Type	N	Duration	Agent	Comparator	Efficacy results[a]
Lavender							
[19]	Akhondzadeh et al. (2003)	DBRCT	MDD = 45	4 weeks	Lavandula (200 mg) + placebo Lavandula (200 mg) + imipramine (100 mg)	Imipramine (100 mg) + placebo	Lavandula + imipramine > mipramine + placebo ($p<0.001$) > Lavandula + placebo ($p<0.001$).
Herbal compound: FEWP							
[20]	Qin et al. (2011)	Meta-analysis	Total = 14 (unipolar depression, bipolar depression)	4–12 weeks	FEWP	Placebo or Psychotropics	FEWP monotherapy > placebo ($p<0.00001$) and = psychotropics. FEWP combination > psychotropics alone ($p<0.009$).
			Monotherapy = 6 Combination = 8		Existing psychotropics + FEWP	Existing psychotropics	
Herbal compound: Jio-zai							
[21]	Yamada et al. (2005)	Open trial	MDD = 20	4 weeks	Existing antidepressants + Jio-zai (15 g)	None	Clinically significant improvement in 60%, but only 30% were much improved. No p values were reported.
SAM-e							
[22]	Papakostas et al. (2010)	DBRCT	TRD = 73	6 weeks	Existing SSRIs/SNRIs + SAM-e (1,600 mg)	Existing SSRIs/SNRIs + placebo	SAM-e > placebo in response ($p=0.01$) and remission ($p=0.02$).
[23]	Alpert et al. (2004)	Open trial	TRD = 45	6 weeks	Existing SSRIs/SNRIs + SAM-e (800–1,600 mg)	None	Significant improvement ($p<0.0001$).

DHEA							
[24]	Woklowitz et al. (1999)	DBRCT	Total = 22 MDD = 20 Bipolar II depression = 2 Medicated = 15 Unmedicated = 7	6 weeks	DHEA (30–90 mg) Existing antidepressants + DHEA (30–90 mg)	Placebo Existing antidepressants + placebo	Both DHEA groups > placebo groups ($p<0.04$).
Tryptophan							
[25]	Levitan et al. (2000)	DBRCT	MDD = 30	8 weeks	Fluoxetine (20 mg) + l-tryptophan (1–4 g)	Fluoxetine (20 mg) + placebo	Earlier improvement with tryptophan ($p<0.001$), but tryptophan = placebo at end of treatment.
[26]	Lam et al. (1997)	Open trial	Seasonal affective disorder = 16, resistant to previous light therapy	2 weeks	Existing light therapy + l-tryptophan (3 g)	None	Significant improvement ($p<0.001$).
Folate							
[27]	Coppen et al. (1986)	DBRCT	Total = 75 (not clinically depressed, mean baseline BDI = 8) Unipolar depression = 53 Bipolar disorder = 17 Schizoaffective disorder = 5	12 months	Existing lithium + folic acid (200 μg)	Existing lithium + placebo	Folic acid > placebo only for unipolar depression ($p<0.02$). Results limited by non-symptomatic patient sample.
[28]	Godfrey et al. (1990)	DBRCT	Total = 41 MDD = 24 Schizophrenia = 17	6 months	Existing TCAs/MAOIs + methylfolate (15 mg)	Existing TCAs/ MAOIs + placebo	Folate > placebo ($p<0.01$).

(continued)

Table 11.2 (continued)

Refs.	Study	Type	N	Duration	Agent	Comparator	Efficacy results[a]
[29]	Coppen and Bailey (2000)	DBRCT	MDD = 127	10 weeks	Fluoxetine (20 mg) + folic acid (500 μg)	Fluoxetine (20 mg) + placebo	Folic acid > placebo for female patients ($p<0.005$).
[30]	Alpert et al. (2002)	Open trial	TRD = 22	8 weeks	Existing SSRIs + folinic acid (15–30 mg)	None	Significant improvement ($p<0.01$), but low response (27%) and remission (18%) rates.
[31]	Resler et al. (2008)	DBRCT	MDD = 27	6 weeks	Fluoxetine (20 mg) + folic acid (10 mg)	Fluoxetine (20 mg) + placebo	Folic acid > placebo ($p=0.04$).
[32]	Basoglu et al. (2009)	Open trial, randomized	MDD = 35	6 weeks	Escitalopram (10 mg) + folic acid (2.5 mg)	Escitalopram (10 mg)	Escitalpram alone > folic acid combination ($p=0.016$).
[33]	Ginsberg et al. (2011)	Retrospective analysis	MDD = 242 Monotherapy = 147 Combination = 95	Variable	SSRIs/SNRIs + l-methylfolate (7.5 mg or 15 mg)	SSRIs/SNRIs	Methylfolate combination > SSRIs/SNRIs alone in response ($p<0.01$), onset of improvement ($p<0.03$) and discontinuation due to side effects ($p<0.0078$).
Inositol							
[34]	Taylor et al. (2004)	Meta-analysis	Total = 4 (unipolar depression, bipolar depression)	4–6 weeks	Inositol	Placebo	Inositol groups = placebo groups.
			Monotherapy = 1 Augmentation = 2		Existing SSRIs + inositol	Existing SSRIs + placebo	
[35]	Levine et al. (1999)	DBRCT	MDD = 27	4 weeks	SSRIs + inositol (12 g)	SSRIs + placebo	Inositol = placebo.
[36]	Nemets et al. (1999)	DBRCT	MDD = 42	4 weeks	Existing SSRIs + inositol (12 g)	Existing SSRIs + placebo	Inositol = placebo.

Zinc							
[37]	Lai et al. (2012)	Meta-analysis	Total = 4	10–12 weeks	Multivitamins with zinc	Multivitamins	Mixed results for zinc in healthy subjects. Zinc > placebo for depression ($p < 0.00001$).
			Combination = 2 (healthy volunteers) + 2 (unipolar depression)		Existing antidepressants + zinc	Existing antidepressants + placebo	
[38]	Novak et al. (2003)	DBRCT	MDD = 14	12 weeks	SSRIs/TCAs + zinc (25 mg)	SSRIs/TCAs + placebo	Zinc > placebo ($p < 0.05$).
[39]	Siwek et al. (2009)	DBRCT	MDD = 60	12 weeks	Imipramine (40 mg) + zinc (25 mg)	Imipramine (40 mg) + placebo	Zinc = placebo. Zinc > placebo for TRD subgroup only at midpoint ($p < 0.05$), but with trend at endpoint ($p = 0.056$) in TRD subgroup.
Amino acid formulations							
[40]	Ille et al. (2007)	DBRCT	MDD = 40	4 weeks	Mirtazapine (30–60 mg) + amino acid mixture (15 g)	Mirtazapine (30–60 mg) + placebo	Amino acids > placebo in clinical improvement ($p < 0.0001$) and response ($p = 0.002$), but only numerically, not statistically, superior in remission rates.

[a]Results statistically significant at $p < 0.05$

Table 11.3 Evidence for CAM therapies as augmentation in bipolar disorder

Refs.	Study	Type	N	Duration	Agent	Comparator	Efficacy results[a]
Herbal compound: FEWP							
[41]	Zhang et al. (2007a)	DBRCT	Total = 235	12 weeks	CBZ (300 mg) + FEWP (36 mg)	CBZ (300 mg) + placebo	Depression: CBZ + FEWP > CBZ + placebo (p = 0.032) > placebo alone (p = 0.044).
			Bipolar depression = 124			Placebo	Mania: CBZ + FEWP = CBZ + placebo, and > placebo (p < 0.05).
			Bipolar mania = 111				
[42]	Zhang et al. (2007b) (Contination phase of Zhang et al. 2007a)	DBRCT	Total = 188 Bipolar depression = 93 Bipolar mania = 84	26 weeks	CBZ (300 mg) + FEWP (36 mg)	CBZ (300 mg) + placebo	CBZ + FEWP = CBZ + placebo for continued improvement. CBZ + FEWP > CBZ + placebo for discontinuation (p = 0.009).
[20]	Qin et al. (2011)	Meta-analysis	Total = 14 (unipolar depression, bipolar depression)	4–12 weeks	FEWP	Placebo or Psychotropics	FEWP monotherapy > placebo (p < 0.00001), and = psychotropics. FEWP combination > to psychotropics alone (p < 0.009).
			Monotherapy = 6 Combination = 8		Existing psychotropics + FEWP	Existing psychotropics	
Omega-3 fatty acids							
[43]	Sarris et al. (2012)	Meta-analysis	Total = 6 (bipolar depression) Augmentation = 6	4–16 weeks	Existing psychotropics + omega-3 fatty acids	Existing psychotropics + placebo	Omega-3 > placebo for bipolar depression (p < 0.029), but not for mania (p < 0.099).

DHEA							
[24]	Woklowitz et al. (1999)	DBRCT	Total = 22 MDD = 20 Bipolar II depression = 2 Medicated = 15 Unmedicated = 7	6 weeks	DHEA (30–90 mg) Existing antidepressants + DHEA (30–90 mg)	Placebo Existing antidepressants + placebo	Both DHEA groups > placebo groups ($p < 0.04$).
Choline							
[44]	Lyoo et al. (2003)	DBRCT	Rapid cycling bipolar disorder = 8	12 weeks	Existing lithium + choline bitartrate (15–30 g)	Existing lithium + placebo	No treatment effects on depression or mania.
[45]	Stoll et al. (1996)	Open case series	Rapid cycling bipolar disorder = 6	Not well reported. Potentially 1–16 weeks	Existing lithium + choline bitartrate (15–30 g)	None	Clinically significant improvement in depression and mania, but no p values reported.
Folate							
[27]	Coppen et al. (1986)	DBRCT	Total = 75 (not clinically depressed, mean baseline BDI = 8) Unipolar depression = 53 Bipolar disorder = 17 Schizoaffective disorder = 5	12 months	Existing lithium + folic acid (200 μg)	Existing lithium + placebo	Folic acid > placebo only for unipolar depression ($p < 0.02$). Results limited by non-symptomatic patient sample.

(continued)

Table 11.3 (continued)

Refs.	Study	Type	N	Duration	Agent	Comparator	Efficacy results[a]
[46]	Behzadi et al. (2009)	DBRCT	Mania = 88	3 weeks	Valproate (900–1,600 mg) + folic acid (3 g)	Valproate (900–16 mg) + placebo	Both groups improved ($p<0.0001$); folic acid > placebo only at week 3 ($p=0.005$).
Inositol							
[34]	Taylor et al. (2004)	Meta-analysis	Total = 4 (unipolar depression, bipolar depression)	4–6 weeks	Inositol	Placebo	Inositol groups = placebo groups.
			Monotherapy = 1 Augmentation = 2		Existing SSRIs + inositol	Existing SSRIs + placebo	
[47]	Chengappa et al. (2000)	DBRCT	Bipolar depression = 24	6 weeks	Existing mood stabilizers + inositol (12 g)	Existing mood stabilizers + placebo	Inositol = placebo.
[48]	Eden Evins et al. (2006)	Two phases: DBRCT, then open label continuation	Bipolar depression = 17	RCT: 6 weeks	RCT: Existing mood stabilizers + inositol (9.5–16.5 g)	RCT: Existing mood stabilizers + placebo	DBRCT: Inositol = placebo; with trend for inositol ($p=0.053$).
				Open: 8 weeks	Open: Existing mood stabilizers + inositol (9.5–16.5 g)		Open: Generally positive results with inositol, but no significance values reported.

[49]	Nierenberg et al. (2006)	Open trial, randomization	Bipolar depression = 66	Up to 16 weeks	Existing psychotropics (mood stabilizers + at least 1 antidepressant) + inositol (10–25 g)	Existing psychotropics + lamotrigine (150–250 mg) Existing psychotropics + risperidone (1–6 mg)	Inositol = lamotrigine = risperidone.
Magnesium							
[50]	Heiden et al. (1999)	Open case series	Bipolar mania = 10	1–3 weeks	Existing mood stabilizers or benzodiazepines + IV magnesium sulfate (200 mg/h)	None	Clinically significant improvement, but no p values reported.
[51]	Giannini et al. (2000)	DBRCT	Bipolar mania = 20	16 weeks	Existing verapamil + magnesium oxide (375 mg)	Existing verapamil + placebo	Magnesium > placebo ($p=0.02$)
Amino acid formulations							
[52]	Scarna et al. (2003)	DBRCT	Bipolar mania = 25	1 week	Existing psychotropics (antipsychotics and/or mood stabilizers and/or benzodiazepines) + branched-chain amino acid drink (60 g)	Existing psychotropics + placebo	Amino acid = placebo at end of treatment. However, amino acid > placebo for early onset of action ($p=0.02$), and at 1-week follow-up ($p<0.01$).

(continued)

Table 11.3 (continued)

Refs.	Study	Type	N	Duration	Agent	Comparator	Efficacy results[a]
NAC							
[53]	Berk et al. (2008)	DBRCT, maintenance study	Bipolar disorder = 75 Euthymic = 37 Depressed = 27 Manic = 11	6 months	Existing psychotropics + NAC (2 g)	Existing psychotropics + placebo	NAC > placebo for depression ($p=0.002$), quality of life ($p=0.006$) and functioning ($p=0.002$), but only a trend for NAC in mania ($p=0.079$). NAC = placebo for time to mood episode.
[54]	Berk et al. (2011)	Two-phase maintenance study:	Bipolar depressed	Open: 2 months	Open: Existing psychotropics + NAC (2 g)	RCT: Existing psychotropics + placebo	Open: Significant improvement in depressive symptoms ($p<0.001$) and quality of life ($p<0.05$), with trend in mania ($p=0.078$).
		Open label, then DBRCT Only open data currently published	Open = 149 RCT = pending	RCT: 6 months	RCT: Existing medications + NAC (2 g)		DBRCT: Results pending.
Nutraceutical compound: EMP+							
[55]	Kaplan et al. (2000)	Open case series	Bipolar disorder = 11 Medicated = 10 Unmedicated = 1	6 months	Existing psychotropics + EMP + (32 capsules) EMP + (32 capsules)	None	Significant improvement in depressive ($p<0.01$) and mania ($p<0.01$), and medication use reduced by >50% ($p<0.01$).

[56]	Popper (2001)	Open case series	Bipolar disorder = 22 (10 adults, 12 children and adolescents) Medicated = 15 Unmedicated = 7	Up to 6–9 months	Existing psychotropics + EMP + (32 capsules) EMP + (32 capsules)	None	Clinically significant improvement in 45%; 73% of medicated patients discontinued psychotropics. No p values reported.
[57]	Simmons (2003)	Open case series	Bipolar disorder = 19 (treatment-resistant) Medicated = 16 Unmedicated = 3	Up to 13 months	Existing psychotropics + EMP + (32 capsules) EMP + (32 capsules)	None	Clinically significant improvement in 63%; 69% of medicated patients discontinued psychotropics. No p values reported.
[58]	Rucklidge et al. (2010)	Database analysis	Bipolar disorder = 120 (children and adolescents) Medicated = 95 Unmedicated = 25	3–6 months	Existing psychotropics + EMP + (32 capsules) EMP + (32 capsules)	None	Significant improvement ($p < 0.001$); 52% of medicated patients stopped psychotropics while the rest reduced medication use by 74%.

[a]Results statistically significant at $p < 0.05$

Table 11.4 Evidence for CAM therapies as augmentation in anxiety disorders

Refs.	Study	Type	*N*	Duration	Agent	Comparator	Efficacy results[a]
Generalized anxiety disorder							
Kava kava							
[59]	De Leo et al. (2001)	DBRCT	GAD = 40	6 months	HRT (50 μg) + kava kava (100 mg)	HRT (50 μg) + placebo	Kava groups > placebo groups
					ERT (50 μg) + kava kava (100 mg)	ERT (50 μg) + placebo	($p < 0.05$).
Magnesium							
[60]	Hanus et al. (2004)	DBRCT	GAD = 264	3 months	Elemental magnesium + hawthorn + California poppy (375 mg)	Placebo (375 mg)	Magnesium combination > placebo ($p = 0.005$).
Obsessive-compulsive disorder							
Omega-3 fatty acids							
[61]	Fux et al. (2004)	DBRCT, cross-over design	OCD = 11	12 weeks	Existing SSRIs + Omega-3 fatty acids (EPA 2 g)	Existing SSRIs + placebo	EPA = placebo.
Inositol							
[62]	Fux et al. (1999)	DBRCT, cross-design	OCD = 10	12 weeks	Existing SRIs + inositol (18 g)	Existing SRIs + placebo	Inositol = Placebo.
[63]	Seedat and Stein (1999)	Open trial	OCD = 10	6 weeks	Existing SRIs + inositol (18 g)	None	No significant improvement.
Post-traumatic stress disorder							
Omega-3 fatty acids							
[64]	Zeev et al. (2005)	Open trial	PTSD = 6	3 months	Existing SSRIs + Omega-3 fatty acids (EPA 2 g)	None	No improvement with EPA.
			Medicated = 4 Unmedicated = 2		Omega-3 fatty acids alone (EPA 2 g)		

[a]Results statistically significant at $p < 0.05$

A number of randomized controlled trials (RCTs) and meta-analyses have supported the efficacy of St. John's wort as a monotherapy for mild to moderate unipolar depression, against both placebo and antidepressant comparators [e.g. 69, 70]. Surprisingly, it has not yet been evaluated as add-on to psychotropic medications, but the literature does report on two studies of St. John's wort in combination with other herbs for MDD and co-morbid anxiety. Among these, one small cross-over placebo-controlled RCT evaluated the combination of kava kava (*Piper methysticum*), a leafy plant though to have similar mood modulating effects [71], with St. John's wort. The St. John's Wort + kava kava combination was significantly superior to placebo alone in reducing depressive symptoms in the initial phase, but there were no group differences in the second phase, after cross-over [16]. Neither treatment improved anxiety symptoms, and though no serious side effects were reported, drop out rates were high, likely due to lack of efficacy. In a second, large open trial, patients were randomized to low-dose or high-dose valerian (*Valeriana officinalis*), another flowering plant with putative antidepressant and anxiolytic properties [72], combined with St. John's Wort [17]. Depressive and anxiety symptoms improved significantly and comparably in both treatment groups, though exact significance values were not reported [17]. The combination was well tolerated.

St. John's wort has been evaluated only to a limited extent in anxiety conditions. Small placebo-controlled RCTs found no benefit to St. John's wort monotherapy in SAD or OCD subjects [73, 74], though a small positive open trial in OCD [75] and case reports in GAD [76, 77] have suggested some benefits. No studies were found of St. John's wort as augmentation or combination for anxiety disorders.

Thus, St. John's wort has only preliminary evidence as add-on to valerian for the treatment of depression and co-morbid anxiety, though it can be questioned whether the lack of a placebo control influenced results. As well, despite its seeming tolerability in these studies, caution has been advised in its use in clinical practice. Adverse effects include photosensitivity and drug interactions, leading to reduced efficacy of immunoregulatory compounds, anticoagulants, anti-infective agents, and oral contraceptives, which is attributed in part to its effect on cytochrome P450 enzymes [78]. As well, serotonin syndrome when used in combination with antidepressants [79] and induction of mania and hypomania have also been reported in the literature [80].

11.2.1.2 Lavender

Lavender (*Lavandula angustifolia*) is a flowering plant from the mint family, and is popularly used for extraction of essential oils for perfumes and aromatherapy. In herbal medicine, it is used as a relaxant, appetite stimulant and an anti-spasmodic [81]. Its active ingredients include linalool and linalyl acetate and its potential neuropsychiatric action is thought to be multimodal, via its effects on gamma-aminobutyric acid (GABA) receptors, as well as glutaminergic and cholinergic systems and ion channel functioning [81].

Monotherapy trials of lavender in depressive disorders are lacking, but one augmentation study was found. A small, 3-arm, placebo-controlled RCT found significant benefit in MDD symptoms with all treatments, but impramine + lavender was superior to imipramine + placebo, with lavender + placebo showing least efficacy [19]. Reported side effects were mild and transient.

In anxiety disorders, a recent small review of the few available monotherapy trials found lavender superior to placebo (for subsyndromal anxiety), as effective as benzodiazepines (in GAD), and well tolerated see review [81]. However, there are no published studies of lavender as augmentation or combination for anxiety conditions.

Lavender shows preliminary evidence of benefit in combination with medication for MDD, which needs confirmation through larger RCTs. It has also generally been well tolerated, except for a few reported cases of allergic reaction (dermatitis) and gastrointestinal symptoms after excessive intake [81, 82].

11.2.1.3 Kava Kava

Kava kava (*Piper methysticum*) is a leafy plant whose roots are ground for herbal medicine purposes, primarily for mental and physical relaxation [83]. Its active ingredients are proposed to be several kavalactones, which are still being individually isolated [68, 83]. The kavalactones are proposed to act on GABAergic and ß-adrenergic systems, and on monoamine oxidase B (MAO-B) activity, mediating its neuropsychiatric effects [68]. In addition, effects on several monoaminergic systems have also been proposed, all of which suggests it may benefit both depressive and anxiety conditions [71].

Kava kava has not been evaluated as monotherapy or augmentation to medications in depressive disorders. However, it has been investigated in combination with other herbs in two studies of unipolar depression with co-morbid anxiety. One small placebo-controlled RCT, with a St. John's wort + kava kava combination (previously described), had inconclusive results [16]. In a small open trial, patients randomized to calcium combined with high-dose or low-dose kava kava showed significantly greater benefit for anxiety than those on calcium alone, but all three groups showed significant and similar reduction in depression [18]. Side effects were mild and tolerable. A limitation of the study is that patients were included based only on self-reported moderate anxiety and subsyndromal depressive symptoms, and not evaluated by objective ratings.

Though placebo-controlled RCTs in anxiety disorders have had mixed results with kava kava monotherapy [66], a single open label monotherapy trial had positive results [84] and the only medication comparator RCT found it as effective as conventional anxiolytics [85]. Small meta-analyses of six monotherapy RCTs each have found it superior to placebo in reducing anxiety, though effect sizes were small [86, 87]. No studies have evaluated kava kava as add-on to pharmacotherapy in anxiety disorders, but one study has investigated its benefit in combination with non-psychotropics. In a small RCT, GAD symptoms in menopausal women improved significantly more with the combination of hormone replacement therapy (progesterone included [HRT] or excluded [ERT]), with kava kava, than with HRT + placebo or ERT + placebo [59]. Subjects did not report any side effects.

The limited literature suggests that kava kava's proposed utility in depression has not been substantiated, but it may have some potential benefit as a combination agent for anxiety conditions. No serious side effects were reported in the above studies, however, recent case reports of liver toxicity have raised concerns about its long-term use, and have led to its being withdrawn from markets in several countries [83, 88]. Excessive intake has also been linked to skin and neurological disorders, and rare cases of drug-drug interactions, including with psychotropics, anticonvulsants, and drugs for neurological, kidney or liver function, have been reported [88, 89].

11.2.1.4 Herbal Compounds

Herbal compounds consist of herbs with individual health-promoting properties, which are thought to have synergistic effects when combined into a single product. Several reports have evaluated herbal compounds as adjunct in depressive disorders, but there are no such studies in anxiety conditions.

Among available publications, two large RCTs evaluated the efficacy of a well-established Chinese polyherbal compound called Free and Easy Wanderer Plus (FEWP) in bipolar disorder. Its 11 ingredients are reported to act on multiple monoaminergic and benzodiazepine receptors, as well as neurosteroid and cytokine function, accounting for its antidepressant and anxiolytic effects [90–92]. A three-arm RCT found the combination of carbamazepine (CBZ) and FEWP more effective than CBZ + placebo in improving bipolar depressive symptoms, with placebo alone being least useful [41]. The CBZ combination groups also improved mania significantly, compared to placebo. Reported side effects were mild, with CBZ + FEWP better tolerated than CBZ + placebo, suggesting that FEWP may alleviate some of the adverse effects of CBZ. A continuation phase included only the CBZ combination groups and found that further symptom improvement was comparable between groups, but that discontinuation rates were much lower with CBZ + FEWP [42]. It should be noted that FEWP has been investigated in several RCTs in depressive disorders published only in Chinese, which are therefore not reviewed in this chapter; Results from these mostly positive studies were included in a recent large systematic review of 26 studies [93] and a meta-analysis of 14 studies (which included 8 augmentation studies) [20]. While the former included small studies with methodological issues [94], publications for the meta-analysis were selected more rigorously [20]. Both reports found FEWP to be effective and tolerable as monotherapy and augmentation to medication in various depressive disorders, including major depression, dysthymia and bipolar depression [20, 93], and was also better tolerated (as monotherapy or augmentation) than conventional agents alone [20]. FEWP has no published reports as monotherapy or augmentation in anxiety disorders.

Among other reports, a small open trial augmentation of current antidepressants with a Japanese herbal compound, Jio-zai (a combination of two other well-established compounds, Rokumigan and Hachimijiogan), was found to reduce residual symptoms in MDD, but only a small percentage of patients were reported to be "much improved" [21]. Statistical significance of efficacy was not reported. Side effects were few and tolerable. The mechanism of antidepressant action of the compound, or its ingredients, is unclear. There are no reports of Jio-zai as monotherapy in depressive, nor any reports (as monotherapy or augmentation) in anxiety conditions.

While FEWP has reasonable evidence of benefit as an augmentation agent in both unipolar and bipolar depression, there is insufficient evidence to evaluate Jio-zai. Though both compounds were well tolerated, the sparse safety data available in English publications, and their limited use outside their countries of origin, would encourage caution in clinical use.

11.2.2 Nutraceuticals

Nutraceuticals are non-prescription, natural health products that are usually concentrated forms of naturally occurring substances, such as vitamins and minerals. They are often used individually or in combination to support good nutrition and general wellness. A literature search on the use of nutraceuticals as adjunctive agents found information relating to omega-3 fatty acids, S-adenosylmethionine (SAM-e), Dehydroepiandrosterone (DHEA), tryptophan, the B vitamins, inositol, magnesium, zinc, amino acid formulations, and proprietary vitamin-mineral formulations.

Several other nutraceuticals that have been evaluated only as monotherapy in depressive and anxiety disorders, and are therefore not reviewed in this chapter, include alpha-lactalbumin (a tryptophan-rich protein fraction), acetyl-L-carnitine (a modified amino acid and acetyl ester of quaternary ammonium compound, L-carnitine) and lysine (an amino acid and precursor of L-carnitine) see reviews [9, 66, 67].

11.2.2.1 Omega-3 Fatty Acids

Omega-3 fatty acids are polyunsaturated fatty acids involved in multiple biological systems, including the nervous system. Omega-3 fatty acid formulations include highly purified estyl esters of eicosapentanoic acid (EPA) or docosahexaenoic acid (DHA) or a combination of both. Their possible neuropsychiatric effect may result from modulation of neuronal communication and their impact on monoaminergic neural systems [94, 95]. A large meta-analysis of 14 studies recently noted a correlation between low omega-3 levels and depressive disorders [96], and low omega-3 levels have also been linked to anxiety conditions [97–99].

The efficacy of omega-3 fatty acids as monotherapy or augmentation in depressive disorders has been the subject of several medium-size meta-analyses that included seven to nine studies each. In both unipolar and bipolar depression, results from several meta-analyses that included both monotherapy and augmentation studies have been inconclusive, with significant heterogeneity between studies noted, as well as speculation about publication bias, with positive results more likely to be reported than negative ones [e.g. 100–102]. The meta-analyses included studies from a range of diagnostic categories, e.g. unipolar and bipolar depression, schizophrenia, as well as other psychiatric or medical conditions in which depressed mood was exhibited, which may have affected results. However, a recent meta-analysis that focused only on six augmentation studies in bipolar disorder reported clear benefit for omega-3 as add-on to antidepressants or mood stabilizers for bipolar depression, but only a trend favouring it as augmentation in mania [43]. The study populations were more homogeneous, and the likelihood of publication bias was noted to be low, though effect sizes were larger in studies with smaller samples. In all studies, omega-3 fatty acids were well tolerated, with reported side effects being mild.

The question has also been raised about which of the omega-3 fatty acids is more useful in depression. Meta-analyses suggest that EPA may be more effective than DHA or EPA + DHA, but due to confounding factors (i.e. degree of baseline depressive severity and variability of omega-3 formulation used), definitive conclusions could not be reached [103, 104].

There are no monotherapy trials of omega-3 fatty acids in anxiety disorders. Data on their use as augmentation is limited to two studies. In one small cross-over RCT, there was no reduction in OCD symptoms with either EPA or placebo augmentation of SSRIs, though EPA was well tolerated [61]. Similar non-efficacy but good tolerability of EPA (as monotherapy or augmentation to SSRIs) was seen in a small open-label case series in PTSD [64].

In conclusion, omega-3 fatty acids have moderate evidence of benefit in depressive disorders, with more robust effects seen in bipolar samples. There is no current evidence for its benefit in anxiety disorders. The mild side effects reported with omega-3 use include diarrhoea, nausea and a fishy aftertaste, but these rarely lead to discontinuation [105, 106]. While there is also evidence to support its cardioprotective benefits [107], it has been noted to increase bleeding tendencies among patients on the anticoagulant, coumadin (warfarin) and anti-platelet medications (acetylsalicylic acid, clopidogrel), with a need for monitoring [108]. Induced hypomania has been reported in a few cases, but this risk has not been noted in systematic reviews or meta-analyses of studies in bipolar depression [e.g. 43, 101, 109].

11.2.2.2 S-Adenosylmethionine (SAM-e)

SAM-e is a naturally occurring molecule found in the body and a derivative of the amino acid, methionine. It serves as a methyl donor in many biological processes [110]. As with several other CAM agents, its benefits has been attributed to its enhancement of monoaminergic neurotransmission [110]. However, studies that examined the association between low SAM-e levels and depression have had mixed results [111–113]. Synthetic SAM-e is available as a non-prescription oral natural health product in North America, but requires medical prescription in Europe.

While several systematic reviews and meta-analyses support the benefit of SAM-e as monotherapy in unipolar depression (as superior to placebo and comparable to TCAs) [e.g. 114–116], only two studies of adjunctive SAM-e in depressive disorders were found, and none in anxiety. In one small RCT in treatment-resistant major depression (TRD), SAM-e augmentation of SSRIs or selective norepinephrine reuptake inhibitors (SNRIs) produced significantly higher response and remission than placebo add-on [22]. Side effects were mild, and discontinuation due to adverse effects was similar between groups, but that due to lack of efficacy was higher with placebo. Similar efficacy and tolerability were noted in a small open trial of oral SAM-e augmentation to SSRIs/SNRIs in TRD [23].

No data was found for SAM-e as monotherapy or augmentation in anxiety disorders.

The limited data above offers only preliminary support for SAM-e as augmentation in TRD, but further investigation is encouraged by the evidence for its benefit as monotherapy. SAM-e is generally well tolerated with few adverse events, which include nausea, jitteriness, and loose stools [106]. Case reports suggests the risk of induction of manic episodes in vulnerable patients, and of serotonin syndrome when it is added to first-line antidepressants [117], though neither have been reported in systematic reviews or in the studies described above.

11.2.2.3 Dehydroepiandrosterone (DHEA)

DHEA is a natural adrenosteroid that converts to the sex hormones, testosterone and estrogen, in the body. Often used as an anti-aging supplement (though with uncertain benefits) [118], it is thought to modulate monoaminergic and glutaminergic neurotransmission, as well as provide neuroprotective and anti-oxidant benefits [119–121]. The association between DHEA levels and affective symptomatology is unclear; some studies have linked low DHEA levels to depressive symptoms [122, 123], while others have found an association with high DHEA levels [124, 125]. Curiously, both low and high DHEA levels have been linked to depressive symptoms in women [126, 127]. High levels of DHEA have also found in anxiety conditions [128, 129].

The literature on the use of DHEA in depressive disorders is very small. The few published monotherapy studies have reported benefits in MDD and dysthymia [130–132]. Only one augmentation study in depressive disorders was found. In that small RCT, DHEA (either as monotherapy or augmentation to antidepressants) significantly improved depressive symptoms in unipolar and bipolar patients, compared to placebo, and was also well tolerated [24]. Of note, the bipolar sample was limited to two patients.

No published data was found for DHEA as monotherapy or augmentation in anxiety disorders.

This pilot data suggest that further investigation of DHEA an augmenting agent in mood disorders may be fruitful. Though no serious side effects were reported in the above studies, DHEA, as a precursor of more potent sex hormones, has potential for side effects that may include acne and hirsutism, and several studies have excluded patients with prostatism or family history of breast cancer [130, 131]. Safety data also suggest monitoring for potential effects of DHEA on blood clotting, liver damage, induction of mania in vulnerable individuals, and dose-related increase in adverse effects [133, 134].

11.2.2.4 Tryptophan

Tryptophan is a dietary amino acid that is converted to 5-hydroxy tryptophan (5-HTP) and then into serotonin (5-HT), both centrally and peripherally. Thus, it is thus thought to enhance serotonergic neurotransmission through "precursor loading" [135]. It is a prescription drug in Canada, and recently was reintroduced in the US. Tryptophan depletion is associated with worsening of mood and cognitive functioning both in patients with a history of depression and those at risk for depression [136, 137]. In studies, tryptophan has been used in both 5-HTP and l-tryptophan formulations.

Several early studies have evaluated 5-HTP as monotherapy or augmentation to SSRIs and TCAs in unipolar and bipolar depression, with generally positive results seen in the mostly monotherapy open trials, but equivocal results in 'blinded' RCTs see review [138]. However, a small monotherapy meta-analysis [135] and a large review (that included six augmentation studies) [138] noted the many methodological flaws in the included studies (all published prior to 1992) and reported inconclusive efficacy of 5-HTP [135, 138]. More recently, a small placebo-controlled RCT found fluoxetine + l-tryptophan combination produced early onset of improvement in MDD, but which was not sustained to endpoint, though the combination was well tolerated [25]. A small open CAM study found l-tryptophan augmentation significantly improved depressive symptoms in patients with seasonal affective disorder who did not initially respond to light therapy, and it was also well tolerated [26]. However, due to the lack of a comparison group, it can be questioned whether longer treatment with light therapy alone might have produced a similar result.

In anxiety disorders, the data on tryptophan is very sparse. One early RCT found 5-HTP monotherapy no different from placebo and inferior to TCAs for PD [139]. There are no studies of tryptophan as add-on in anxiety conditions.

The preliminary support for tryptophan as an augmenting agent in depressive disorders needs verification through further RCTs. It has no evidence of benefit in anxiety disorders at this time. Side effects usually reported with tryptophan include drowsiness, dry mouth, nausea, and other gastrointestinal symptoms, but reports of serotonin syndrome are relatively rare in RCTs [135, 138]. In 1989, tryptophan ingestion was associated with an outbreak of Eosinophilia-Myalgia Syndrome that resulted in significant mortality, but this was attributed to a contaminated batch from a single manufacturer, and no such reports have emerged since then [135, 138].

11.2.2.5 The B Vitamins

The water-soluble B vitamins are found in foods and are vital to the growth, division and metabolism of cells, as well as for immune and nervous system functioning. They consist of thiamine (B1), riboflavin (B2), niacin (B3), pantothenic acid (B5), pyridoxine (B6), biotin (B7), folic acid or folate (B9) and assorted cobalamins (B12). Vitamin B9 (folate) is implicated in monoaminergic synthesis [140], and is the most studied as a CAM therapy, but Vitamins B6 and B12 have also been investigated. Folate and Vitamin B12 are both necessary for production of homocysteine which is converted to methionine, a precursor to S-adenosyl methionine, which is a methyl donor involved in neurotransmitter function [140, 141]. Several studies have noted low levels of folate (in particular) and Vitamin B12 in depressed patients [e.g. 142, 143], though others have failed to confirm this association [e.g. 144, 145]. Similarly, studies evaluating the association between low Vitamin B6 levels and depression have had both positive [e.g. 146, 147] and negative [e.g. 144, 145] results. No associations have been noted between these B vitamins and anxiety disorders, thus far. Other research has focused on choline, a nutrient in the B vitamin family that is a precursor for the neurotransmitter, acetylcholine, and which also supports phosphate production in the brain [44]. Low levels of acetylcholine and of phosphates have been linked to mania [44, 148], as have low levels of choline [45, 149], but the data is not robust. Elevated choline levels have been found in depression [150, 151], while low levels have been correlated with anxiety [152, 153].

Folate: Several investigations have evaluated the efficacy of folate in depressive disorders. In an early placebo-controlled RCT, folic acid augmentation significantly improved depressive symptoms in unipolar depressed patients, but not in bipolar or schizophrenia patients [27]. However, the patients were only marginally depressed at the start of the study, which was a limitation. Side effects were comparable and tolerable across groups. Another early placebo-controlled RCT found methylfolate augmentation of tricyclic antidepressants (TCAs) or monoamine oxidase inhibitors (MAOIs) significantly superior to placebo in improving depressive symptoms in MDD and schizophrenia, though tolerability data was not reported and sample size was small [28]. Subsequently, an adequately-sized RCT found fluoxetine + folic acid combination superior to fluoxetine + placebo in MDD, but only among female patients, and it was also better tolerated than the placebo combination [29]. This was followed by a small open trial that found folinic acid augmentation of SSRIs to be significantly effective in improving TRD and well tolerated, but only a small percentage of patients achieved response or remission levels [30]. The findings of these four studies were included in recent small systematic reviews of folate in unipolar depression, which found it effective as both monotherapy and augmentation [154, 155], and well tolerated [154]. More recently, folic acid augmentation of fluoxetine was found significantly superior to placebo augmentation in a small RCT in MDD; tolerability data is unknown [31]. Paradoxically, a small open randomized trial found escitalopram monotherapy significantly superior to escitalopram + folic acid combination in MDD, but with tolerability data not reported [32]. A recent large retrospective analysis of 242 cases, which compared the efficacy of l-methylfolate co-initiated with antidepressant therapy to antidepressant therapy alone in MDD, found that the folate combination was associated with significantly better treatment response, faster onset of improvement and less discontinuation due to side effects than antidepressants alone [33]. In the only study in bipolar disorder, an adequate-sized RCT found that both valproate + folic acid and valproate +placebo combinations significantly improved manic symptoms and were well tolerated; the folic acid combination showed statistical superiority to placebo only at end of the brief treatment period [46]. There is no data on folate as monotherapy or augmentation in anxiety disorders.

Vitamin B12: Literature on the use of Vitamin B12 is very sparse. A single early monotherapy RCT found no difference between Vitamin B12 and placebo in seasonal affective disorder [156]. No augmentation or combination studies were found with Vitamin B12 in other mood and anxiety conditions.

Vitamin B6: A recent small systematic review of the efficacy of Vitamin B6 as monotherapy or augmentation in unipolar depression found no benefit for its use, and noted limitations of small sample size and heterogeneity of patient populations [157]. The only published augmentation study, a small placebo-controlled RCT which used a B complex vitamin (comprised of Vitamins B1, B2 and B6), as add-on to TCAs, was included in the review, and also had negative results [158]. There are no reports of Vitamin B6 as monotherapy or augmentation in anxiety conditions.

Choline: There are no studies of choline monotherapy in depressive disorders. Choline augmentation has been evaluated in bipolar disorder in two studies, with mixed results. In a small open label case series, choline bitartrate augmentation of lithium significantly improved depressive and manic symptoms in most patients and was well tolerated, but important study data was not published, including duration of treatment and statistical significance values [45]. In a small RCT, choline bitartrate or placebo augmentation of lithium had no effect on bipolar depression or mania; no tolerability data was reported [44]. No investigations of choline as monotherapy or augmentation in anxiety conditions are currently available.

Thus, evidence is lacking for Vitamin B6, Vitamin B12 or choline as augmentation in depressive disorders. However, there is reasonable evidence for folate as augmentation or combination to medication for MDD. Folate was well tolerated in all reported studies, and there are no known drug interactions or contradictions to the use of methylfolate [140]. However, there is evidence that high folate doses (>800 mcg) may lead to increased levels of unmetabolized serum folic acid, which can lower levels of natural killers cells and brain l-methylfolate and deplete monoamines, and may worsen depression [140, 154]. Folic acid, in high doses (e.g. 15 μg), has been associated with increased depression in some studies, and sleep difficulties, irritability, hyperactivity and discomfort have also been reported in healthy volunteers [140, 159].

11.2.2.6 Vitamin D

Vitamin D is a fat-soluble secosteroid that is found in foods and is also naturally produced by the body during adequate sun exposure. Essential to bone health, it acts through prevention of bone demineralization and promotion of calcium absorption, and is also thought to influence cellular and kidney function [160, 161]. It has been postulated that Vitamin D may affect mood through its modulation of serotonin synthesis and glucocorticoid activity, and may also be neuroprotective [162, 163]. While several epidemiological studies have reported an association between low serum vitamin D levels and depression e.g. [164–166], others have not confirmed such links [167, 168]. It has also been suggested that any relationship may be seasonally influenced [169, 170] and may have a female gender skew [171].

Reviews of the limited research on Vitamin D monotherapy in depression have noted only modest benefit in seasonal affective disorder and methodological weaknesses in many of the studies found, limiting the generalizability of results [161, 167]. Thus, the role of Vitamin D in depressive disorders (as a cause, consequence or associate) also remains unelucidated [157, 167]. No published studies have evaluated Vitamin D as an add-on in depressive disorders, or as monotherapy or augmentation in anxiety conditions.

Evidence is currently lacking to recommend Vitamin D as an agent for depressive or anxiety disorders. However, it continues to be recommended as a dietary supplement for general health benefits at a dosage of up to 2,000 IU per day [172]. Toxicity has been reported at dosages over 20,000 IU per day, and has included gastrointestinal symptoms, low appetite and hypercalcemia [172, 173].

11.2.2.7 Inositol

Inositol is a carboxylic polyol, an isomer of glucose that is integral to the production of cellular secondary messengers, such as inositol triphosphate, that mediates neurotransmitter receptor activity, and in turn, intracellular processes [34]. The association between low inositol levels and depression is equivocal, with some studies noting a correlation [174–176], but others not [177]. Low levels of inositol have also been linked to anxiety in animal models [178, 179].

There is a small body of literature on the use of inositol in depressive disorders. No group differences were noted in two small placebo-controlled RCTs of inositol add-on to SSRIs in MDD [35, 36]. It had comparable tolerability to placebo in the first study [35], but in the other, drop out due to side effects (including one case of serotonin syndrome) was greater with inositol than with placebo [36]. In bipolar disorder, a small RCT failed to find group differences between inositol or placebo augmentation of mood stabilizers in bipolar depression, though it was well tolerated [47]. A small meta-analysis of four studies in depressive disorders, which included these three studies (and one placebo-controlled monotherapy RCT), also found no evidence of benefit for inositol as monotherapy or augmentation in unipolar or bipolar depression [34]. More recently, a two-phase study in bipolar depression failed to note any benefit to inositol augmentation of mood stabilizers in its placebo-controlled RCT phase (though a trend favoured inositol) [48]. The subsequent open label continuation phase supported inositol augmentation, though significance values were not reported. Another small open trial, an arm of the Systematic Treatment Enhancement Program for Bipolar Disorder (STEP-BD) study, found randomized augmentation with lamotrigine, inositol or risperidone to be comparable in efficacy and tolerability in bipolar depression [49].

In anxiety disorders, a small review found modest benefits with inositol monotherapy in PD and OCD, with inositol showing superiority to placebo, comparable efficacy to SSRIs, and good tolerability [67]. However, these benefits were not replicated in the only two augmentation studies with inositol, both in OCD. No significant benefit was noted to inositol augmentation of SSRIs/TCAs in either a cross-over placebo-controlled RCT [62], or an open trial [63]. Side effect data, available for only one of the studies, found inositol to be well tolerated [63].

Thus, overall, there is insufficient evidence to recommend inositol as an augmenting agent in either depressive or anxiety disorders. It appears to be well tolerated, but induction of mania or hypomania, and hospitalization due to worsening of psychiatric symptoms, have been reported in case reports, as well as in some patients in clinical trials [35, 47, 48, 180].

11.2.2.8 Magnesium

Magnesium is an essential mineral that is integral to cellular and neuronal functioning in the brain [181]. It modulates both N-methyl-D-aspartic acid (NMDA) and GABA neurotransmission, suggesting a possible route of antidepressant action, but is also thought to modulate HPA axis activity, and thus stress and anxiety pathways [182–184]. Magnesium deficiency is associated with increased vulnerability to stress reactivity, depression and anxiety in animal models [181, 185], and to postpartum depression in humans [186].

Data on magnesium supplementation in mood and anxiety disorders is limited. A recent small review of mostly early studies noted that monotherapy with magnesium supplements appeared to benefit depression, mania and anxiety, but heterogeneity of study populations, variation in formulations used and lack of RCT data limit the value of the findings [187]. Only two augmentation studies were found in depressive disorders, both in bipolar patients. In the first, a small open case series, intravenous (IV) magnesium sulfate augmentation of existing mood stabilizers or benzodiazepines improved refractory mania, though no statistical significance values were reported [50]. Significant side effects of brachycardia (frequent) and burning sensation in the veins (rare) were resolved with reduction in IV dosage. In the other, a small RCT, magnesium oxide augmentation of verapamil was found significantly superior to placebo augmentation for mania, but tolerability data was not reported [51].

Any published evidence for magnesium monotherapy for anxiety symptoms is challenged by methodological flaws, particularly the lack of distinct syndromal anxiety patient samples [187]. In the only add-on study available, a large RCT in GAD combined hawthorn (*Crataegus oxyacantha*; a fruit-bearing shrub), and California poppy (*Eschscholtzia californica*; a flowering plant), both thought to have anxiolytic properties [188, 189], with elemental magnesium and found the combination to be significantly superior to placebo in improving GAD symptoms [60]. Side effects were mild with both treatments.

This preliminary data is promising, but there is currently insufficient evidence to recommend magnesium augmentation for depressive or anxiety disorders. Though magnesium is generally well tolerated in over-the-counter formulations, the absence of long-term safety data is also a cautionary note, in particular as excess intake of magnesium has been linked to gastrointestinal upset and cardiac arrhythmia [186, 190].

11.2.2.9 Zinc

Zinc is an essential mineral that is involved in ribonucleic acid (RNA) and deoxyribonucleic acid (DNA) metabolism, signal transduction, and gene expression, and is a component in enzymes, amino acids and proteins [191]. Its exact role in the pathophysiology of mood and anxiety disorders remains unclear. One hypothesis is that deficiency of zinc (found in highest concentrations in the hippocampus and amygdala) [192], leads to reduced hippocampal neurogenesis [193], and in turn to the decreased hippocampal volumes reported with depression and anxiety [194, 195]. Zinc is also suggested to modulate NMDA-receptor activity, pharmacological antagonists of which have been shown to benefit both depression and anxiety [196, 197]. It is also posited to support serotonergic signaling [198, 199], and to improve neuroplasticity by increasing BDNF gene expression [200, 201] and glutathione levels [202], an effect similar to that of antidepressants [203, 204]. Thus, it may have several modes of antidepressant and anxiolytic action. Zinc deficiency is associated with anxiety in animal models [205, 206], while human studies have noted a correlation between zinc deficiency and depression [e.g. 207, 208].

There are no monotherapy studies of zinc as intervention in depressive disorders. A recent small meta-analysis of four studies (two monotherapy studies in healthy subjects and two augmentation RCTs in depressed subjects) found zinc to be superior to placebo as augmentation to SSRIs/TCAs in unipolar depression [37]. However, methodological flaws restrict generalizability of the results. Both RCTs had small MDD samples [38, 39]. Furthermore, in one RCT, the zinc combination was superior to placebo add-on only in the antidepressant-resistant subgroup and only at midpoint, with only a trend to superiority in this subgroup at endpoint [39]. Zinc was well tolerated in both studies.

There are no published studies of zinc as monotherapy or augmentation in anxiety disorders.

This limited but promising data suggest that more and larger placebo-controlled RCTs would be useful to help determine the utility of zinc for depression. In the above studies, zinc supplementation was well tolerated and no drug-drug interactions were reported. However, there are reports of excess zinc consumption being associated with ataxia, lethargy, iron and copper deficiency, and cerebral ischemia [209–211].

11.2.2.10 Other Dietary Supplements

Additional studies on adjunctive use of other dietary supplements in mood and anxiety disorders have reported on the benefits of several amino acid formulations or proprietary vitamin-mineral formulations.

While several amino acids are produced by the body, others are only found in foods. Though mostly known for their key role in protein synthesis, amino acids are also important in many physiological processes, including synthesis of neurotransmitters, by which effect they may influence affective state [212, 213]. Disturbances in amino acid levels have been reported with depression, and improvement in amino acid levels has been seen with antidepressant treatment response [214, 215]. Among individual amino acids, a few small and mostly early RCTs found acetyl-L-carnitine as monotherapy to be superior to placebo and comparable to atypical antipsychotics in unipolar depression, and to be well tolerated [216–219]. However, there is no published data to support its benefit as augmentation. On the other hand, while amino acid formulations have not been evaluated as monotherapy in depressive disorders, there are two augmentation studies in the literature. In a small RCT with an amino acid mixture (comprised of ten amino acids, 11 vitamins and three minerals), response in severe MDD was significantly greater with mirtazapine + amino acid mixture than mirtazapine + placebo, though remission rates and tolerability were similar [40]. Another small RCT found augmentation with a branched-chain amino acid drink (consisting of three amino acids) produced faster onset of improvement in bipolar mania than placebo; group differences disappeared by end of treatment, but re-emerged in favour of amino acids at 1-week follow-up [52]. The amino acid drink was well tolerated. There are no studies of amino acids as monotherapy or augmentation in anxiety disorders.

N-acetylcysteine (NAC) is acetylated derivative of the amino acid, cysteine, which is the precursor of glutathione, the main antioxidant in the brain [220]. Impaired glutathione metabolism is linked to increased oxidative stress, which, in turn, is thought to underl the pathophysiology of several psychiatric disorders, including depression [220, 221]. NAC has no monotherapy data in depressive disorders, but there are two maintenance augmentation studies in bipolar disorder. A small placebo-controlled maintenance RCT found NAC augmentation to existing psychotropics (antidepressants, mood stabilizers, antipsychotics, etc.) produced significant improvement in bipolar depressive symptoms, quality of life and functioning; a trend to improvement in manic symptoms may have been moderated by the low mania scores at study onset [53]. There were no group differences in time to mood episode, and NAC was generally well tolerated. Similar benefits with NAC augmentation of existing psychotropics were also noted in the results from the large open trial stage of a two-phase maintenance RCT by the same research group, though side effect data were not reported [54]. Results of the subsequent double-blind phase are pending. No studies were found with NAC as monotherapy in anxiety disorders, but a single case report suggests its benefit as augmentation to SSRIs [222].

A proprietary nutritional supplement made up of 36 chelated trace vitamins and minerals, called E. M. Power Plus (EMP+), has also been investigated in bipolar disorder. It is thought to alleviate bipolar-like symptoms by correcting nutritional deficiencies that may contribute to metabolic dysfunction [55]. Three case series with adult patients have noted significant improvement in bipolar depressive and manic symptoms with EMP + (as monotherapy or augmentation), leading to significant reduction in psychotropic medication use [55–57]. Only one of the case series reported significance values, but it had a small sample and almost all patients were male, limiting generalizability [55]. In general, EMP + was well tolerated in these studies, with few side effects. Hypomanic switch was reported in two cases, as well as symptom recurrence in some subjects post-study, needing resumption of psychotropics [57]. A recent large database analysis of open label EMP + monotherapy or augmentation in child and adolescent bipolar patients noted similar efficacy and tolerability with EMP+, but lack of RCTs hinder definitive conclusions [58]. A systematic review of the safety and tolerability of EMP + found that it was well tolerated in both adult and youth populations, with mild and transitory GI symptoms and headache most reported, no abnormal lab results or toxicity, and fewer adverse events and lower weight gain than with psychotropics [223]. There is no data on the use of EMP + as monotherapy or augmentation in anxiety conditions.

There is only preliminary evidence for the benefit of amino acid compounds, and due to the variability in formulation between studies, data is insufficient to make recommendations. The pilot data on NAC augmentation for bipolar depression appears promising and if the pending data from the double-blind phase of the latest study [54] is positive, it may support the use of NAC in this disorder. While the preliminary efficacy data with EMP + in bipolar disorder also appears to warrant further placebo-controlled investigations, it must be noted that the only such trial registered on clinicaltrials.gov was discontinued due to recruitment difficulties, large expectancy effects and uninformative results [224]. Side effects reported with the above supplements appear to be mild and tolerable, for most part. However, due to the general paucity of evidence, their utility in clinical practice remains undefined.

11.3 Conclusions and Future Directions

Although clinical trials of herbal and dietary supplements as augmentation or combination in mood and anxiety disorders are being increasingly reported, they are still significantly fewer than those with conventional pharmacological agents. As this review has also shown, research on the supplementary use of these compounds is much more common for depressive disorders than for anxiety conditions.

It is of note that despite the general dearth of efficacy and tolerability data with the CAM agents reviewed in this chapter, there is relatively good information on the basic physiological mechanism of action of many of them. Enhancement of monoaminergic and glutaminergic neurotransmission, impact on HPA axis functioning, and enhanced neurogenesis, have been reported to result from the use of several of these agents, as with conventional antidepressants. Large head-to-head effectiveness trials against first-line antidepressants may prove to be valuable.

Based on the evidence from available studies, the herbal and dietary supplements that appear to hold most promise as adjunctive agents to pharmacotherapy include the herbal supplement, FEWP (in unipolar depression, bipolar depression or mania), and the nutraceuticals, omega-3 fatty acids (in bipolar depression) and folate (in MDD). There is also preliminary evidence of benefit for combination with some other herbal remedies, such as lavandula (in MDD), and dietary supplements, such as SAM-e (in TRD), DHEA (in MDD), magnesium (in mania), zinc (in MDD), amino acid formulations (in unipolar depression and mania), NAC (as maintenance in bipolar depression), and EMP + (in bipolar disorder). Among the other supplements reviewed, St. John's wort (for depression and co-morbid anxiety), kava (for anxiety symptoms), and tryptophan (for seasonal affective disorder) only have data in combination with non-pharmacological agents, thus far. Currently, there is insufficient evidence to support other herbal and nutraceutical agents (i.e. Jio-zai, inositol and Vitamin D) as augmentation for depressive and anxiety disorders.

While these agents were frequently effective and usually well tolerated in published studies, limited numbers of good quality RCTs and/or limited familiarity of use in clinical practice has meant that most guidelines would recommend their use usually as augmentation, and often later in the treatment algorithm. In particular, there is sparse information on their potential interaction with conventional psychiatric drugs, and as such, longer-term efficacy and safety data may help to increase support for wider clinical application.

References

1. Andrade L, Caraveo-Anduaga JJ, Berglund P et al (2000) Cross-national comparisons of the prevalences and correlates of mental disorders. WHO international consortium in psychiatric epidemiology. Bull World Health Organ 78:413–426
2. Demyttenaere K, Bruffaerts R, Posada-Villa J et al (2004) WHO world mental health survey consortium. Prevalence, severity, and unmet need for treatment of mental disorders in the World Health Organization world mental health surveys. JAMA 291:2581–2590
3. Goldberg JF, Garno JL, Harrow M (2005) Long-term remission and recovery in bipolar disorder: a review. Curr Psychiatry Rep 7:456–461
4. Rush AJ, Fava M, Wisniewski SR et al (2004) Sequenced treatment alternatives to relieve depression (STAR*D): rationale and design. Control Clin Trials 25:119–142
5. Yonkers KA, Bruce SE, Dyck IR et al (2003) Chronicity, relapse, and illness—course of panic disorder, social phobia, and generalized anxiety disorder: findings in men and women from 8 years of follow-up. Depress Anxiety 17:173–179
6. Keller MB, McCullough JP, Klein DN et al (2000) A comparison of nefazodone, the cognitive behavioral-analysis system of psychotherapy, and their combination for the treatment of chronic depression. N Engl J Med 342:1462–1470
7. Zivin K, Madden JM, Graves AJ et al (2009) Cost-related medication nonadherence among beneficiaries with depression following Medicare Part D. Am J Geriatr Psychiatry 17:1068–1076

8. Andreescu C, Mulsant BH, Emanuel JE (2008) Complementary and alternative medicine in the treatment of bipolar disorder—a review of the evidence. J Affect Disord 110:16–26
9. Ravindran AV, Lam RW, Filteau MJ et al (2009) Canadian Network for Mood and Anxiety Treatments (CANMAT). Canadian Network for Mood and Anxiety Treatments (CANMAT) clinical guidelines for the management of major depressive disorder in adults. V. Complementary and alternative medicine treatments. J Affect Disord 117(Suppl 1):S54–S64
10. van der Watt G, Laugharne J, Janka A (2008) Complementary and alternative medicine in the treatment of anxiety and depression. Curr Opin Psychiatry 21:37–42
11. Kessler RC, Soukup J, Davis RB et al (2001) The use of complementary and alternative therapies to treat anxiety and depression in the United States. Am J Psychiatry 158:289–294
12. Wahlström M, Sihvo S, Haukkala A et al (2008) Use of mental health services and complementary and alternative medicine in persons with common mental disorders. Acta Psychiatr Scand 118:73–80
13. da Silva TL, Ravindran LN, Ravindran AV (2009) Yoga in the treatment of mood and anxiety disorders. Asian J Psychiatry 2:6–16
14. Ströhle A (2009) Physical activity, exercise, depression and anxiety disorders. J Neural Transm 116:777–784
15. Tuunainen A, Kripke DF, Endo T (2004) Light therapy for non-seasonal depression. Cochrane database Syst Rev (2):CD004050
16. Sarris J, Kavanagh DJ, Deed G et al (2009) St. John's wort and Kava in treating major depressive disorder with comorbid anxiety: a randomised double-blind placebo-controlled pilot trial. Hum Psychopharmacol 24:41–48
17. Müller D, Pfeil T, von den Driesch V (2003) Treating depression comorbid with anxiety—results of an open, practice-oriented study with St John's wort WS 5572 and valerian extract in high doses. Phytomedicine 10(Suppl 4):25–30
18. Cagnacci A, Arangino S, Renzi A et al (2003) Kava-Kava administration reduces anxiety in perimenopausal women. Maturitas 44:103–109
19. Akhondzadeh S, Kashani L, Fotouhi A et al (2003) Comparison of Lavandula angustifolia Mill. tincture and imipramine in the treatment of mild to moderate depression: a double-blind, randomized trial. Prog Neuropsychopharmacol Biol Psychiatry 27:123–127
20. Qin F, Wu XA, Tang Y et al (2011) Meta-analysis of randomized controlled trials to assess the effectiveness and safety of Free and easy wanderer plus, a polyherbal preparation for depressive disorders. J Psychiatr Res 45:1518–1524
21. Yamada K, Yagi G, Kanba S (2005) Effectiveness of herbal medicine (Rokumigan and Hachimijiogan) for fatigue or loss of energy in patients with partial remitted major depressive disorder. Psychiatry Clin Neurosci 59:610–612
22. Papakostas GI, Mischoulon D, Shyu I et al (2010) S-adenosyl methionine (SAMe) augmentation of serotonin reuptake inhibitors for antidepressant nonresponders with major depressive disorder: a double-blind, randomized clinical trial. Am J Psychiatry 167:942–948
23. Alpert JE, Papakostas G, Mischoulon D et al (2004) S-adenosyl-L-methionine (SAMe) as an adjunct for resistant major depressive disorder: an open trial following partial or nonresponse to selective serotonin reuptake inhibitors or venlafaxine. J Clin Psychopharmacol 24:661–664
24. Wolkowitz OM, Reus VI, Keebler A et al (1999) Double-blind treatment of major depression with dehydroepiandrosterone. Am J Psychiatry 156:646–649
25. Levitan RD, Shen JH, Jindal R et al (2000) Preliminary randomized double-blind placebo-controlled trial of tryptophan combined with fluoxetine to treat major depressive disorder: antidepressant and hypnotic effects. J Psychiatry Neurosci 25:337–346
26. Lam RW, Levitan RD, Tam EM et al (1997) L-tryptophan augmentation of light therapy in patients with seasonal affective disorder. Can J Psychiatry 42:303–306
27. Coppen A, Chaudhry S, Swade C (1986) Folic acid enhances lithium prophylaxis. J Affect Disord 10:9–13
28. Godfrey PS, Toone BK, Carney MW et al (1990) Enhancement of recovery from psychiatric illness by methylfolate. Lancet 336:392–395

29. Coppen A, Bailey J (2000) Enhancement of the antidepressant action of fluoxetine by folic acid: a randomised, placebo controlled trial. J Affect Disord 60:121–130
30. Alpert JE, Mischoulon D, Rubenstein GE, Bottonari K, Nierenberg AA, Fava M (2002) Folinic acid (Leucovorin) as an adjunctive treatment for SSRI-refractory depression. Ann Clin Psychiatry 14:33–38
31. Resler G, Lavie R, Campos J et al (2008) Effect of folic acid combined with fluoxetine in patients with major depression on plasma homocysteine and vitamin B12, and serotonin levels in lymphocytes. Neuroimmunomodulation 15:145–152
32. Basoglu C, Ates MA, Algul A et al (2009) Adjuvant folate with escitalopram treatment and homocystein, folate, vitamin B-12 levels in patients with major depressive disorder. Bull Clin Psychopharmacol 19:135–142
33. Ginsberg LD, Oubre AY, Daoud YA (2011) L-methylfolate Plus SSRI or SNRI from treatment initiation compared to SSRI or SNRI monotherapy in a major depressive episode. Innov Clin Neurosci 8:19–28
34. Taylor MJ, Wilder H, Bhagwagar Z, et al (2004) Inositol for depressive disorders. Cochrane Database Syst Rev (2):CD004049
35. Levine J, Mishori A, Susnosky M et al (1999) Combination of inositol and serotonin reuptake inhibitors in the treatment of depression. Biol Psychiatry 45:270–273
36. Nemets B, Mishory A, Levine J et al (1999) Inositol addition does not improve depression in SSRI treatment failures. J Neural Transm 106:795–798
37. Lai J, Moxey A, Nowak G et al (2012) The efficacy of zinc supplementation in depression: systematic review of randomised controlled trials. J Affect Disord 136:e31–e39
38. Nowak G, Siwek M, Dudek D et al (2003) Effect of zinc supplementation on antidepressant therapy in unipolar depression: a preliminary placebo-controlled study. Pol J Pharmacol 55:1143–1147
39. Siwek M, Dudek D, Paul IA et al (2009) Zinc supplementation augments efficacy of imipramine in treatment resistant patients: a double blind, placebo-controlled study. J Affect Disord 118:187–195
40. Ille R, Spona J, Zickl M et al (2007) "Add-On"-therapy with an individualized preparation consisting of free amino acids for patients with a major depression. Eur Arch Psychiatry Clin Neurosci 257:222–229
41. Zhang ZJ, Kang WH, Tan QR et al (2007a) Adjunctive herbal medicine with carbamazepine for bipolar disorders: a double-blind, randomized, placebo-controlled study. J Psychiatr Res 41:360–369
42. Zhang ZJ, Kang WH, Li Q et al (2007b) The beneficial effects of the herbal medicine Free and Easy Wanderer Plus (FEWP) for mood disorders: double-blind, placebo-controlled studies. J Psychiatr Res 41:828–836
43. Sarris J, Mischoulon D, Schweitzer I (2012) Omega-3 for bipolar disorder: meta-analyses of use in mania and bipolar depression. J Clin Psychiatry 73:81–86
44. Lyoo IK, Demopulos CM, Hirashima F et al (2003) Oral choline decreases brain purine levels in lithium-treated subjects with rapid-cycling bipolar disorder: a double-blind trial using proton and lithium magnetic resonance spectroscopy. Bipolar Disord 5:300–306
45. Stoll AL, Sachs GS, Cohen BM et al (1996) Choline in the treatment of rapid-cycling bipolar disorder: clinical and neurochemical findings in lithium-treated patients. Biol Psychiatry 40:382–388
46. Behzadi AH, Omrani Z, Chalian M et al (2009) Folic acid efficacy as an alternative drug added to sodium valproate in the treatment of acute phase of mania in bipolar disorder: a double-blind randomized controlled trial. Acta Psychiatr Scand 120:441–445
47. Chengappa KN, Levine J, Gershon S et al (2000) Inositol as an add-on treatment for bipolar depression. Bipolar Disord 2:47–55
48. Eden Evins A, Demopulos C, Yovel I et al (2006) Inositol augmentation of lithium or valproate for bipolar depression. Bipolar Disord 8:168–174
49. Nierenberg AA, Ostacher MJ, Calabrese JR et al (2006) Treatment-resistant bipolar depression: a STEP-BD equipoise randomized effectiveness trial of antidepressant augmentation with lamotrigine, inositol, or risperidone. Am J Psychiatry 163:210–216

50. Heiden A, Frey R, Presslich O et al (1999) Treatment of severe mania with intravenous magnesium sulphate as a supplementary therapy. Psychiatry Res 89:239–246
51. Giannini AJ, Nakoneczie AM, Melemis SM et al (2000) Magnesium oxide augmentation of verapamil maintenance therapy in mania. Psychiatry Res 93:83–87
52. Scarna A, Gijsman HJ, McTavish SF et al (2003) Effects of a branched-chain amino acid drink in mania. Br J Psychiatry 182:210–213
53. Berk M, Copolov DL, Dean O et al (2008) N-acetyl cysteine for depressive symptoms in bipolar disorder—a double-blind randomized placebo-controlled trial. Biol Psychiatry 64:468–475
54. Berk M, Dean O, Cotton SM et al (2011) The efficacy of N-acetylcysteine as an adjunctive treatment in bipolar depression: an open label trial. J Affect Disord 135:389–394
55. Kaplan B, Simpson J, Ferre R et al (2001) Effective mood stabilization with a chelated mineral supplement: an open-label trial in bipolar disorder. J Clin Psychiatry 62:936–944
56. Popper CW (2001) Do vitamins or minerals (apart from lithium) have mood-stabilizing effects? J Clin Psychiatry 62:933–935
57. Simmons M (2003) Nutritional approach to bipolar disorder. J Clin Psychiatry 64:338
58. Rucklidge JJ, Gately D, Kaplan BJ (2010) Database analysis of children and adolescents with bipolar disorder consuming a micronutrient formula. BMC Psychiatry 10:74
59. De Leo V, la Marca A, Morgante G et al (2001) Evaluation of combining kava extract with hormone replacement therapy in the treatment of postmenopausal anxiety. Maturitas 39:185–188
60. Hanus M, Lafon J, Mathieu M (2004) Double-blind, randomised, placebo-controlled study to evaluate the efficacy and safety of a fixed combination containing two plant extracts (Crataegus oxyacantha and Eschscholtzia californica) and magnesium in mild-to-moderate anxiety disorders. Curr Med Res Opin 20:63–71
61. Fux M, Benjamin J, Nemets B (2004) A placebo-controlled cross-over trial of adjunctive EPA in OCD. J Psychiatr Res 38:323–325
62. Fux M, Benjamin J, Belmaker RH (1999) Inositol versus placebo augmentation of serotonin reuptake inhibitors in the treatment of obsessive-compulsive disorder: a double-blind cross-over study. Int J Neuropsychopharmacol 2:193–195
63. Seedat S, Stein DJ (1999) Inositol augmentation of serotonin reuptake inhibitors in treatment-refractory obsessive-compulsive disorder: an open trial. Int Clin Psychopharmacol 14:353–356
64. Zeev K, Michael M, Ram K et al (2005) Possible deleterious effects of adjunctive omega-3 fatty acids in post-traumatic stress disorder patients. Neuropsychiatr Dis Treat 1:187–190
65. Lam RW, Kennedy SH, Grigoriadis S et al (2009) Canadian Network for Mood and Anxiety Treatments (CANMAT). Canadian Network for Mood and Anxiety Treatments (CANMAT) clinical guidelines for the management of major depressive disorder in adults. III. Pharmacotherapy. J Affect Disord 117(Suppl 1):S26–S43
66. Lakhan SE, Vieira KF (2010) Nutritional and herbal supplements for anxiety and anxiety-related disorders: systematic review. Nutr J 9:42
67. Saeed SA, Bloch RM, Antonacci DJ (2007) Herbal and dietary supplements for treatment of anxiety disorders. Am Fam Physician 76:549–556
68. Sarris J, Kavanagh DJ (2009) Kava and St. John's Wort: current evidence for use in mood and anxiety disorders. J Altern Complement Med 15:827–836
69. Kasper S, Dienel A (2002) Cluster analysis of symptoms during antidepressant treatment with hypericum extract in mildly to moderately depressed out-patients. A meta-analysis of data from three randomized, placebo-controlled trials. Psychopharmacology (Berl) 164:301–308
70. Linde K, Berner MM, Kriston L (2008) St John's wort for major depression. Cochrane Database Syst Rev (4):CD000448
71. Baum SS, Hill R, Rommelspacher H (1998) Effects of kava extract and individual kavapyrones on neurotransmitter levels in the nucleus accumbens of rats. Prog Neuropsychopharmacol Biol Psych 22:1105–1120

72. Hattesohl M, Feistel B, Sievers H et al (2008) Extracts of Valeriana officinalis L. s.l. show anxiolytic and antidepressant effects but neither sedative nor myorelaxant properties. Phytomedicine 15:2–15
73. Kobak KA, Taylor LV, Bystritsky A et al (2005) St John's wort versus placebo in obsessive-compulsive disorder: results from a double-blind study. Int Clin Psychopharmacol 20:299–304
74. Kobak KA, Taylor LV, Warner G et al (2005) St. John's wort versus placebo in social phobia: results from a placebo-controlled pilot study. J Clin Psychopharmacol 25:51–58
75. Taylor LH, Kobak KA (2000) An open-label trial of St. John's wort (Hypericum perforatum) in obsessive-compulsive disorder. J Clin Psychiatry 61:575–578
76. Davidson JR, Connor KM (2001) St. John's wort in generalized anxiety disorder: three case reports. J Clin Psychopharmacol 21(6):635–636
77. Kobak KA, Taylor L, Futterer R et al (2003) St. John's wort in generalized anxiety disorder: three more case reports. J Clin Psychopharmacol 23:531–532
78. Golan DE, Tashjian AH, Armstrong EJ et al (2007) Principles of pharmacology: the pathophysiologic basis of drug therapy. Lippincott Williams & Wilkins, New York, pp 49–62
79. Knuppel L, Linde K (2004) Adverse effects of St. John's wort: a systematic review. J Clin Psychiatry 65:1470–1479
80. Rodriguez-Landa JF, Contreras CM (2003) A review of clinical and experimental observations about antidepressant actions and side effects produced by Hypericum perforatum extracts. Phytomedicine 10:688–699
81. Kasper S, Gastpar M, Müller WE et al (2010) Efficacy and safety of silexan, a new, orally administered lavender oil preparation, in subthreshold anxiety disorder – evidence from clinical trials. Wien Med Wochenschr 160:547–556
82. Cavanagh H, Wilkinson J (2005) Lavender essential oil: a review. Austr Infect Coun 10:35–37. Available at: http://www.publish.csiro.au/?act=view_file&file_id=HI05035.pdf. Accessed May 1, 2012
83. Bilia AR, Gallon S, Vincieri FF (2002) Kava-kava and anxiety: growing knowledge about the efficacy and safety. Life Sci 70:2581–2597
84. Scherer J (1998) Kava-kava extract in anxiety disorders: an outpatient observational study. Adv Ther 15:261–269
85. Boerner RJ, Sommer H, Berger W et al (2003) Kava-Kava extract LI 150 is as effective as Opipramol and Buspirone in Generalised Anxiety Disorder – an 8-week randomized, double-blind multi-centre clinical trial in 129 out-patients. Phytomedicine 10:38–49
86. Pittler MH, Ernst E (2003) Kava extract for treating anxiety. Cochrane Database Syst Rev (1):CD003383
87. Witte S, Loew D, Gaus W (2005) Meta-analysis of the efficacy of the acetonic kava-kava extract WS1490 in patients with non-psychotic anxiety disorders. Phytother Res 19:183–188
88. Gounder R (2006) Kava consumption and its health effects. Pac Health Dialog 13:131–135
89. Stevinson C, Huntley A, Ernst E (2002) A systematic review of the safety of kava extract in the treatment of anxiety. Drug Saf 25:251–261
90. Liao JF, Jan YM, Huang SY et al (1995) Evaluation with receptor binding assay on the water extracts of ten CNS-active Chinese herbal drugs. Proc Natl Sci Coun Repub China 19:151–158
91. Mizowaki M, Toriizuka K, Hanawa T (2001) Anxiolytic effect of Kami-Shoyo-San (TJ-24) in mice: possible mediation of neurosteroid synthesis. Life Sci 69:2167–2177
92. Sugiyama K, Muteki T, Kano T (1996) The Japanese herbal medicine 'saikokeishi- to' activates GABAA receptors of rat sensory neurons in culture. Neurosci Lett 216:147–150
93. Zhang Y, Han M, Liu Z, et al. (2012) Chinese herbal formula xiao yao san for treatment of depression: a systematic review of randomized controlled trials. Evid Based Complement Alternat Med 2012;931636. Available at: http://www.ncbi.nlm.nih.gov/pmc/articles/PMC3159992/pdf/ECAM2012-931636.pdf
94. Glen AIM, Ross BM (2004) Eicosanoids in the central nervous system. In: Curtis-Prior P (ed) The eicosanoids. Wiley, London, pp 210–220

95. Stahl SM (2000) Essential psychopharmacology: neuroscientific basis and practical applications, 2nd edn. Cambridge University Press, Cambridge
96. Lin PY, Huang SY, Su KP (2010) A meta-analytic review of polyunsaturated fatty acid compositions in patients with depression. Biol Psychiatry 68:140–147
97. Green P, Hermesh H, Monselise A et al (2006) Red cell membrane omega-3 fatty acids are decreased in nondepressed patients with social anxiety disorder. Eur Neuropsychopharmacol 16:107–113
98. Ross BM (2009) Omega-3 polyunsaturated fatty acids and anxiety disorders. Prostaglandins Leukot Essent Fatty Acids 81:309–312
99. Yehuda S, Rabinovitz S, Mostofsky DI (2005) Mixture of essential fatty acids lowers test anxiety. Nutr Neurosci 8:265–267
100. Appleton KM, Rogers PJ, Ness AR (2010) Updated systematic review and meta-analysis of the effects of n-3 long-chain polyunsaturated fatty acids on depressed mood. Am J Clin Nutr 91:757–770
101. Bloch MH, Hannestad J (2011) Omega-3 fatty acids for the treatment of depression: systematic review and meta-analysis. Mol Psychiatry Sep 20. doi:10.1038/mp.2011.100. [Epub ahead of print]
102. Kraguljac NV, Montori VM, Pavuluri M et al (2009) Efficacy of omega-3 fatty acids in mood disorders—a systematic review and metaanalysis. Psychopharmacol Bull 42:39–54
103. Martins JG, Bentsen H, Puri BK (2012) Eicosapentaenoic acid appears to be the key omega-3 fatty acid component associated with efficacy in major depressive disorder: a critique of Bloch and Hannestad and updated meta-analysis. Mol Psychiatry Apr 10. doi:10.1038/mp.2012.25. [Epub ahead of print]
104. Ross BM, Seguin J, Sieswerda LE (2007) Omega-3 fatty acids as treatments for mental illness: which disorder and which fatty acid? Lipids Health Dis 6:21
105. Freeman MP, Fava M, Lake J et al (2010) Complementary and alternative medicine in major depressive disorder: the American psychiatric association task force report. J Clin Psychiatry 71(6):669–681
106. Nahas R, Sheikh O (2011) Complementary and alternative medicine for the treatment of major depressive disorder. Can Fam Physician 57:659–663
107. Gruppo Italiano per lo Studio della Sopravvivenza nell'Infarto miocardico (GISSI) (1999) Dietary supplementation with n-3 polyunsaturated fatty acids and vitamin E after myocardial infarction: results of the GISSI-Prevenzione trial. Lancet 354:447–455
108. Freeman MP, Hibbeln JR, Wisner KL et al (2006) Omega-3 fatty acids: evidence basis for treatment and future research in psychiatry. J Clin Psychiatry 67:1954–1967
109. Montgomery P, Richardson AJ (2008) Omega-3 fatty acids for bipolar disorder. Cochrane Database Syst Rev (2):CD005169
110. Alpert JE, Papakostas GI, Mischoulon D (2008) One-carbon metabolism and the treatment of depression: roles of S-adenosyl-l-methionine and folate. In: Mischoulon D, Rosenbaum J (eds) Natural medications for psychiatric disorders: considering the alternatives, 2nd edn. Lippincott Williams and Wilkins, Philadelphia, pp 68–83
111. Bottiglieri T, Hyland K (1994) S-adenosylmethionine levels in psychiatric and neurological disorders: a review. Acta Neurol Scand Suppl 154:19–26
112. Bottiglieri T, Godfrey P, Flynn T et al (1990) Cerebrospinal fluid S-adenosylmethionine in depression and dementia: effects of treatment with parenteral and oral S-adenosylmethionine. J Neurol Neurosurg Psychiatry 53:1096–1098
113. Maj M, Zizolfi S, Del Vecchio M (1981) Blood levels of S-adenosylmethionine in unmedicated schizophrenic and depressive patients. Neuropsychobiology 7:188–191
114. Papakostas GI (2009) Evidence for S-adenosyl-L-methionine (SAM-e) for the treatment of major depressive disorder. J Clin Psychiatry 70(Suppl 5):18–22
115. Williams AL, Girard C, Jui D, Sabina A, Katz DL (2005) S-adenosylmethionine (SAMe) as treatment for depression: a systematic review. Clin Invest Med 28:132–139
116. Bressa GM (1994) S-adenosyl-l-methionine (SAMe) as antidepressant: meta-analysis of clinical studies. Acta Neurol Scand Suppl 154:7–14

117. Natural Medicines Comprehensive Database (2009) SAMe monograph. Available at: http://www.naturaldatabase.com/(S(e4rus0neempxru55g2cipjqg))/nd/Search.aspx?cs=&s=ND&pt=100&id=786&ds=&name=SAMe. Accessed 1 May 2012
118. Bhagra S, Nippoldt TB, Nair KS (2008) Dehydroepiandrosterone in adrenal insufficiency and ageing. Curr Opin Endocrinol Curr Opin Endocrinol Diabetes Obes 15:239–243
119. Maninger N, Wolkowitz OM, Reus VI et al (2009) Neurobiological and neuropsychiatric effects of dehydroepiandrosterone (DHEA) and DHEA sulfate (DHEAS). Front Neuroendocrinol 30:65–91
120. Pérez-Neri I, Méndez-Sánchez I, Montes S et al (2008) Acute ehydroepiandrosterone treatment exerts different effects on dopamine and serotonin turnover ratios in the rat corpus striatum and nucleus accumbens. Prog Neuropsychopharmacol Biol Psychiatry 32:1584–1589
121. Pérez-Neri I, Montes S, Ríos C (2009) Inhibitory effect of dehydroepiandrosterone on brain monoamine oxidase activity: in vivo and in vitro studies. Life Sci 85:652–656
122. Markianos M, Tripodianakis J, Sarantidis D et al (2007) Plasma testosterone and dehydroepiandrosterone sulfate in male and female patients with dysthymic disorder. J Affect Disord 101:255–258
123. Morsink LF, Vogelzangs N, Nicklas BJ et al (2007) Health ABC study. Associations between sex steroid hormone levels and depressive symptoms in elderly men and women: results from the health ABC study. Psychoneuroendocrinology 32:874–883
124. Assies J, Visser I, Nicolson NA et al (2004) Elevated salivary dehydroepiandrosterone-sulfate but normal cortisol levels in medicated depressed patients: preliminary findings. Psychiatry Res 128:117–122
125. Goodyer IM, Herbert J, Tamplin A (2003) Psychoendocrine antecedents of persistent first-episode major depression in adolescents: a community-based longitudinal enquiry. Psychol Med 33:601–610
126. Morrison MF, Freeman EW, Lin H et al (2011) Higher DHEA-S (dehydroepiandrosterone sulfate) levels are associated with depressive symptoms during the menopausal transition: results from the PENN ovarian aging study. Arch Womens Ment Health 14:375–382
127. Morrison MF, Ten Have T, Freeman EW et al (2001) DHEA-S levels and depressive symptoms in a cohort of African American and Caucasian women in the late reproductive years. Biol Psychiatry 50:705–711
128. Gill J, Vythilingam M, Page GG (2008) Low cortisol, high DHEA, and high levels of stimulated TNF-alpha, and IL-6 in women with PTSD. J Trauma Stress 21:530–539
129. Hsiao CC (2006) Positive correlation between anxiety severity and plasma levels of dehydroepiandrosterone sulfate in medication-free patients experiencing a major episode of depression. Psychiatry Clin Neurosci 60:746–750
130. Bloch M, Schmidt PJ, Danaceau MA, Adams LF, Rubinow DR (1999) Dehydroepiandrosterone treatment of midlife dysthymia. Biol Psychiatry 45:1533–1541
131. Schmidt PJ, Daly RC, Block M et al (2005) Dehydroepiandrosterone monotherapy in midlife-onset major and minor depression. Arch Gen Psychiatry 62:154–162
132. Wolkowitz OM, Reus VI, Roberts E et al (1997) Dehydroepiandrosterone (DHEA) treatment of depression. Biol Psychiatry 41:311–318
133. Natural Medicines Comprehensive Database. DHEA monograph (2009) Available at: http://www.naturaldatabase.com/(S(e4rus0neempxru55g2cipjqg))/nd/Search.aspx?cs=&s=ND&pt=100&id=331&ds=&name=DHEA. Accessed 1 May 2012
134. Natural Standard. DHEA professional monograph (2009) Available at: http://www.naturalstandard.com/monographs/monoframeset.asp?monograph=/monographs/herbssupplements/dhea.asp%3Fprintversion%3Dtrue. Accessed 1 May 2012
135. Shaw K, Turner J, Del Mar C (2002) Are tryptophan and 5-hydroxytryptophan effective treatments for depression? A meta-analysis. Aust N Z J Psychiatry 36:488–491
136. Booij L, Van der Does AJ, Haffmans PM et al (2005) The effects of high-dose and low-dose tryptophan depletion on mood and cognitive functions of remitted depressed patients. J Psychopharmacol 19:267–275

137. Feder A, Skipper J, Blair JR et al (2011) Tryptophan depletion and emotional processing in healthy volunteers at high risk for depression. Biol Psychiatry 69:804–807
138. Turner EH, Loftis JM, Blackwell AD (2006) Serotonin a la carte: supplementation with the serotonin precursor 5-hydroxytryptophan. Pharmacol Ther 109:325–338
139. Kahn RS, Westenberg HG, Verhoeven WM et al (1987) Effect of a serotonin precursor and uptake inhibitor in anxiety disorders; a double-blind comparison of 5-hydroxytryptophan, clomipramine and placebo. Int Clin Psychopharmacol 2:33–45
140. Farah A (2009) The role of l-methylfolate in depressive disorders. CNS Spectr 14(1 Suppl 2):2–7
141. Bottiglieri T (2005) Homocysteine and folate metabolism in depression. Prog Neuro-Psychopharmacol Biol Psychiatry 29:1103–1112
142. Coppen A, Bolander-Gouaille C (2005) Treatment of depression: time to consider folic acid and vitamin B12. J Psychopharmacol 19:59–65
143. Ng TP, Feng L, Niti M et al (2009) Folate, vitamin B12, homocysteine, and depressive symptoms in a population sample of older Chinese adults. J Am Geriatr Soc 57:871–876
144. Kamphuis MH, Geerlings MI, Grobbee DE et al (2008) Dietary intake of B(6-9-12) vitamins, serum homocysteine levels and their association with depressive symptoms: the Zutphen elderly study. Eur J Clin Nutr 62:939–945
145. Watanabe H, Suganuma N, Hayashi A, Hirowatari Y, Hirowatari T, Ohsawa M (2010) No relation between folate and homocysteine levels and depression in early pregnant women. Biosci Trends 4:344–350
146. Hvas AM, Juul S, Bech P et al (2004) Vitamin B6 level is associated with symptoms of depression. Psychother Psychosom 73:340–343
147. Skarupski KA, Tangney C, Li H et al (2010) Longitudinal association of vitamin B-6, folate, and vitamin B-12 with depressive symptoms among older adults over time. Am J Clin Nutr 92:330–335
148. Leiva DB (1990) The neurochemistry of mania: a hypothesis of etiology and rationale for treatment. Prog Neuropsychopharmacol Biol Psychiatry 14:423–429
149. DelBello MP, Cecil KM, Adler CM et al (2006) Neurochemical effects of olanzapine in first hospitalization manic adolescents: a proton magnetic resonance spectroscopy study. Neuropsychopharmacology 31:1264–1273
150. Kumar A, Thomas A, Lavretsky H et al (2002) Frontal white matter biochemical abnormalities in late-life major depression detected with proton magnetic resonance spectroscopy. Am J Psychiatry 159:603–636
151. Steingard RJ, Yurgelun-Todd DA, Hennen J et al (2000) Increased orbitofrontal cortex levels of choline in depressed adolescents as detected by in vivo proton magnetic resonance spectroscopy. Biol Psychiatry 48:1053–1061
152. Bjelland I, Tell GS, Vollset SE et al (2009) Choline in anxiety and depression: the Hordaland health study. Am J Clin Nutr 90:1056–1060
153. Coplan JD, Mathew SJ, Mao X et al (2006) Decreased choline and creatine concentrations in centrum semiovale in patients with generalized anxiety disorder: relationship to IQ and early trauma. Psychiatry Res 147:27–39
154. Fava M, Mischoulon D (2009) Folate in depression: efficacy, safety, differences in formulations, and clinical issues. J Clin Psychiatry 70(suppl 5):12–17
155. Morris DW, Madhukar HT, Rush AJ (2008) Folate and unipolar depression. J Altern Comp Med 14:277–285
156. Oren DA, Teicher MH, Schwartz PJ et al (1994) A controlled trial of cyanocobalamin (vitamin B12) in the treatment of winter seasonal affective disorder. J Affect Disord 32:197–200
157. Williams AL, Cotter A, Sabina A et al (2005) The role for vitamin B-6 as treatment for depression: a systematic review. Fam Pract 22:532–537
158. Bell IR, Edman JS, Morrow FD et al (1992) Brief communication. Vitamin B1, B2, and B6 augmentation of tricyclic antidepressant treatment in geriatric depression with cognitive dysfunction. J Am Coll Nutr 11:159–163

159. Lazarou C, Kapsou M (2010) The role of folic acid in prevention and treatment of depression: An overview of existing evidence and implications for practice. Comp Ther Clin Pract 16:161–166
160. Christakos S, Dhawan P, Benn B et al (2007) Vitamin D: molecular mechanism of action. Ann N Y Acad Sci 1116:340–348
161. Parker G, Brotchie H (2011) ‘D’ for depression: any role for vitamin D? ‘Food for thought’ II. Acta Psychiatr Scand 124:243–249
162. Gaines S (2005) The saddest season. Minnesota Med 88:25–32
163. Obradovic D, Gronemeyer H, Lutz B et al (2006) Cross-talk of vitamin D and glucocorticoids in hippocampal cells. J Neurochem 96:500–509
164. Ganji V, Milone C, Cody MM et al (2010) Serum vitamin D concentrations are related to depression in young adult US population: the third national health and nutrition examination survey. Int Arch Med 3:29
165. Hoang MT, Defina LF, Willis BL et al (2011) Association between low serum 25-hydroxyvitamin D and depression in a large sample of healthy adults: the cooper center longitudinal study. Mayo Clin Proc 86:1050–1055
166. Hoogendijk WJ, Lips P, Dik MG et al (2008) Depression is associated with decreased 25-hydroxyvitamin D and increased parathyroid hormone levels in older adults. Arch Gen Psychiatry 65:508–512
167. Bertone-Johnson ER (2009) Vitamin D, and the occurrence of depression: causal association or circumstantial evidence? Nutr Rev 67:481–492
168. Chan R, Chan D, Woo J et al (2011) Association between serum 25-hydroxyvitamin D and psychological health in older Chinese men in a cohort study. J Affect Disord 130:251–259
169. Berk M, Sanders KM, Pasco JA et al (2007) Vitamin D deficiency may play a role in depression. Med Hypotheses 69:1316–1319
170. Nanri A, Mizoue T, Matsushita Y et al (2009) Association between serum 25-hydroxyvitamin D and depressive symptoms in Japanese: analysis by survey season. Eur J Clin Nutr 63:1444–1447
171. Milaneschi Y, Shardell M, Corsi AM et al (2010) Serum 25-hydroxyvitamin D and depressive symptoms in older women and men. J Clin Endocrinol Metab 95:3225–3233
172. Heaney RP (2008) Vitamin D: criteria for safety and efficacy. Nutr Rev 66(10 Suppl 2):S178–S181
173. Penckofer S, Kouba J, Byrn M et al (2010) Vitamin D and depression: where is all the sunshine? Issues Ment Health Nurs 31:385–393
174. Barkai AI, Dunner DL, Gross HA et al (1978) Reduced myo-inositol levels in cerebrospinal fluid from patients with affective disorder. Biol Psychiatry 13:65–72
175. Coupland NJ, Ogilvie CJ, Hegadoren KM et al (2005) Decreased prefrontal myoinositol in major depressive disorder. Biol Psychiatry 57:1526–1534
176. Shimon H, Agam G, Belmaker RH et al (1997) Reduced frontal cortex inositol levels in postmortem brain of suicide victims and patients with bipolar disorder. Am J Psychiatry 154:1148–1150
177. Levine J, Kurtzman L, Rapoport A et al (1996) CSF inositol does not predict antidepressant response to inositol. J Neural Transm 103:1457–1462
178. Einat H, Belmaker RH (2001) The effects of inositol treatment in animal models of psychiatric disorders. J Affect Disord 62:113–121
179. Kofman O, Einat H, Cohen H et al (2000) The anxiolytic effect of chronic inositol depends on the baseline level of anxiety. J Neural Transm 107:241–253
180. Levine J, Barak Y, Gonzalves M et al (1995) Double-blind, controlled trial of inositol treatment of depression. Am J Psychiatry 152:792–794
181. Sartori SB, Whittle N, Hetzenauer A et al (2012) Magnesium deficiency induces anxiety and HPA axis dysregulation: modulation by therapeutic drug treatment. Neuropharmacology 62: 304–312

182. Haddad JJ (2005) N-methyl-D-aspartate (NMDA) and the regulation of mitogenactivated protein kinase (MAPK) signaling pathways: a revolving neurochemical axis for therapeutic intervention? Prog Neurobiol 77:252–282
183. Murck H (2002) Magnesium and affective disorders. Nutr Neurosci 5:375–389
184. Murck H, Steiger A (1998) Mg2þ reduces ACTH secretion and enhances spindle power without changing delta power during sleep in men—possible therapeutic implications. Psychopharmacology (Berl) 137:247–252
185. Siwek M, Wróbel A, Dudek D et al (2005) The role of copper and magnesium in the pathogenesis and treatment of affective disorders. Psychiatr Pol 39:911–920
186. Eby GA, Eby KL (2006) Rapid recovery from major depression using magnesium treatment. Med Hypotheses 67:362–370
187. Eby GA, Eby KL (2010) Magnesium for treatment-resistant depression: a review and hypothesis. Med Hypoth 74:649–660
188. Schäfer HL, Schafer H, Schneider W et al (1955) Sedative action of extract combination of *Eschscholtzia California* and *Corydalis cava*. Arzneimittelforschung 45:124–126
189. Walker AF, Marakis G, Morris AP et al (2002) Promising hypotensive effect of hawthorn extract: a randomised doubleblind pilot study of mild, essential hypotension. Phytother Res 16:48–54
190. Delva P (2003) Magnesium and cardiac arrhythmias. Mol Aspects Med 24(1–3):53–62
191. Hambidge KM, Krebs NF (2007) Zinc deficiency: a special challenge. J Nutr 137:1101–1105
192. Takeda A, Tamano H (2009) Insight into zinc signaling from dietary zinc deficiency. Brain Res Rev 62:33–44
193. Suh SW, Won SJ, Hamby AM et al (2009) Decreased brain zinc availability reduces hippocampal neurogenesis in mice and rats. J Cereb Blood Flow Metab 29:1579–1588
194. Revest JM, Dupret D, Koehl M et al (2009) Adult hippocampal neurogenesis is involved in anxiety-related behaviors. Mol Psychiatry 14:959–967
195. Sahay A, Hen R (2007) Adult hippocampal neurogenesis in depression. Nat Neurosci 10:1110–1115
196. Dziedzicka-Wasylewska M, Rogóż Z, Solich J et al (2002) Effect of joint administration of imipramine and amantadine on binding of [3H]7-OH-DPAT to dopamine D3 receptors in peripheral blood lymphocytes of the patients with drug-resistant unipolar depression. Pol J Pharmacol 54:703–706
197. Pittenger C, Coric V, Banasr M et al (2008) Riluzole in the treatment of mood and anxiety disorders. CNS Drugs 22:761–786
198. Cichy A, Sowa-Kućma M, Legutko B et al (2009) Zinc-induced adaptive changes in NMDA/glutamatergic and serotonergic receptors. Pharmacol Rep 61:1184–1191
199. Szewczyk B, Poleszak E, Wlaź P et al (2009) The involvement of serotonergic system in the antidepressant effect of zinc in the forced swim test. Prog Neuropsychopharmacol Biol Psychiatry 33:323–329
200. Nowak G, Legutko B, Szewczyk B et al (2004) Zinc treatment induces cortical brain-derived neurotrophic factor gene expression. Eur J Pharmacol 492:57–59
201. Shimizu E, Hashimoto K, Okamura N et al (2003) Alterations of serum levels of brain-derived neurotrophic factor (BDNF) in depressed patients with or without antidepressants. Biol Psychiatry 54:70–75
202. Franco JL, Posser T, Brocardo PS et al (2008) Involvement of glutathione, ERK1/2 phosphorylation and BDNF expression in the antidepressant-like effect of zinc in rats. Behav Brain Res 188:316–323
203. Schmidt HD, Duman RS (2007) The role of neurotrophic factors in adult hippocampal neurogenesis, antidepressant treatments and animal models of depressive-like behaviour. Beh Pharmacol 18:391–418
204. Slamon ND, Pentreath VW (2000) Antioxidant defense against antidepressants in C6 and 1321N1 cells. Chem Biol Interact 127:181–199

205. Cope EC, Levenson CW (2010) Role of zinc in the development and treatment of mood disorders. Curr Opin Clin Nutr Metab Care 13:685–689
206. Joshi M, Akhtar M, Najmi A, et al (2012) Effect of zinc in animal models of anxiety, depression and psychosis. Hum Exp Toxicol May 1. [Epub ahead of print]
207. Salimi S, Kianpoor M, Abassi MR et al (2008) Lower total serum protein, albumin and zinc in depression in an Iranian population. J Med Sci 8:587–590
208. Siwek M, Dudek D, Schlegel-Zawadzka M et al (2010) Serum zinc level in depressed patients during zinc supplementation of imipramine treatment. J Affect Disord 126:447–452
209. Fosmire GJ (1990) Zinc toxicity. Am J Clin Nutr 51:225–227
210. Shuttleworth CW, Weiss JH (2011) Zinc: new clues to diverse roles in brain ischemia. Trends Pharmacol Sci 32:480–486
211. Sommerville RB, Baloh RH (2011) Anemia, paresthesias, and gait ataxia in a 57-year-old denture wearer. Clin Chem 57:1103–1106
212. Fernstrom JD (2005) Branched-chain amino acids and brain function. J Nutr 135 (6 Suppl):1539S–1546S
213. Markus CR (2008) Dietary amino acids and brain serotonin function; implications for stress-related affective changes. Neuromolecular Med 10:247–258
214. Altamura C, Maes M, Dai J et al (1995) Plasma concentrations of excitatory amino acids, serine, glycine, taurine and histidine in major depression. Eur Neuropsychopharmacol 5(Suppl):71–75
215. Maes M, Verkerk R, Vandoolaeghe E et al (1998) Serum levels of excitatory amino acids, serine, glycine, histidine, threonine, taurine, alanine and arginine in treatment-resistant depression: modulation by treatment with antidepressants and prediction of clinical responsivity. Acta Psychiatr Scand 97:302–308
216. Bella R, Biondi R, Raffaele R et al (1990) Effect of acetyl-L-carnitine on geriatric patients suffering from dysthymic disorders. Int J Clin Pharmacol Res 10:355–360
217. Garzya G, Corallo D, Fiore A et al (1990) Evaluation of the effects of L-acetylcarnitine on senile patients suffering from depression. Drugs Exp Clin Res 16:101–106
218. Tempesta E, Casella L, Pirrongelli C et al (1987) L-acetylcarnitine in depressed elderly subjects. A cross-over study vs placebo. Drugs Exp Clin Res 13:417–423
219. Zanardi R, Smeraldi E (2006) A double-blind, randomised, controlled clinical trial of acetyl-L-carnitine vs. amisulpride in the treatment of dysthymia. Eur Neuropsychopharmacol 16:281–287
220. Berk M, Ng F, Dean O et al (2008) Glutathione: a novel treatment target in psychiatry. Trends Pharmacol Sci 29:346–351
221. Bilici M, Efe H, Köroğlu MA et al (2001) Antioxidative enzyme activities and lipid peroxidation in major depression: alterations by antidepressant treatments. J Affect Disord 64:43–51
222. Lafleur DL, Pittenger C, Kelmendi B et al (2006) N-acetylcysteine augmentation in serotonin reuptake inhibitor refractory obsessive-compulsive disorder. Psychopharmacology (Berl) 184:254–256
223. Simpson JS, Crawford SG, Goldstein ET et al (2011) Systematic review of safety and tolerability of a complex micronutrient formula used in mental health. BMC Psychiatry 11:62
224. ClinicalTrials.gov (n.d.). Clinical trial of a nutritional supplement in adults with bipolar disorder. Investigators: Kaplan BJ, Goldstein E. Study registered in April 2005, updated to August 2011. Available at: http://www.clinicaltrials.gov/ct/show/NCT00109577?order=1. Accessed 1 May 2012

Chapter 12
Obsessive-Compulsive Syndromes in Schizophrenia: A Case for Polypharmacy?

Frederike Schirmbeck and Mathias Zink

Abstract Obsessive-compulsive symptoms (OCS) are often associated with schizophrenia. So far no single pathogenetic theory was able to convincingly explain this co-occurrence, due to heterogeneous subgroups within the comorbid sample. Based on long-term case observations, one hypothesis assumes that second-onset OCS in the course of schizophrenia might be a side effect of second generation antipsychotics (SGA), most importantly clozapine (CLZ). This review summarizes the supporting epidemiological and pharmacological evidence and defines several open questions regarding pathogenetic influence of genetic factors, differential neurocognitive profiles, affective comorbidity and interactions of serotonergic, dopaminergic and glutamatergic neurotransmission. Treatment of comorbid patients might involve cognitive behavioural therapy (CBT) with graduated exposure and response prevention (ERP). However, so far no controlled clinical trials confirmed efficacy and tolerability of psychotherapy for this specific indication. Strategies of polypharmacy are often preferred, although based on similarly scarce systematic evidence. The combination of amisulpride or aripipirazole with pro-obsessive, antiserotonergic antipsychotics in minimally sufficient dose levels yielded favourable effects. Adding serotonergic antidepressants or mood stabilizers resemble augmentation approaches. In perspective, individual psychotherapeutic and pharmacological strategies have to be further evaluated. Head to head trials of different approaches as well as combinations of the mentioned strategies promise therapeutic progress and will help to improve treatment options for schizophrenia patients suffering from comorbid OCS.

F. Schirmbeck, Dipl.-Psych. • M. Zink, M.D. (✉)
Department of Psychiatry and Psychotherapy, Medical Faculty Mannheim,
Central Institute of Mental Health, University of Heidelberg, Mannheim, Germany
e-mail: frederike.schirmbeck@zi-mannheim.de; mathias.zink@zi-mannheim.de

M.S. Ritsner (ed.), *Polypharmacy in Psychiatry Practice, Volume II: Use of Polypharmacy in the "Real World"*, DOI 10.1007/978-94-007-5799-8_12,

Abbreviations

AD	Antidepressant
AMS	Amisulpride
APZ	Aripiprazole
ARMS	At risk mental state
CBT	Cognitive behavioural therapy
CDSS	Calgary depression scale for schizophrenia
CGI-S	Clinical global impression, severity of illness
CLZ	Clozapine
ERP	Exposure and response prevention
FEP	First episode schizophrenic patients
FGA	First generation antipsychotics
HAL	Haloperidole
OCD	Obsessive compulsive disorder
OCS	Obsessive compulsive symptoms
OLZ	Olanzapine
PANSS	Positive and negative syndrome scale
PP	Per protocol
PSP	Personal and social performance scale
RCT	Randomised *placebo*-controlled trial
SA	Schizoaffective disorder
SANS	Scale for the assessment of negative symptoms
SCH	Schizophrenia
SGA	Second generation antipsychotics
SIPS	Structured interview for prodromal symptoms
SZ	Schizophrenia and schizophrenia spectrum disorders
UHR	Ultra high risk
Y	Years
YBOCS	Yale-Brown-Obsessive-Compulsive Scale

12.1 Introduction

The relations between schizophrenia and obsessive compulsive symptoms (OCS) have interested scientists since Carl Friedrich Otto Westphal in the nineteenth century [1]. Authors in the middle of the twentieth century even assumed protective effects of comorbid OCS against psychotic desintegration and beneficial consequences on the course of schizophrenia [1–5]. Indeed, somatic obsessions and hoarding might compensate psychotic anxiety and disorganization [6]. However, the general assumption of an antagonism between OCS and schizophrenia has been disproved by larger epidemiological investigations. Comorbid OCS in schizophrenia is linked with higher and often treatment resistant global, positive, and negative psychotic symptoms [7], greater service utilization [8], heightened levels of anxiety and depression [9], resulting in poorer social and vocational function [10–13]. In summary, these additional impairments lead to a less favourable overall prognosis [5]. Several important aspects need further scientific attention regarding the comorbidity of schizophrenia and OCS: The interplay of pathogenetic factors has not been unravelled and only very limited evidence concerning therapeutic treatment approaches exists, since controlled clinical trials are still missing [14].

This review summarizes the current state of pathogenetic theories and therapeutic implications with a main focus on pharmacological augmentation and combination strategies.

12.2 Epidemiology: Prevalence of Obsessive-Compulsive Symptoms in Schizophrenia

Schizophrenia patients have a high lifetime risk for comorbid OCS. Recent epidemiological investigations estimate that about 12% of schizophrenia patients also fulfil the criteria for obsessive compulsive disorder, while almost every fourth patient reports comorbid OCS [9, 14–19]. In contrast, primary OCD-patients most frequently present comorbid affective or anxiety disorders and only 1.7% suffer from comorbid psychotic symptoms [20]. On the level of clinical psychopathology, the differentiation between obsessions and delusions merits high importance: Obsessions are recurrent, intrusive, ego-dystonic thoughts that are accompanied by the insight that they are senseless, whereas delusions carry subjective conviction and cannot be affected by rational arguments or evidence to the contrary. Comorbid OCS in schizophrenia is associated with pronounced and treatment resistant positive and negative symptoms [21], in particular if recent concepts of response, remission and recovery [22, 23] are integrated.

12.3 Pathogenesis: Heterogeneous Subgroups

Specific neurobiological factors seem to dispose schizophrenia patients to comorbid OCS. So far, no single theory was able to convincingly explain the observed high comorbidity rates. It might be taken for granted that several different factors interact and the comorbid sample comprises heterogeneous subgroups [24]. A small minority of patients might coincidently suffer from both schizophrenia and OCS, representing random associations of two common disorders. Within the spectrum of OCD, the concept of "schizotypic OCD" has been described [25, 26] integrating the assumption that primary OCD-patients present cognitions that migrate on a spectrum between obsessions and delusions. A similar concept of "obsessions without insight" was integrated into current diagnostic systems making the differentiation between obsessions and delusions more difficult. OCD-patients without insight might represent a subgroup with genetic, phenotypic and therapeutic vicinity to the schizophrenia-spectrum [27, 28]. Using stepwise regression models, Guillem et al. [6] showed positive correlations between delusions and obsessions, as well as hallucinations and compulsions suggesting that common pathogenetic mechanisms should be considered. Within the spectrum of schizophrenia, a so-called "schizo-obsessive" subtype of psychosis has been proposed [29–33]; specific subtypes of OCS were perceived as part of the basic symptom cluster in the early course of schizophrenia [34, 35]. Furthermore, catatonic symptoms of schizophrenia overlap with the obsessive-compulsive phenotype [36]. This circumstance limits the precision of psychometric scales such as the catatonia rating scale (CRS) [37] and the Yale-Brown-Obsessive-Compulsive Scale (YBOCS) [38, 39]. However, descriptions of the natural long-term course of schizophrenia, for instance published by Karl Leonhard [40], allow clear discrimination between OCS and catatonic symptoms most importantly in patients with so-called "manieristic catatonia" and do not support the view that OCS might be a part of the residual state.

The summarized pathogenetic concepts are matters of current discussion. For scientific purposes, it seems strongly recommendable to use a dimensional rather than a categorial perspective on OCS and psychotic symptoms and to assume a certain degree of heterogeneity within the comorbid sample. Progress in pathogenetic understanding appears very difficult until homogeneous subgroups are defined for neurobiological research. Based on the expected results of these investigations the development of specific therapeutic interventions might be possible. A remarkably simple clinical assessment of three important events allows a rough, but useful subgrouping of comorbid patients:

1. When did the first psychotic manifestation occur?
2. When was antipsychotic treatment initiated?
3. When did OCS develop or showed – if pre-existing – a marked aggravation?

12.4 Second-Onset OCS Induced by Antiserotonergic Antipsychotics

Applying the above mentioned characterization by clinical events, another subgroup of comorbid patients can be identified: These patients experienced the *de novo*-onset of OCS or a marked aggravation of OCS severity after treatment initiation with second generation antipsychotics (SGA), most importantly clozapine (CLZ), representing an 1-2-3-order of the above mentioned events. This clinical observation is linked to SGAs and has rarely been reported under first generation antipsychotics (FGA). Noteworthy, SGAs carry the important pharmacodynamic feature of balanced antidopaminergic and antiserotonergic properties that markedly exceed 5HT-receptor blockade by FGAs [41, 42]. Starting with the observations of Baker et al. [43] and

De Haan et al. [44] the hypothesis of SGA-induced OCS was formulated [45]. Since then several studies support this assumption, especially for the association between CLZ treatment and the de-novo occurrence of OCS [24, 46–48].

The pioneer SGA CLZ must be considered a necessary and indispensable part of the antipsychotic armament [49, 50]. In 1988, Kane et al. provided first evidence that CLZ might improve treatment resistant psychoses [51]. Today several investigations [52] including the CATIE-study [53] have demonstrated its superior antipsychotic efficacy in the treatment of refractory schizophrenia. Therefore, CLZ is used as the antipsychotic of first choice in treatment resistant schizophrenia. In addition, the substance embarks important protective effects against suicidal behaviour resulting in low mortality rates of schizophrenia patients as has been documented in the large, naturalistic FIN11-study [54]. However, the *de novo* occurrence or exacerbation of OCS under antipsychotic treatment has most often been observed during the administration of CLZ [24, 45, 47]. Several epidemiological and pharmacological arguments support the assumption of pro-obsessive effects of clozapine (see Tables 12.1 and 12.2). Noteworthy, direct causal interactions remain difficult to proof according to the general criteria suggested by Bradford Hill [71].

12.5 Epidemiological Evidence

Quantitative estimations on OCS comorbidity in schizophrenia vary to a high degree as a consequence of differences in sample characteristics, applied psychometric procedures and diagnostic criteria, as summarized by Mukhopadhaya et al. [18]. Furthermore, a potential publication bias and change of the general awareness of this topic have to be considered. Nevertheless, the careful analysis of epidemiological studies over time leads to several conclusions:

12.5.1 Increase of OCS Prevalence After Market Approval of SGAs

Despite early descriptions on clinical interactions of psychotic disorders and OCS [1], notable concern about this problem arose not before the last decades of the twentieth century [18]. As mentioned above, only a small number of investigations reported comorbidity rates in samples treated with FGA [8, 10, 72, 73]. After market approval of SGAs, most importantly CLZ in the 1970s in Europe and the late 1980s in the USA [49, 74], prevalence estimations of comorbid OCS simultaneously rose up to 30% [9, 15, 17, 18] and the awareness and clinical concern increased. CLZ differed from FGAs due to pharmacodynamic properties as a potent antiserotonergic and weak antidopaminergic agent [41, 42].

Table 12.1 Epidemiological arguments

Argument		References	Number of patients and clinical characterization	Design	Main findings
Increase of prevalence from prodromal states over first episode samples to chronic course of schizophrenia	At risk mental state samples	Shioiri et al. [55]	219 FEP	Retrospective assessment of OCS-prevalence	Before onset of schizophrenia 1.5% had been diagnosed with OCD, and 9.2% showed OCS
		Rubino et al. [56]	197 schizophrenia patients	Retrospective assessment of morbidity before the age of 18	8% of schizophrenic patients suffer from OCD before age of 18
		Niendam et al. [57]	64 UHR-patients	Cross-sectional survey using SIPS and Padua-inventory	14% of UHR patients suffer from OCD according to SCID I, another 6% report OCS (selfrating), none of them experiences conversion into psychosis
		Fontanelle et al. [58]	396 UHR-patients	Cross-sectional and longitudinal assessments of OCS	8.1% of UHR patients suffer from comorbid OCS. 1.9% show persistent OCS
		Bechdolf et al. [59]	135 patients at risk of psychosis	Cross-sectional assessment of OCS	3.7% of at risk patients suffer from OCD according to SCID I
	First episode patients	De Haan et al. [48]	196 FEP	Retrospective chart study	7% of FEPs showed OCS at first manifestation.
		Shioiri et al. [55]	219 FEP	Retrospective assessment of OCS-prevalence	1.5% of FEPs fulfill diagnostic criteria for OCD at first manifestation
		Poyurovsky et al. [60]	50 FEP	Cross-sectional assessment of OCD comorbidity	At first manifestation of psychosis, 14% fulfill criteria for OCD
		Sterk et al. [61]	194 FEP	Cross-sectional assessment of OCS comorbidity	At first manifestation of psychosis, 9.3% show OCS. Criteria for OCD met in 1.5% patients

Schizophrenic patient	Mukhopadhaya et al. [18]	1,972	Review of studies reporting on OCS prevalence in schizophrenia	High variability. Mean prevalence of 22% reviewing data on 1,972 patients
	Buckley et al. [17]	3,656	Review of studies reporting on OCS prevalence in schizophrenia	Mean prevalence of 23%
	Lysaker et al. [9]	Not specified	Review of studies reporting on OCS prevalence in schizophrenia	Amongst schizophrenic patients, more than one third suffers from clinically significant OCS, 10–25% meet diagnostic criteria of OCD
De novo onset or exacerbation of OCS during antipsychotic treatment	Case reports (Zink et al. [62, 63]) and Case series (Englisch et al. [64])	Nine SCH patients	Longitudinal observation of course of illness	First manifestation and start of antipsychotic treatment precede onset of OCS
	De Haan et al. [44]	121 recent-onset SCH patients	Longitudinal observation of course of illness	Emergence or increase of OCS in 1.3% of non-clozapine treated and 20.6% of clozapine-treated patients
	Lykouras et al. [45]	55 SCH patients	Systematic review of published case reports	Until 2003, a *de novo* onset or exacerbation of OCS had been published regarding clozapine (N=30), risperidone (N=16), olanzapine (N=8) and quetiapine (N=1)
	De Haan et al. [48]	200 recent-onset SCH patients	Longitudinal observation of course of illness	Emergence or increase of OCS in 0% of non-clozapine treated and 9.8% of clozapine-treated patients

(continued)

Table 12.1 (continued)

Argument	References	Number of patients and clinical characterization	Design	Main findings
Proportion of SGA-induced OCS within the complete comorbid sample	Lin et al. [65]	CLZ: 102	Cross-sectional: Stratification for CLZ-treatment with or without OCS	Within 39 clozapine-treated patients with OCS, 29 were classified as clozapine-induced
	Lim et al. [66]	Total sample: 209, comorbid subsample: 26	Cross-sectional. Stratification for SZ with or without OCS	Within 26 SGA-associated schizophrenics with OCS, only 3 had a history of transient OCS before the onset of psychosis
	Schirmbeck et al. [67]	CLZ: 26 OLZ: 13	Cross-sectional. Stratification for treatment with SGAs in monotherapy	Within 39 patients, 28 showed OCS, but only 3 reported OCS before or at onset of psychosis

Epidemiological studies show an increase of OCS- and OCD-prevalence during course of illness suggesting the *de novo*-onset of an SGA-induced side effect
FEP first episode schizophrenic patients, *FGA* first generation antipsychotics, *OCD* obsessive compulsive disorder, *OCS* obsessive compulsive symptoms, *OLZ* olanzapine, *SCH* schizophrenia, *SG* second generation antipsychotics, *SIPS* Structured interview for prodromal symptoms, *SZ* schizophrenia and schizophrenia spectrum disorders, *UHR* Ultra high risk

Table 12.2 Pharmacological arguments

Argument	References	Number of patients	Design	Main findings
Association of CLZ with comorbid OCS	Lim et al. [66]	Total sample: 209, comorbid subsample: 26	Cross-sectional. Stratification for SZ with or without OCS	CLZ-treatment in 35.9% of the total sample, but in 76.9% of the comorbid patients
Association of OCS with OLZ or CLZ	Sa et al. [21]	CLZ: 40 HAL: 20	Cross-sectional. Stratification for treatment with CLZ or HAL	Prevalence of OCS 20% (CLZ) vs. 10% (HAL). Higher severity of OCS with CLZ
	Ertugrul et al. [68]	CLZ: 50	Cross-sectional. Stratification of treatment with CLZ	Within 50 patients treated with CLZ, 76% showed OCS. 20% reported retrospectively *de novo* onset and 18% an exacerbation
	Schirmbeck et al. [67]	CLZ: 26 OLZ: 13 AMS: 15 APZ:16	Cross-sectional. Stratification for treatment with SGAs in monotherapy	Prevalence of OCS 71.8% in CLZ or OLZ vs. 9.7% in AMS or APZ. Highest severity of OCS with CLZ
Correlation of OCS with duration of treatment	Lin et al. [65]	CLZ: 102	Cross-sectional: Stratification for CLZ-treatment with or without OCS	Duration of CLZ-treatment significantly longer in CLZ-OCS-patients (82 vs 56 months), no difference in duration of illness
	Schirmbeck et al. [67]	CLZ: 26	Cross-sectional: Stratification for CLZ-monotherapy	Duration of CLZ-treatment correlates positively with OCS severity (YBOCS, $R=0.59$)
Correlation of OCS with CLZ-dosage or plasma concen-tration	Reznik et al. [47]	N=15	Cross-sectional: Stratification for CLZ-therapy	Dosage-related, pro-obsessive influence of CLZ
	Mukhopadhaya et al. [18]	N=59	Cross-sectional: Stratification for CLZ-therapy	Higher CLZ-dosage in patients with comorbid OCS (432 mg/day) than without (351 mg/day)

(continued)

Table 12.2 (continued)

Argument	References	Number of patients	Design	Main findings
	Schirmbeck et al. [67]	CLZ: 26	Cross-sectional: Stratification for CLZ-monotherapy	CLZ-dosage correlates positively with OCS severity (YBOCS, $R = 0.50$)
	Lin et al. [65]	CLZ: 102	Cross-sectional: Stratification for CLZ-treatment with or without OCS	Higher plasma concentrations in CLZ-treated patients with OCS (595 ng/L) than without OCS (434 ng/L)
Improvement after CLZ dose-reduction	Rocha et al. [69]	Three	Longitudinal observation of OCS severity	Reduction of OCS severity after CLZ down-tapering in combination with APZ
	Zink et al. [62]	One	Longitudinal observation of OCS severity	Reduction of OCS severity from YBOCS 24 to 19 after reduction of CLZ from 500 to 250 mg/die and combination with APZ (30 mg)
	Englisch et al. [64]	Seven	Longitudinal observation of OCS severity	Reduction of OCS severity from YBOCS 19 to 12 after reduction of CLZ from 364 to 293 mg/die and combination with APZ (23 mg)
Increase of OCS severity during treatment with CLZ or OLZ	Schirmbeck et al. [70]	75	Longitudinal observation of OCS severity	CLZ progressively aggravates OCS. A significant time effect discriminates betweens groups treated with CLZ/OLZ or AMS/APZ

Pharmacological evidence in favour of an association between clozapine-treatment and OCS
AMS Amisulpride, *APZ* Aripiprazole, *CLZ* Clozapine, *FGA* First generation antipsychotics, *HAL* Haloperidol, *OCS* Obsessive compulsive symptoms, *OLZ* Olanzapine, *SGA* Second generation antipsychotics, *SZ* Schizophrenia and schizophrenia spectrum disorders, *vs* versus, *YBOCS* Yale-Brown-Obsessive-Compulsive Scale

12.5.2 *Increase of OCS Prevalence Between Prodromal Stages, First Manifestation and Chronic Course*

Prevalence estimations of OCS in samples at ultra high risk (UHR) for psychosis [56–59] or in first episode patients (FEP) [60] are considerably lower than in patients with established diagnosis of schizophrenia. The comorbidity rates range from 1.5% [55] or 3.7% [59] in the at risk mental state (ARMS) to 7–14% in FEPs [48, 60, 61]. Even lower comorbidity rates were reported by Shioiri et al. where only three of 219 patients were diagnosed with OCD at onset of psychosis [55]. Similarly in another sample of recent onset psychotic disorders only 1.3% showed OCS under antipsychotic treatment (excluding CLZ) [44]. Low prevalence rates in early stages of the disease markedly contrast with cross-sectional studies of later or mixed disease stages, suggesting that a significant proportion develops OCS during or even as a consequence of antipsychotic treatment.

12.5.3 *Onset of De Novo OCS During Antipsychotic Treatment*

Several case reports [62, 63], cases series [64] and systematic evaluations [44, 45, 48] describe this *de novo* emergence of OCS during the treatment with atypical antipsychotics (see Table 12.1). De Haan et al. reported OCS development within several months after treatment initiation with CLZ in 20.6% of recent-onset patients [44]. In a study by Ertugrul et al. 20% reported new onset of OCS while 18% showed exacerbation of their preexisting symptoms after the initiation of clozapine [68]. Poyurovski et al. estimated that up to 70% of schizophrenics treated with antiserotonergic SGAs such as CLZ, olanzapine or risperidone develop secondary OCS [16], while Lykouras et al. reviewed published data and even reported de-novo OCS in 77% of CLZ treated patients [15, 26]. In line with these results, independent studies reported high proportions of SGA-induced OCS within samples of comorbid patients: 25 of 28 (89%) [67], 29 of 39 (74%) [65] and 23 of 26 (88%) [66].

Extending the perspective from epidemiology to pharmacology, further arguments for pro-obsessive effects of antiserotonergic SGA have to be considered (see Table 12.2 for summary).

12.6 Pharmacological Evidence

12.6.1 *Higher Prevalence of OCS in Samples Treated with CLZ*

The risk for comorbid OCS markedly differs if patients are stratified according to their mode of antipsychotic treatment. While high prevalences of comorbid OCS of up to 76% were reported in clozapine-treated patients [68], these results markedly contrast with lower rates and less severity of OCS in patients treated with the FGA haloperidol (HAL) [21] or other SGAs. Within SGAs, specific pharmacodynamic properties markedly differ, in particular regarding inherent serotonergic blockade, monoaminergic reuptake inhibition or even partial serotonergic agonism [75–79]. The partial dopaminergic and serotonergic agonist aripiprazole per se was associated with an inherent anti-obsessive potency in schizophrenia patients with OCS [62, 64, 80–82], quite similar to amisulpride, a substance with nearly exclusive affinity to dopamine D3/D2 receptors [83, 84]. In a recent cross-sectional study 70 schizophrenia patients under antipsychotic monotherapy were stratified into two groups with either antiserotonergic SGAs (CLZ or olanzapine (OLZ); group I) or mainly dopaminergic SGAs (amisulpride (AMS) or aripiprazole (APZ); group II). The comparison revealed that 71.8% of group-I-patients suffered from OCS while only 9.7% of patients in group-II reported OCS. In group I, 16 of 39 investigated patients (41%) reported YBOCS scores above 16 representing clinically meaningful severity of OCS [67]. Vice versa, a stratification according to presence or absence of comorbid OCS revealed "CLZ treatment" in 76.9% of comorbid patients versus 35.9% in schizophrenia patients without OCS [66]. These results clearly suggest an association between CLZ treatment and comorbid OCS. As a limitation, confounding effects due to the selection of specific SGAs for specific subgroups should be considered.

12.7 Evidence for a Dose-Effect-Relation

In order to gain further evidence in favour of causal interactions between a pharmacological agent and a clinical effect, correlation analyses between the clinical variable and duration of treatment, dosage and serum levels were performed.

12.7.1 Effects of Duration of Treatment with Antiserotonergic SGAS on OCS

Lin et al. [65] compared CLZ-treated patients with and without comorbid OCS and found significantly longer CLZ treatment, despite no difference in duration of illness. In concert with this study, a positive correlation of OCS severity with duration of treatment was found for the subgroup of CLZ treated schizophrenics by Schirmbeck et al. [67]. Similar observations were reported by De Haan et al. [85] regarding the closely related SGA olanzapine, where the severity of OC symptoms significantly correlated with the duration of olanzapine treatment.

12.7.2 Effects of Dosage and Blood Serum Levels of CLZ on OCS Severity

Independent studies were able to demonstrate positive correlations between dose or serum levels of CLZ and severity of OCS [18, 47, 65]. The stratification of schizophrenia patients according to specific SGA treatment revealed positive correlations between the daily dose of CLZ and OCS severity [67].

12.7.3 Reduction of OCS Severity After Reduction of CLZ Treatment Dosage

If CLZ exerts dose-dependent pro-obsessive effects, a reduction of daily dosage might lead to OCS improvement. Indeed, OCS alleviation was reported after dose reduction of CLZ, for instance due to combinations with other SGAs such as aripiprazole [62, 64, 69] (see also Table 12.4). This might be an indirect hint towards a suggested dose-related side effect of CLZ. However, because aripiprazole itself exerts anti-obsessive effects due to its partial dopaminergic and serotonergic agonism, evidence from combination trials is limited.

12.7.4 OCS Aggravate During Treatment with CLZ

A recent longitudinal observation of 75 schizophrenia patients in SGA monotherapy over a period of 12 months revealed differential effects of antipsychotic agents on comorbid obsessive-compulsive symptoms. Repeated measure analyses of variance (ANOVAs) showed significant interaction effects representing differential YBOCS-changes between the two SGA treatment groups (CLZ/OLZ versus AMS/APZ) over time (per protocol sample; PP): $p = 0.006$; last observation carried forward sample: $p = 0.007$). While patients under CLZ/OLZ showed stable or slightly increasing OCS severity, the other group showed further decrease of the initially low OCS [70].

In summary, comorbid OCS in schizophrenia is clearly associated with antiserotonergic SGAs, most importantly CLZ. Published evidence strongly suggests causal interactions. The question arises, if specific characteristics, such as genetic factors (see below), subtype of schizophrenia, stage of the illness, any affective comorbidity or a family history for anxiety disorders might modify the liability to develop OCS during CLZ treatment.

It should be mentioned that conflicting results reporting an alleviation of OCS severity in schizophrenia after the addition of CLZ [95] or after an increase in dosage [45] have been reported. Explanation for these contradicting findings of casuistic observations might lay in mentioned diagnostic difficulties to differentiate between OCS and delusional or catatonic symptoms of schizophrenia and the heterogeneity within comorbid clinical samples. Furthermore, favourable therapeutic effects of antipsychotics in the treatment of primary OCD, exhibiting treatment-resistance to serotonergic antidepressants, should be mentioned [96–99]. Nevertheless, even in treatment-resistant OCD current treatment guidelines do not recommend CLZ as an augmentation strategy.

12.8 Directions of Further Research on OCS in Schizophrenia

12.8.1 *Causality: De Novo OCS as a Side Effect of CLZ?*

Although the reported evidence strongly suggests that substances such as CLZ or OLZ bear an inherent pro-obsessive potency due to pronounced antiserotonergic pharmacodynamic properties, a randomized-controlled trial would be necessary to prove causal interactions [71]. Since ethical and legal conditions preclude this obvious design of a randomized trial involving CLZ, longitudinal observations seem indicated to substantiate hypothesized *de novo* emergence or aggravation of OCS during SGA treatment [24, 44]. So far, two prospective studies focussed on first episode patients and a more general perspective of schizophrenia and OCS comorbidity [11] or reported a rather short follow-up period [85]. Another longitudinal perspective was able to show significant group-specific time-effects of CLZ-treatment on OCS-severity [70].

12.8.2 *Mechanism of Action*

As a neurochemical and functional explanation of obsessions and compulsions, a dysregulation of serotonergic neurotransmission in a network comprising cortical, striatal and thalamic centres has been proposed [100]. Therefore, CLZ might induce OCS due to its strong inherent antiserotonergic properties [49, 50, 101], most importantly the antagonism at 5-HT1C, 5-HT2A and 5HT2C receptors [78, 102, 103]. Corresponding evidence is provided by the therapeutic effects of SSRIs (serotonin specific reuptake inhibitors) and changes of serotonergic neurotransmission after successful cognitive behavioural therapy (CBT) in OCD [104, 105]. In addition, reciprocal interactions of antipsychotics with dopaminergic and serotonergic receptors leading to altered glutamatergic neurotransmission must also be considered [77]. First insight into a specific neurogenetic disposition was provided by Kwon et al. [46]. The independently replicated candidate polymorphism associated with a genetic risk for OCD is located in the gene *SLC1A1* (solute carrier family member 1A1, former nomenclature EAAC1: excitatory amino acid carrier 1) encoding the neuronal glutamate transporter [106–108]. Kwon et al. [46] reported significant associations of specific SNPs (single nucleotide polymorphisms) with the development of

OCS during treatment with SGAs, but a replication approach in a Caucasian sample was unable to confirm these results [109]. Future research should investigate, if polymorphisms in several genes interact resulting in an increased liability to SGA-induced OCS in schizophrenia [110]. Recently, an association between the Val66Met polymorphism in the BDNF gene and OCS in schizophrenia has been observed [111].

12.8.3 Neurocognitive Characterization of Schizophrenia Patients With or Without OCS

Preliminary results showed that patients at high risk for psychosis and comorbid OCS seem to be less impaired in some neurocognitive domains compared to UHR-patients without OCS [112]. In contrast to these findings, studies investigating individuals with manifest schizophrenia and comorbid OCS reported domain specific higher deficits especially in executive functioning and visuo-spatial memory, compared to schizophrenia patients without OCS [9, 31, 113–118]. Schirmbeck et al. described marked impairment in CLZ- or OLZ-treated, OCS-positive patients in visual memory, impulse inhibition, perseveration and set-shift abilities [67]. These pronounced cognitive deficits appeared stable over a 1 year observational period and correlated significantly with OCS severity [70]. A specific neurocognitive profile might therefore be linked to the pathomechanism of OCS in schizophrenia. In the future, neurocognitive assessment prior to SGA treatment might help to define patients at risk for secondary OCS and should be considered for differential treatment decisions. During SGA treatment, monitoring of deficits in the mentioned domains might facilitate early recognition of OCS even in subclinical stages. Careful multimodal assessments seem necessary, since up to 50% of schizophrenia patients with comorbid OCS are currently undiagnosed during routine psychiatric treatment [18].

12.8.4 Treatment of OCS in Schizophrenia

Several modes of anti-obsessive treatment in schizophrenia follow a neurobiological rationale, but highly differ regarding the levels of currently available evidence.

12.8.5 Psychotherapy

Cognitive behavioral therapy is a core component of general schizophrenia treatment according to international consensus guidelines [119, 120]. Efficacy and tolerability have been proven regarding cognitive remediation, treatment resistant positive and negative symptoms, as well as comorbid depressive episodes [121–127].

For OCD, CBT including exposure and response prevention (ERP) is considered treatment of first choice with remarkable effect sizes of $d=0.998$ (CI:0.559–1.437) [128–131]. Exposure seems to be essential [128], however the effects of massive vs.

graduated procedures have not been compared so far. While a series of CBT treatment manuals exists [132–135] only the one by Fricke et al. provides recommendations for comorbid OCS in schizophrenia based on a detailed case report by Rufer and Watzke [136].

A comprehensive screening of public available databases (PubMed, PsychInfo, Google Scholar) revealed only a hand full of reports investigating the effect of CBT on comorbid OCS in schizophrenia (Table 12.3). Of the nine single case reports, the majority reported a decrease in OCS [136–139, 141], while some treatment attempts failed to show an improvement [93, 140]. In addition, Tundo et al. [142] published a case series of 21 index patients with severe, comorbid OCS (YBOCS scores on average 31.6) receiving CBT with ERP. Despite a dropout rate of 24% and one psychotic exacerbation the severity of OCS decreased significantly, while the insight of the patients into their illness increased. These results are however limited, due to missing information concerning the methods of exposure, the demarcation between delusions and obsessions, the course of the psychotic symptoms during CBT and applied antipsychotic pharmacotherapy.

One reason for scarce application of CBT including ERP to schizophrenia patients might lay in the apprehension of imminent psychotic exacerbations as a reaction to stress accompanying exposure. In addition, schizotypic personality traits have been defined as predicting less favorable treatment outcome in OCD [136, 143, 144]. Further research seems highly desirable. In summary, CBT with gradual exposure for OCS in schizophrenia seems recommendable in cases with sufficient remission of psychotic symptoms under stable antipsychotic pharmacotherapy. Psychoeducation and the elaboration of an individualized emergency plan according to early signs of psychotic deterioration should be included [136].

12.8.6 Polypharmacy

Combination and augmentation strategies in schizophrenia might be perceived as the clinical answers to high rates of treatment resistance [145]. The population of most severely affected patients carries the highest probability for clozapine treatment and in consequence the risk for second-onset OCS. Several recent reviews and the chapters volume I, part 1, 3 and 5 as well as chapters volume II, part 1, 7 in this book summarized guidelines towards an optimized clozapine treatment by polypharmacy [146–148]. Accordingly, evidence suggesting polypharmacy in the treatment of comorbid OCS in schizophrenia can be subdivided into combination as well as augmentation strategies.

12.8.7 Combination Approaches

In contrast to potent antiserotonergic SGAs such as CLZ and OLZ, mainly dopaminergic SGAs are able to supplement the profile of receptor interactions and

Table 12.3 Treatment of OCS in schizophrenia with psychotherapy

References	Number of patients	Patients' or sample characteristics	CBT methods	Outcome and main findings
Ganesan et al. [137]	Three (within a sample of 15 comorbid patients)	Male, 33 y, Female, 25 y Male, 31 y	Retrospective analysis, SGA and SSRI treatment plus CBT with ERP	Marked improvement of OCS in all three patients
McCabe et al. [138]	One	Male 50 y with CLZ-induced OCS	CBT with ERP	YBOCS improved
Ekers et al. [139]	One	Male, 31 y, SCH and OCD,	CBT with ERP	Successful treatment of OCD without significant deterioration of psychotic symptoms.
Peasley-Miklus et al. [140]	One	Male, 22 y, OCD and schizophrenia	CBT	Complicated course regarding OCS and psychotic symptoms
Fricke et al. [136]	One	Female ("young")	Importance of the therapeutic alliance, motivation, ERP	Marked and sustainable improvement
Kobori et al. [141]	One	Second-onset OCS after remission of psychotic symptoms	Psychoeducation, case formulation, cognitive restructuring, EPR, behavioral experiments	Improvement of compulsive behaviors
Rodriguez et al. [93]	One	Male, 19 y, coincident psychotic symptoms and OCS, treatment with CLZ	Few sessions of CBT with ERP	Resistance to clomiramine and SSRIs, dropout from CBT, improvement after augmentation with lamotrigine
Tundo et al. [142]	21	13 males, eight females, ~29.3 y, (SCH, N=9) and schizoaffective disorder (SA, N=12), duration of OCD: ~6.8 y, severity:	CBT over ~34.3 h (SA) or 31.1 h (SCH) including imaginal and in vivo exposure, ritual prevention and/or delay, cognitive therapy and other ad hoc interventions	16 patients improved (YBOCS and CGI-S), five dropouts, three hospitalizations, one exacerbation of psychotic disorder.

(continued)

Table 12.3 (continued)

References	Number of patients	Patients' or sample characteristics	CBT methods	Outcome and main findings
Schirmbeck et al. (unpublished data)	Six within a sample of 32 OCS-positive SCH patients	Six males, ~ 39.3 y, duration of OCS: 9 y. Severity of OCS: 18.3 YBOCS	Four received CBT, Two psychodynamic therapy, Mean 32.4 h	CBT: two improved, one unchanged, one dropped out Psychodynamic therapy: no changes regarding OCS

Reports on psychotherapy, most often CBT with ERP, in cases with OCS and schizophrenia. Screening of public databases (PsychInfo, Google-Scholar, PubMed) revealed report about in total 36 heterogeneous cases

CBT Cognitive behavioural therapy, *CGI-S* Clinical Global Impression, Severity Scale, *ERP* Exposure and Response Prevention, *OCS* Obsessive Compulsive Symptoms, *SA* Schizoaffective Disorder, *SGA* Second Generation Antipsychotics, *SSRI* Selective Serotonin Reuptake Inhibitors, *y* years, *YBOCS* Yale Brown Obsessive Compulsive Scale

were associated with favourable effects on comorbid OCS or as augmentation to selective serotonin reuptake inhibitors (SSRIs) in primary OCD. Here, AMS [149] and APZ [150] seem to be beneficial or at least neutral regarding OCS [62, 64, 80, 82, 83, 99, 151]. These two substances are therefore frequently used in clinical practice, if due to comorbid OCS switching from other SGAs is indicated [83]. In clinical practice, patients treated with CLZ often cannot be successfully treated with alternative SGAs [152–154], therefore it is more recommendable to reduce CLZ- or OLZ-dosages to minimal sufficient levels (Table 12.4) [80]. Preliminary evidence showed marked improvement of OCS under combination treatment with CLZ and APZ, in cases with subsequent CLZ dose reductions [62, 64, 69, 88] as well as under constant CLZ- [81] or OLZ-dosages [87].

12.8.8 Augmentation Approaches

In analogy to the efficacy of serotonergic antidepressants (AD) in primary OCD, schizophrenia patients with comorbid OCS have been treated with the tricyclic antidepressant clomipramine or SSRI, most often fluvoxamine (see [94] and Table 12.4). In summary, findings have been heterogenous and some studies failed to observe the intented effects. In general, side effects and pharmacokinetic interactions have to be considered: Adding clomipramine to SGAs such as CLZ or OLZ might result in additive, anticholinergic effects and increase side effects in the cardiovascular system. The SSRIs fluoxetin or fluvoxamine are slowly metabolised involving the hepatic cytochrom P450 system. In consequence, an antagonism with the CLZ-metabolism explains marked pharmacokinetic interactions resulting in increased CLZ-serum levels. Unintendedly, this fact might even increase antiserotonergic effects and prohibit anti-obsessive effects.

Table 12.4 Polypharmacy for OCS in schizophrenia

	References	Patients'or sample characteristics	Procedure	Main findings
Combination				
Add-on of Aripiprazole to SGAs	Rocha et al. [69]	Three male SCH patients	Add-on of 15 mg APZ to CLZ	Improved OCS and dose reductions of CLZ
	Zink et al. [62]	One male SCH patient (30 y)	Add-on of 30 mg APZ	YBOCS-decrease from 24 to 16, dose reduction of CLZ by 50%
	Glick et al. [86]	Seven (Six male) SCH patients with YBOCS ≥ 16	Add-on of APZ to previous FGA or SGA-treatment	YBOCS-decrease by ~13 points
	Chang et al. [81]	29 (22 male) SCH patients (RCT)	Add-on of 15.5 ± 7.1 mg APZ to 304.3 ± 104.8	YBOCS-decrease from 14.5 to 12.0 points.
	Englisch et al. [64]	Seven (Six male) schizophrenia patients	Add-on of 22.9 mg APZ to CLZ	YBOCS-decrease from 18.7 to 12.4, CLZ dose reduction by 19.6%
	Schönfelder et al. [87]	One female schizophrenia patient (58 y)	Add-on of 20 mg APZ to OLZ	Improved OCS
	Villari et al. [88]	Two male schizophrenia patients	Add-on of APZ	Improved OCS
Augmentation				
Add-on of clomipramine	Berman et al. [72]	Six SCH with OCS.	Double-blind, randomized cross-over design with placebo	Significantly more improvement of PANSS and YBOCS with clomipramine
Add-on of fluvoxamine	Poyurovsky et al. [89]	Ten (five males) SCH patients with YBOCS ≥ 7.	Open label add-on of 150 mg fluvoxamine to antipsychotic agents	Significant improvement of obsessions
	Reznik et al. [90]	14 (ten males) SCH patients (RCT)	Add-on of 200 mg fluvoxamine to antipsychotic agents	Significant reduction of OCS severity (YBOCS) compared to placebo.

(continued)

Table 12.4 (continued)

	References	Patients'or sample characteristics	Procedure	Main findings
Add-on of valproic acid	Zink et al. [63]	Male SCH patient, 32 y, CLZ-aggravated OCS	CBT and SSRI-treatment failed. Add-on of 1,300 mg valproic acid and reduction of CLZ	Improvement of OCS severity from YBOCS 24 to 6.
	Canan et al. [91]	Male SCH patient, 51 y, CLZ-induced OCS	Add-on of 1,000 mg valproic acid to 500 mg CLZ	Improvement of OCS
Add-on of lamotrigine	Poyurovsky et al. [92]	11 patients with YBOCS ≥ 16	Add-on of lamotrigine (200 mg/day) to antipsychotic agents	Improvement of OCS severity (YBOCS from 22.9 to 17.4)
	Rodriguez et al. [93]	One male, 19 y, coincident psychotic symptoms and OCS, treatment with CLZ	Resistance to clomipramine, SSRI, dropout from CBT. Add-on of lamotrigine 200 mg/day to CLZ 300 mg/day.	Psychosis in remission and OCS-improvement by about 40%

Overview about pharmacological interventions in cases with schizophrenia and comorbid OCS. In addition to the option of switching to for instance amisulpride [83], several strategies imply polypharmacy, in detail combinations of SGAs with different pharmacokinetic properties and augmentations of SGAs with antidepressants (for review see [94]) or mood stabilizers
APZ Aripiprazole, *CBT* cognitive behavioural therapy, *CGI-S* Clinical Global Impression, Severity Scale, *CLZ* Clozapine, *FGA* First Generation Antipsychotics, *OCS* Obsessive Compulsive Symptoms, *OLZ* Olanzapine, *PANSS* Positive and negative syndrome scale, *RCT* Randomized Controlled Trial, *SCH* Schizophrenia, *SGA* Second Generation Antipsychotics, *SSRI* Selective Serotonin Reuptake Inhibitors, *y* years, *YBOCS* Yale Brown Obsessive Compulsive Scale

Mood stabilizers have also been added to SGA in order to alleviate comorbid OCS, but the evidence derived from these mainly casuistic reports does not allow final conclusions and therapeutic recommendations (see Table 12.4) as is generally true for these add-on strategies in treatment-resistant schizophrenia [148, 155]. The augmentation of valproic acid in schizophrenia showed beneficial impact on aggressive symptoms as well as on tardive dyskinesia, but regarding psychotic symptoms it appeared not to be superior to *placebo* when added to SGAs [156]. However, with regard to comorbid OCS, casuistic evidence suggests an anti-obsessive potency of valproic acid in schizophrenia [63, 91]. Lamotrigine might confer some benefit to

CLZ-treatment resistant schizophrenic patients [157] and preliminary results suggest favourable effects on OCS in schizophrenia [92, 93].

So far, efficacy and tolerability of the mentioned therapeutic interventions have not been evaluated in head-to-head clinical trials. In addition, a combination of pharmacological and non-pharmacological interventions seems well possible. Finally, specific and so far incompletely understood neurobiological characteristics of the patients might influence the treatment response.

12.9 Conclusions and Future Directions

Comorbid OCS in schizophrenia is a common clinical problem. For a subgroup of these heterogeneous patients, several lines of evidence strongly suggest an induction of second-onset OCS through antiserotonergic effects of SGAs, most importantly CLZ. Forthcoming pathogenetic research on well-defined, homogeneous samples will facilitate the neurobiological factors leading to OCS in schizophrenia. Multimodal projects will have to involve methods of psychopathology, neuropsychology, neurogenetics and functional imaging. In terms of therapeutic implications CBT with ERP as well as several pharmacological combination and augmentation approaches are still awaiting clinical evaluation to a sufficient degree. In the future, early recognition and intervention, differential indications and combinations of the proposed strategies should be investigated in well-designed, controlled clinical trials.

Acknowledgments F.S. was supported by a research grant of the Evangelisches Studienwerk. M.Z. receives unrestricted scientific grants of ERAB (European Research Advisory Board), German Research Foundation (DFG), Servier, Pfizer Pharma GmbH, Bristol-Myers Squibb GmbH & CoKGaA, further speaker and travel support from Pfizer Pharma GmbH, Bristol-Myers Squibb GmbH & CoKGaA, Astra Zeneca, Eli-Lilly and Janssen Cilag.

References

1. Westphal K (1878) Ueber zwangsvorstellungen. Archiv für Psychiatrie und Nervenkrankheiten 8:734–750
2. Stengel E (1945) A study on some clinical aspects of the relationship between obsessional neurosis and psychotic reaction types. J Ment Sci 91:166–187
3. Rosen I (1957) The clinical significance of obsessions in schizophrenia. J Ment Sci 103:773–785
4. Dowling FG, Pato MT, Pato CN (1995) Comorbidity of obsessive-compulsive and psychotic symptoms: a review. Harv Rev Psychiatry 3:75–83
5. Zink M, Englisch S, Dressing H (2008) Neurobiology confirms psychopathology: on the antagonism of psychosis and obsessive-compulsive syndromes. Psychopathology 41:279–285
6. Guillem F, Satterthwaite J, Pampoulova T, Stip E (2009) Relationship between psychotic and obsessive compulsive symptoms in schizophrenia. Schizophr Res 115:358–362
7. Cunill R, Castells X, Simeon D (2009) Relationships between obsessive-compulsive symptomatology and severity of psychosis in schizophrenia: a systematic review and meta-analysis. J Clin Psychiatry 70:70–82

8. Berman I, Kalinowski A, Berman SM, Lengua J, Green AI (1995) Obsessive and compulsive symptoms in chronic schizophrenia. Compr Psychiatry 36:6–10
9. Lysaker PH, Whitney KA (2009) Obsessive-compulsive symptoms in schizophrenia: prevalence, correlates and treatment. Expert Rev Neurother 9:99–107
10. Fenton WS, McGlashan TH (1986) The prognostic significance of obsessive-compulsive symptoms in schizophrenia. Am J Psychiatry 143:437–441
11. de Haan L, Sterk B, Wouters L, Linszen DH (2011) The 5-year course of obsessive-compulsive symptoms and obsessive-compulsive disorder in first-episode schizophrenia and related disorders. Schizophr Bull. doi:10.1093/schbul/sbr077
12. Lysaker PH, Lancaster RS, Nees MA, Davis LW (2004) Patterns of obsessive-compulsive symptoms and social function in schizophrenia. Psychiatry Res 125:139–146
13. Öngür D, Goff DC (2005) Obsessive-compulsive symptoms in schizophrenia: associated clinical features, cognitive function and medication status. Schizophr Res 75:349–362
14. Hadi E, Greenberg Y, Sirota P (2011) Obsessive-compulsive symptoms in schizophrenia: prevalence, clinical features and treatment. A literature review. World J Biol Psychiatry 13:2–13
15. Achim AM, Maziade M, Raymond E, Olivier D, Merette C, Roy MA (2011) How prevalent are anxiety disorders in schizophrenia? A meta-analysis and critical review on a significant association. Schizophr Bull 37:811–821
16. Poyurovsky M, Weizman A, Weizman R (2004) Obsessive-compulsive disorder in schizophrenia: clinical characteristics and treatment. CNS Drugs 18:989–1010
17. Buckley PF, Miller BJ, Lehrer DS, Castle DJ (2009) Psychiatric comorbidities and schizophrenia. Schizophr Bull 35:383–402
18. Mukhopadhaya K, Krishnaiah R, Taye T, Nigam A, Bailey AJ, Sivakumaran T et al (2009) Obsessive-compulsive disorder in UK clozapine-treated schizophrenia and schizoaffective disorder: a cause for clinical concern. J Psychopharmacol 23:6–13
19. Poyurovsky M, Zohar J, Glick I, Koran LM, Weizman R, Tandon R, et al (2012) Obsessive-compulsive symptoms in schizophrenia: implications for future psychiatric classifications. Compr Psychiatry 53(5):480–483. http://dx.doi.org/10.1016/j.comppsych.2011.08.009.
20. de Haan L, Dudek-Hodge C, Verhoeven Y, Denys D (2009) Prevalence of psychotic disorders in patients with obsessive-compulsive disorder. CNS Spectrums 14:415–417
21. Sa AR, Hounie AG, Sampaio AS, Arrais J, Miguel EC, Elkis H (2009) Obsessive-compulsive symptoms and disorder in patients with schizophrenia treated with clozapine or haloperidol. Compr Psychiatry 50:437–442
22. Andreasen NC, Carpenter WT Jr, Kane JM, Lasser RA, Marder SR, Weinberger DR (2005) Remission in schizophrenia: proposed criteria and rationale for consensus. Am J Psychiatry 162:441–449
23. Jaeger M, Messer T, Laux G, Pfeiffer H, Naber D, Schmidt LG et al (2008) Standardized remission criteria in schizophrenia: descriptive validity and comparability with previously used outcome measures. Pharmacopsychiatry 41:190–195
24. Schirmbeck F, Zink M (2012) Clozapine-induced obsessive-compulsive symptoms in schizophrenia: a critical review. Curr Neuropharmacol 10:88–95
25. Poyurovsky M, Faragian S, Pashinian A, Heidrach L, Fuchs C, Weizman R et al (2008) Clinical characteristics of schizotypal-related obsessive-compulsive disorder. Psychiatry Res 159:254–258
26. Poyurovsky M, Koran LM (2005) Obsessive-compulsive disorder (OCD) with schizotypy vs. schizophrenia with OCD: diagnostic dilemmas and therapeutic implications. J Psychiatr Res 39:399–408
27. Catapano F, Perris F, Fabrazzo M, Cioffi V, Giacco D, De S V et al (2010) Obsessive-compulsive disorder with poor insight: a three-year prospective study. Prog Neuro-Psychopharmacol Biol Psychiatry 34:323–330
28. Tumkaya S, Karadag F, Oguzhanoglu NK, Tekkanat C, Varma G, Ozdel O et al (2009) Schizophrenia with obsessive-compulsive disorder and obsessive-compulsive disorder with poor insight: a neuropsychological comparison. Psychiatry Res 165:38–46

29. Rajkumar RP, Reddy YC, Kandavel T (2008) Clinical profile of "schizo-obsessive" disorder: a comparative study. Compr Psychiatry 49:262–268
30. Reznik I, Kotler M, Weizman A (2005) Obsessive and compulsive symptoms in schizophrenia patients – from neuropsychology to clinical typology and classification. J Neuropsychiatry Clin Neurosci 17:254–255
31. Hwang MY, Morgan JE, Losconzcy MF (2000) Clinical and neuropsychological profiles of obsessive-compulsive schizophrenia: a pilot study. J Neuropsychiatry Clin Neurosci 12:91–94, see comment
32. Bottas A, Cooke RG, Richter MA (2005) Comorbidity and pathophysiology of obsessive-compulsive disorder in schizophrenia: is there evidence for a schizo-obsessive subtype of schizophrenia. J Psychiatry Neurosci 30:187–193
33. Sevincok L, Akoglu A, Arslantas H (2006) Schizo-obsessive and obsessive-compulsive disorder: comparison of clinical characteristics and neurological soft signs. Psychiatry Res 145:241–248
34. Ebel H, Gross G, Klosterkotter J, Huber G, Ebel H, Gross G et al (1989) Basic symptoms in schizophrenic and affective psychoses. Psychopathology 22:224–232
35. Sullwold L, Huber G (1986) Basic schizophrenic disorders. Monographien aus dem gesamtgebiete der psychiatrie. Psychiatry Ser 42:1–177
36. Fink M, Taylor MA (2001) The many varieties of catatonia. Eur Arch Psychiatry Clin Neurosci 251(Suppl 1):I 8–13
37. Bräunig P, Krüger S, Shugar G, Höffler J, Börner I (2000) The catatonia rating scale I – development, reliability, and use. Compr Psychiatry 41:147–158
38. Woody SR, Steketee G, Chambless DL (1995) Reliability and validity of the Yale-brown obsessive-compulsive scale. Behav Res Ther 33:597–605
39. de Haan L, Hoogeboom B, Beuk N, Wouters L, Dingemans PM, Linszen DH (2006) Reliability and validity of the Yale-brown obsessive-compulsive scale in schizophrenia patients. Psychopharmacol Bull 39:25–30
40. Beckmann H, Bartsch AJ, Neumärker K-J, Pfuhlmann B, Verdaguer MF, Franzek E (2000) Schizophrenias in the Wernicke-Kleist-Leonhard school. Am J Psychiatry 157:1024–1025
41. Meltzer HY (1995) Role of serotonin in the action of atypical antipsychotic drugs. Clin Neurosci 3:64–75
42. Meltzer HY, Li Z, Kaneda Y, Ichikawa J (2003) Serotonin receptors: their key role in drugs to treat schizophrenia. Prog Neuro-Psychopharmacol Biol Psychiatry 27:1159–1172
43. Baker RW, Chengappa KN, Baird JW, Steingard S, Christ MA, Schooler NR (1992) Emergence of obsessive compulsive symptoms during treatment with clozapine. J Clin Psychiatry 53:439–442
44. de Haan L, Linszen DH, Gorsira R (1999) Clozapine and obsessions in patients with recent-onset schizophrenia and other psychotic disorders. J Clin Psychiatry 60:364–365
45. Lykouras L, Alevizos B, Michalopoulou P, Rabavilas A (2003) Obsessive-compulsive symptoms induced by atypical antipsychotics. A review of the reported cases. Prog Neuro-Psychopharmacol Biol Psychiatry 27:333–346
46. Kwon JS, Joo YH, Nam HJ, Lim M, Cho EY, Jung MH et al (2009) Association of the glutamate transporter gene SLC1A1 with atypical antipsychotics-induced obsessive-compulsive symptoms. Arch Gen Psychiatry 66:1233–1241
47. Reznik I, Yavin I, Stryjer R, Spivak B, Gonen N, Strous R et al (2004) Clozapine in the treatment of obsessive-compulsive symptoms in schizophrenia patients: a case series study. Pharmacopsychiatry 37:52–56
48. de Haan L, Oekeneva A, Van AT, Linszen D (2004) Obsessive-compulsive disorder and treatment with clozapine in 200 patients with recent-onset schizophrenia or related disorders. Eur Psychiatry J Assoc Eur Psychiatrists 19:524
49. Kang X, Simpson GM (2010) Clozapine: more side effects but still the best antipsychotic. J Clin Psychiatry 71:982–983
50. Joober R, Boksa P (2010) Clozapine: a distinct, poorly understood and under-used molecule. J Psychiatry Neurosci 35:147–149

51. Kane J, Honigfeld G, Singer J, Meltzer H (1988) Clozapine for the treatment-resistant schizophrenic. A double-blind comparison with chlorpromazine. Arch Gen Psychiatry 45:789–796
52. Asenjo Lobos C, Komossa K, Rummel-Kluge C, Hunger H, Schmid F, Schwarz S et al (2010) Clozapine versus other atypical antipsychotics for schizophrenia. Cochrane Database Systemat Rev 11:CD006633
53. McEvoy JP, Lieberman JA, Stroup TS, Davis SM, Meltzer HY, Rosenheck RA et al (2006) Effectiveness of clozapine versus olanzapine, quetiapine, and risperidone in patients with chronic schizophrenia who did not respond to prior atypical antipsychotic treatment. Am J Psychiatry 163:600–610, see comment
54. Tiihonen J, Lonnqvist J, Wahlbeck K, Klaukka T, Niskanen L, Tanskanen A et al (2009) 11-year follow-up of mortality in patients with schizophrenia: a population-based cohort study (FIN11 study). Lancet 374:620–627, see comment
55. Shioiri T, Shinada K, Kuwabara H, Someya T (2007) Early prodromal symptoms and diagnoses before first psychotic episode in 219 in patients with schizophrenia. Psychiatry Clin Neurosci 61:348–354
56. Rubino IA, Frank E, Croce NR, Pozzi D, di Lanza ST, Siracusano A (2009) A comparative study of axis I antecedents before age 18 of unipolar depression, bipolar disorder and schizophrenia. Psychopathology 42:325–332
57. Niendam TA, Berzak J, Cannon TD, Bearden CE (2009) Obsessive compulsive symptoms in the psychosis prodrome: correlates of clinical and functional outcome. Schizophr Res 108:170–175
58. Fontenelle LF, Lin A, Pantelis C, Wood SJ, Nelson B, Yung AR (2011) A longitudinal study of obsessive-compulsive disorder in individuals at ultra-high risk for psychosis. J Psychiatr Res 45:1140–1145
59. Bechdolf A, Mueller H, Stoetzer H, Wagner M, Maier W, Lautenschlager M et al (2011) Rationale and baseline characteristics of PREVENT: a second-generation intervention trial in subjects at-risk (Prodromal) of developing first-episode psychosis evaluating cognitive behavior therapy, aripiprazole, and placebo for the prevention of psychosis. Schizophr Bull 37:S111–S121
60. Poyurovsky M, Fuchs C, Weizman A (1999) Obsessive-compulsive disorder in patients with first-episode schizophrenia. Am J Psychiatry 156:1998–2000
61. Sterk B, Lankreijer K, Linszen DH, de Haan L (2011) Obsessive-compulsive symptoms in first episode psychosis and in subjects at ultra high risk for developing psychosis; onset and relationship to psychotic symptoms. Aust NZ J Psychiatry 45:400–405
62. Zink M, Knopf U, Kuwilsky A (2006) Management of clozapine-induced obsessive compulsive symptoms in a man with schizophrenia. Aust NZ J Psychiatry 41:293–294
63. Zink M, Englisch S, Knopf U, Kuwilsky A, Dressing H (2007) Augmentation of clozapine with valproic acid for clozapine-induced obsessive compulsive symptoms. Pharmacopsychiatry 40:202–203
64. Englisch S, Esslinger C, Inta D, Weinbrenner A, Peus V, Gutschalk A et al (2009) Clozapine-induced obsessive compulsive syndromes improve in combination with aripiprazole. Clin Neuropharmacol 32:227–229
65. Lin SK, Su SF, Pan CH (2006) Higher plasma drug concentration in clozapine-treated schizophrenic patients with side effects of obsessive/compulsive symptoms. Ther Drug Monit 28:303–307
66. Lim M, Park DY, Kwon JS, Joo YH, Hong KS (2007) Prevalence and clinical characteristics of obsessive-compulsive symptoms associated with atypical antipsychotics. J Clin Psychopharmacol 27:712–713
67. Schirmbeck F, Esslinger C, Rausch F, Englisch S, Meyer-Lindenberg A, Zink M (2011) Antiserotonergic antipsychotics are associated with obsessive-compulsive symptoms in schizophrenia. Psychol Med 41:2361–2374
68. Ertugrul A, nil Yagcioglu AE, Eni N, Yazici KM (2005) Obsessive-compulsive symptoms in clozapine-treated schizophrenic patients. Psychiatry Clin Neurosci 59:219–222

69. Rocha FL, Hara C (2006) Benefits of combining aripiprazole to clozapine: three case reports. Prog Neuro-Psychopharmacol Biol Psychiatry 30:1167–1169
70. Schirmbeck F, Rausch F, Englisch S, Eifler S, Esslinger C, Meyer-Lindenberg A, et al (2012) Stable cognitive deficits in schizophrenia patients with comorbid obsessive-compulsive symptoms: a 12 months longitudinal study. Schizophrenia Bulletin. doi:10.1093/schbul/sbs123
71. Bradford HA (2011) The environment and disease: association or causation. Bull World Health Org 83:295–300
72. Berman I, Sapers BL, Chang HH, Losonczy MF, Schmildler J, Green AI (1995) Treatment of obsessive-compulsive symptoms in schizophrenic patients with clomipramine. J Clin Psychopharmacol 15:206–210
73. Nolfe G, Milano W, Zontini G, Petrella C, De RM, Rundle-Smith S et al (2010) Obsessive-compulsive symptoms in schizophrenia: their relationship with clinical features and pharmacological treatment. J Psychiatr Pract 16:235–242
74. Hippius H (1989) The history of clozapine. Psychopharmacology 99(Suppl):S3–S5
75. Shapiro DA, Renock S, Arrington E, Chiodo LA, Liu LX, Sibley DR et al (2003) Aripiprazole, a novel atypical antipsychotic drug with a unique and robust pharmacology. Neuropsychopharmacology 28:1400–1411
76. Meltzer HY, Sumiyoshi T (2008) Does stimulation of 5-HT(1A) receptors improve cognition in schizophrenia. Behav Brain Res 195:98–102
77. Lopez-Gil X, Artigas F, Adell A (2010) Unraveling monoamine receptors involved in the action of typical and atypical antipsychotics on glutamatergic and serotonergic transmission in prefrontal cortex. Curr Pharm Des 16:502–515
78. Meltzer HY, Huang M (2008) In vivo actions of atypical antipsychotic drug on serotonergic and dopaminergic systems. Prog Brain Res 172:177–197
79. Remington G (2008) Alterations of dopamine and serotonin transmission in schizophrenia. Prog Brain Res 172:117–140
80. Englisch S, Zink M (2008) Combined antipsychotic treatment involving clozapine and aripiprazole. Prog Neuro-Psychopharmacol Biol Psychiatry 32:1386–1392
81. Chang JS, Ahn Y-M, Park HJ, Lee KY, Kim SH, Kang UG et al (2008) Aripiprazole augmentation in clozapine-treated patients with refractory schizophrenia: an 8-week, randomized, double-blind, placebo-controlled trial. J Clin Psychiatry 69:720–731
82. Connor KM, Payne VM, Gadde KM, Zhang W, Davidson JR, Connor KM et al (2005) The use of aripiprazole in obsessive-compulsive disorder: preliminary observations in 8 patients. J Clin Psychiatry 66:49–51
83. Kim SW, Shin IS, Kim JM, Yang SJ, Hwang MY, Yoon JS (2008) Amisulpride improves obsessive-compulsive symptoms in schizophrenia patients taking atypical antipsychotics: an open-label switch study. J Clin Psychopharmacol 28:349–352
84. Pani L, Villagran JM, Kontaxakis VP, Alptekin K (2008) Practical issues with amisulpride in the management of patients with schizophrenia. Clin Drug Invest 28:465–477
85. de Haan L, Beuk N, Hoogenboom B, Dingemans P, Linszen D (2002) Obsessive-compulsive symptoms during treatment with olanzapine and risperidone: a prospective study of 113 patients with recent-onset schizophrenia or related disorders. J Clin Psychiatry 63:104–107
86. Glick ID, Poyurovsky M, Ivanova O, Koran LM (2009) Aripiprazole in schizophrenia patients with comorbid obsessive-compulsive symptoms: an open-label study of 15 patients. J Clin Psychiatry 69:1856–1859
87. Schönfelder S, Schirmbeck F, Waltereit R, Englisch S, Zink M (2011) Aripiprazole improves olanzapine-associated obsessive compulsive symptoms in schizophrenia. Clin Neuropharmacol 34:256–257
88. Villari V, Frieri T, Fagiolini A (2011) Aripiprazole augmentation in clozapine-associated obsessive-compulsive symptoms. J Clin Psychopharmacol 31:375–376
89. Poyurovsky M, Isakov V, Hromnikov S, Modai I, Rauchberger B, Schneidman M et al (1999) Fluvoxamine treatment of obsessivecompulsive symptoms in schizophrenic patients: an add-on open study. Int Clin Psychopharmacol 14:95–100

90. Reznik IM, Sirota PMMP (2000) Obsessive and compulsive symptoms in schizophrenia: a randomized controlled trial with fluvoxamine and neuroleptics. J Clin Psychopharmacol 20:410–416
91. Canas F, Aydinoglu U, Sinani G (2012) Valproic acid augmentation in clozapine-associated hand-washing compulsion. Psychiatry Clin Neurosci (in press)
92. Poyurovsky M, Glick I, Koran LM (2010) Lamotrigine augmentation in schizophrenia and schizoaffective patients with obsessive-compulsive symptoms. J Psychopharmacol 24:861–866
93. Rodriguez CI, Corcoran C, Simpson HB (2010) Diagnosis and treatment of a patient with both psychotic and obsessive-compulsive symptoms. Am J Psychiatry 167:754–761
94. Hwang MY, Kim SW, Yum SY, Opler LA (2009) Management of schizophrenia with obsessive-compulsive features. Psychiatr Clin N Am 32:835–851
95. Peters B, de Haan L (2009) Remission of schizophrenia psychosis and strong reduction of obsessive-compulsive disorder after adding clozapine to aripiprazole. Prog Neuro-Psychopharmacol Biol Psychiatry 33:1576–1577
96. Bloch MH, Landeros-Weisenberger A, Kelmendi B, Coric V, Bracken MB, Leckman JF (2006) A systematic review: antipsychotic augmentation with treatment refractory obsessive-compulsive disorder. Mol Psychiatry 11:622–632
97. Bandelow B, Zohar J, Hollander E, Kasper S, Ller HJ, WFSBP Task Force on Treatment Guidelines for Anxiety O-CaP-TSD et al (2008) World Federation of Societies of Biological Psychiatry (WFSBP) guidelines for the pharmacological treatment of anxiety, obsessive-compulsive and post-traumatic stress disorders. World J Biol Psychiatry 9:248–312, first revision
98. Dold M, Aigner M, Lanzenberger R, Kasper S (2011) Efficacy of antipsychotic augmentation therapy in treatment-resistant obsessive-compulsive disorder – a meta-analysis of double-blind, randomised, placebo-controlled trials. Fortsch Neurol Psychiatr 79:453–466
99. Muscatello MR, Bruno A, Pandolfo G, Mico U, Scimeca G, Romeo VM et al (2011) Effect of aripiprazole augmentation of serotonin reuptake inhibitors or clomipramine in treatment-resistant obsessive-compulsive disorder: a double-blind, placebo-controlled study. J Clin Psychopharmacol 31:174–179
100. Pogarell O, Hamann C, Poepperl G, Juckel G, Chouker M, Zaudig M et al (2003) Elevated brain serotonin transporter availability in patients with obsessive-compulsive disorder. Biol Psychiatry 54:1406–1413
101. Steingard S, Chengappa KNR, Baker R, Schooler NR (1993) Clozapine, obsessive symptoms, and serotonergic mechanisms. Am J Psychiatry 150:1435
102. Meltzer HY (1994) An overview of the mechanism of action of clozapine. J Clinical Psychiatry 55(Suppl B):47–52
103. Coward DM (1992) General pharmacology of clozapine. Br J Psychiatry 160(Suppl 17):5–11
104. Linden DE (2006) How psychotherapy changes the brain – the contribution of functional neuroimaging. Mol Psychiatry 11:528–538
105. Saxena S, Gorbis E, O'Neill J, Baker SK, Mandelkern MA, Maidment KM et al (2009) Rapid effects of brief intensive cognitive-behavioral therapy on brain glucose metabolism in obsessive-compulsive disorder. Mol Psychiatry 14:197
106. Dickel DE, Veenstra-VanderWeele J, Cox NJ, Wu X, Fischer DJ, Van Etten-Lee M et al (2006) Association testing of the positional and functional candidate gene SLC1A1/EAAC1 in early-onset obsessive-compulsive disorder. Arch Gen Psychiatry 63:778–785
107. Arnold PD, Sicard T, Burroughs E, Richter MA, Kennedy JL (2006) Glutamate transporter gene SLC1A1 associated with obsessive-compulsive disorder. Arch Gen Psychiatry 63: 769–776
108. Veenstra-VanderWeele J, Kim SJ, Gonen D, Hanna GL, Leventhal BL, Cook EH Jr (2001) Genomic organization of the SLC1A1/EAAC1 gene and mutation screening in early-onset obsessive-compulsive disorder. Mol Psychiatry 6:160–167
109. Schirmbeck F, Nieratschker V, Frank J, Englisch S, Rausch F, Meyer-Lindenberg A, et al (2012) Polymorphisms in the glutamate transporter gene SLC1A1 and obsessive compulsive symptoms induced by second generation antipsychotic agents. Psychiatr Gen 22:245–252

110. Ryu S, Oh S, Cho EY, Nam HJ, Yoo JH, Park T et al (2011) Interaction between genetic variants of DLGAP3 and SLC1A1 affecting the risk of atypical antipsychotics-induced obsessive-compulsive symptoms. Am J Med Genet 156:949–959
111. Hashim HM, Fawzy N, Fawzi MM, Karam RA (2012) Brain-derived neurotrophic factor Val66Met polymorphism and obsessive-compulsive symptoms in Egyptian schizophrenia patients. J Psychiatr Res. http://dx.doi.org/10.1016/j.jpsychires.2012.03.007
112. Hur JW, Shin NY, Jang JH, Shim G, Park HY, Hwang JY et al (2012) Clinical and neurocognitive profiles of subjects at high risk for psychosis with and without obsessive-compulsive symptoms. Aust NZ J Psychiatry 46:161–169
113. Lysaker PH, Whitney KA, Davis LW (2009) Associations of executive function with concurrent and prospective reports of obsessive-compulsive symptoms in schizophrenia. J Neuropsychiatry Clin Neurosci 21:38–42
114. Berman I, Merson A, Viegner B, Losonczy MF, Pappas D, Green AI (1998) Obsessions and compulsions as a distinct cluster of symptoms in schizophrenia: a neuropsychological study. J Nerv Ment Dis 186:150–156
115. Sliman EB (2007) Differentielle neurokognitive Defizite bei Zwangsstörungen in Ab-hängigkeit vom klinischen Störungsbild und dem Ausprägungsgrad der Symptomatik im Vergleich zu Patienten mit Schizophrenie und gesunden Kontrollen. Dissertation Ruhr University Bochum, 1-169. Ref Type: Generic
116. Lysaker PH, Bryson GJ, Marks KA, Greig TC, Bell MD (2002) Association of obsessions and compulsions in schizophrenia with neurocognition and negative symptoms. J Neuropsychiatry Clin Neurosci 14:449–453
117. Patel DD, Laws KR, Padhi A, Farrow JM, Mukhopadhaya K, Krishnaiah R et al (2010) The neuropsychology of the schizo-obsessive subtype of schizophrenia: a new analysis. Psychol Med 40:921–933
118. Lee M-J, Shin Y-B, Sunwoo Y-K, Jung S-H, Kim W-H, Kang M-H et al (2009) Comparative analysis of cognitive function in schizophrenia with and without obsessive compulsive disorder. Psychiatry Invest 6:286–293
119. Wobrock T, Weinmann S, Falkai P, Gaebel W (2009) Leitlinienbasierte therapie der schizophrenie. Nervenheilkunde: Zeitschrift fuer Interdisziplinaere Fortbildung 28:448–455
120. Puschner B, Vauth R, Jacobi F, Becker T (2011) Bedeutung von psychotherapie in der versorgung von menschen mit schizophrenen störungen in deutschland. Der Nervenarzt 77(11):1301–1309
121. Sarin F, Wallin L, Widerloev B (2011) Cognitive behavior therapy for schizophrenia: a meta-analytical review of randomized controlled trials. Nord J Psychiatry 65:162–174
122. Lincoln T (2006) Kognitive verhaltenstherapie der schizophrenie: ein individuenzentrierter ansatz zur veraenderung von wahn, halluzinationen und negativsymptomatik. Hogrefe, Göttingen
123. Turkington DMD, Kingdon DMD, Weiden PJM (2006) Cognitive behavior therapy for schizophrenia. Am J Psychiatry 163:365–373
124. Wykes T, Steel C, Everitt B, Tarrier N (2008) Cognitive behavior therapy for schizophrenia: effect sizes, clinical models, and methodological rigor. Schizophr Bull 34:523–537
125. Grant PM, Huh GA, Perivoliotis D, Stolar NM, Beck AT (2012) Randomized trial to evaluate the efficacy of cognitive therapy for low-functioning patients with schizophrenia. Arch Gen Psychiatry 69:121–127
126. Bailer J, Takats I, Schmitt A (2002) Individualisierte kognitive verhaltenstherapie bei schizophrenen patienten mit negativsymptomatik und sozialer behinderung: II. Responderanalysen und praediktoren des therapieerfolgs. Verhaltenstherapie 12:192–203
127. Bailer J, Takats I, Westermeier C (2012) Die wirksamkeit individualisierter kognitiver verhaltenstherapie bei schizophrener negativsymptomatik und sozialer behinderung: eine kontrollierte studie. Z Klin Psychol Psychother 30:268–278
128. Rosa-Alcazar AI, Sanchez-Meca J, Gomez-Conesa A, Marin-Martinez F (2008) Psychological treatment of obsessive-compulsive disorder: a meta-analysis. Clin Psychol Rev 28:1310–1325
129. Gava I, Barbui C, Aguglia E, Carlino D, Churchill R, De VM, et al (2007) Psychological treatments versus treatment as usual for obsessive compulsive disorder (OCD). Cochrane Database of Syst Rev CD005333

130. Koran LM, Hanna GL, Hollander E, Nestadt G, Simpson HB (2007) American psychiatric association. Practice guideline for the treatment of patients with obsessive-compulsive disorder. Am J Psychiatry 164:5–53
131. Kuelz AK, Voderholzer U (2011) Psychotherapie der zwangsstörung. Der Nervenarzt 82:308–318
132. Foerstner U, Kuelz AM, Voderholzer U (2011) Störungsspezifische behandlung der zwangsstörungen: ein therapiemanual. Kohlhammer, Stuttgart
133. Lakatos A, Reinecker H (2007) Kognitive verhaltenstherapie bei zwangsstörungen: ein therapiemanual. Hogrefe, Göttingen
134. Oelkers C, Hautzinger M, Bleibel M (2007) Zwangsstoerungen: ein kognitiv-verhaltenstherapeutisches behandlungsmanual. Beltz Psychologie Verlags Union, Weinheim
135. Emmelkamp PMG, van Oppen P (2000) Zwangsstoerungen. Hogrefe, Göttingen
136. Fricke S, Rufer M, Hand I (2006) Verhaltenstherapie bei zwangsstoerungen: fallbasierte therapiekonzepte. Urban & Fischer Elsevier, Muenchen
137. Ganesan V, Kumar TCR, Khanna S (2001) Obsessive-compulsive disorder and psychosis. Can J Psychiatry/La Revue canadienne de psychiatrie 46:750–754
138. MacCabe JH, Marks IM, Murray RM (2002) Behavior therapy attenuates clozapine-induced obsessions and compulsions. J Clin Psychiatry 63:1179–1180
139. Ekers D, Carman S, Schlich T (2004) Successful outcome of exposure and response prevention in the treatment of obsessive compulsive disorder in a patient with schizophrenia. Behav Cogn Psychother 32:375–378
140. Peasley-Miklus C, Massie E, Baslett G, Carmin C (2005) Treating obsessive-compulsive disorder and schizophrenia: the case of Sam. Cogn Behav Prac 12:379–383
141. Kobori O, Sato H, Katsukura R, Harada S (2008) Cognitive behavioural therapy for obsessive compulsive symptoms affected by past psychotic experience of schizophrenia: a case report. Behav Cogn Psychother 36:365–369
142. Tundo A, Salvati L, Di Spigno D, Cieri L, Parena A, Necci R et al (2012) Cognitive-behavioral therapy for obsessive-compulsive disorder as a comorbidity with schizophrenia or schizoaffective disorder. Psychother Psychosom 81:58–60
143. Keeley ML, Storch EA, Merlo LJ, Geffken GR (2008) Clinical predictors of response to cognitive-behavioral therapy for obsessive-compulsive disorder. Clin Psychol Rev 28:118–130
144. Moritz S, Fricke S, Jacobsen D, Kloss M, Wein C, Rufer M et al (2004) Positive schizotypal symptoms predict treatment outcome in obsessive–compulsive disorder. Behav Res Ther 42:217–227
145. Englisch S, Zink M (2011) Combination and augmentation strategies in treatment-resistant schizophrenia. Drug Discov Today Ther Strat 8:17–23
146. Nielsen J, Damkier P, Lublin H, Taylor D (2011) Optimizing clozapine treatment. Acta Psychiatr Scand 123:411–422
147. Kane JM (2011) A user's guide to clozapine. Acta Psychiatr Scand 123:407–408
148. Zink M, Englisch S, Meyer-Lindenberg A (2010) Polypharmacy in schizophrenia. Curr Opin Psychiatry 23:103–111
149. Scatton B, Claustre Y, Cudennec A, Oblin A, Perrault G, Sanger DJ et al (1997) Amisulpride: from animal pharmacology to therapeutic action. Int Clin Psychopharmacol 12(Suppl 2): S29–S36
150. Sparshatt A, Taylor D, Patel MX, Kapur S (2010) A systematic review of aripiprazole – dose, plasma concentration, receptor occupancy, and response: implications for therapeutic drug monitoring. J Clin Psychiatry 71:1447–1456
151. Yang KC, Su TP, Chou YH (2008) Effectiveness of aripiprazole in treating obsessive compulsive symptoms. Prog Neuro-Psychopharmacol Biol Psychiatry 32:585–586
152. Still DJ, Dorson PG, Crismon ML, Pousson C (1996) Effects of switching inpatients with treatment resistant schizophrenia from clozapine to risperidone. Psychiatr Serv 47:1382–1384
153. Gupta S, Daniel DG (1995) Cautions in the clozapine-to-risperidone switch. Ann Clin Psychiatry 7:149

154. Kelly DL, Richardson CM, Tamminga CA, Carpenter WT (2003) The efficacy of high-dose olanzapine versus clozapine in treatment-resistant schizophrenia: a double-blind, crossover study. J Clin Psychopharmacol 23:668–670
155. Citrome L (2009) Adding lithium or anticonvulsants to antipsychotics for the treatment of schizophrenia: useful strategy or exercise in futility? J Clin Psychiatry 70:932–933
156. Casey DE, Daniel DG, Tamminga C, Kane JM, Tran-Johnson T, Wozniak P et al (2009) Divalproex ER combined with olanzapine or risperidone for treatment of acute exacerbations of schizophrenia. Neuropsychopharmacology 34:1330–1338
157. Tiihonen J, Wahlbeck K, Kiviniemi V (2009) The efficacy of lamotrigine in clozapine-resistant schizophrenia: a systematic review and meta-analysis. Schizophr Res 109:10–14

Chapter 13
Polypharmacy and Potentially Inappropriate Medication Use Among Elders with Dementia

Jan Luzny

Abstract Senior patients are at hight risk of polymorbidity which may correspond with hight risk of polypharmacy. Benefit of pharmacotherapy on one hand and risk of pharmacotherapy on the other hand are two different scales of one balance we have to measure on.

The paper shows basic principles of safe and efficient pharmacotherapy in the elderly – including inappropriate psychotropic drugs and drug-drug interactions which should be avoided.

Abbreviations

BZD	benzodiazepines
CYP	cytochrome P450 superfamily
ECG	electrocardiography
MAO inhibitors	monoamine oxidase inhibitors
MASSA	melatonin agonist and selective serotonin antagonist
NASSA	noradrenergic and specific serotonergic antidepressant
NDRI	noradrenergic and dopaminergic reuptake inhibitor
NSAID's	nonsteroid anti-inflammatory drugs
QT	QT interval in electrocardiogram
SARI	serotonin antagonist reuptake inhibitor

J. Luzny, M.D. (✉)
Mental Hospital Kromeriz and Palacky University Olomouc,
Praha, Czech Republic
e-mail: luznyj@plkm.cz

M.S. Ritsner (ed.), *Polypharmacy in Psychiatry Practice, Volume II: Use of Polypharmacy in the "Real World"*, DOI 10.1007/978-94-007-5799-8_13,

SIADH syndrome of inappropriate antidiuretic hormone secretion
SNRI serotonin noradrenaline reuptake inhibitors
SSRI selective serotonin reuptake inhibitors
TCA's tricyclic antidepressants
"Z"-agents zolpidem zopiclone, zaleplone

Prolongation of life expectancy is a matter of fact in well-developped countries. Together with actual demographical trends (decrease in born rate, postponing the morbidity and mortality to the older age) this is leading to new challenges for medicine of nowadays [1]. The population in modern societies is becoming older, those who are older than 65 years will represent 20% of the population according to predictions for the year 2025 [2]. For practical reasons, an age 65 years is used to describe elderly people [3]. In general, purely age-related effects should be distinguished from those of coexisting diseases [4]. Frailty and disease-related alterations are more obvious and less prone to underestimation in the clinical routine [5, 6].

Geriatric medicine is closely associated with modified clinical picture both of somatic and mental disease, polymorbidity, polypharmacy, changes both in pharmacokinetics and pharmacodynamics, higher risk of developping drug interactions and risk of potential harm to a senior patient [1, 7].

13.1 Modified Clinical Picture of Disease in Geriatric Medicine and Geriatric Psychiatry

Diseases of senior citizens usually have a modified clinical picture, accompanied by microsymptomatology (the symptoms of diseases are less expressed than in the general adult population), monosymptomatology or oligosymptomatology (symptoms of diseases can be expressed only by one or several symptoms instead of typical syndromology), non-specific clinical signs (which can be observed in many different conditions), symptoms of secondary deterioration (first clinical signs of a disease comes from the organ with the worst adaptation and the worst functional status, for instance delirious states as cerebral dysfunction caused primarily by bacterial infection), cascades of clinical signs (clinical signs coming from deterioration of more organs – "domino effect" of primary pathological condition), atypical adverse effects of therapy (due to changes in pharmacodynamics and pharmacokinetics of used drugs), risk of acute or emergent deterioration of performance status because of disease, high potential of invalidity caused by a disease (loss of autonomy, loss of independence in activities of daily living), social impact of a disease (risk of hospitalization and institutionalization) [7, 8].

As for mental disorders, alexithymia or somatization are common in elderly [9, 10]. Alexithymia means disability of an individual to perceive and describe correctly feeling of his or her emotional status [11] – it can be described as "misunderstanding of own emotions". Emotional discomfort is expressed via surrogative somatic symptoms such as functional pain, dyspnoe, palpitation, gastrointestinal disturbances or

Table 13.1 Features of morbidity in senior age

Microsymptomatology
Monosymptomatology or oligosymptomatology
Non-specific clinical signs
Symptoms of secondary deterioration
Cascades of clinical signs
Atypical adverse effects of therapy
Risk of acute or emergent deterioration of performance status because of disease
High potential of invalidity caused by a disease
Social impact of a disease
Somatic polymorbidity and psychiatric comorbidity

unexplained weight loss – "language of soul" is replaced by "language of body". Furthermore, somatizations or somatical symptoms of mental disorders in elderly are sometimes better accepted by somatically oriented physicians and even by patient family than psychiatric symptoms [12].

Both alexithymia and somatization in geriatric medicine may lead to clinical misinterpretation of originally psychiatric conditions (depression in elderly or anxiety disorders in senior patients can be misdiagnosed as a gastrointestinal, cardiovascular or musculoskeletal condition) and inappropriate treatment [13] (Table 13.1).

13.2 Polymorbidity in the Elderly

Psychiatric polymorbidity is usually understood as comorbid presence of different psychiatric conditions in an individual. This may lead to new, complex and altered clinical picture. In geriatric psychiatry, for instance substance abuse is often comorbid to geriatric depression or stress-related disorders. Another frequent psychiatric comorbidity in seniors is between depression and stress-related disorders as well as among different types of stress-related disorders (generalized anxiety disorder/obsessive compulsive disorder/specific phobias and agoraphobia/somatophorm disorders/post-traumatic stress and adjustment disorders).

Somatic polymorbidity means the presence of two or more diseases in an individual at the same time. In geriatrics and geriatric psychiatry clusters of both somatic and psychiatric diseases are a typical characteristic feature [14–16]. Non-communicable diseases represent a shift in morbidity in the twenty-first century compared to the morbidity of former centuries. While infectious diseases were threatening conditions in nineteenth century and the beginning of the twentieth century (tuberculosis, poliomyelitis, wound infection, puerperal sepsis), the twenty-first century brings pandemia of new diseases such as obesity, hypertension, diabetes mellitus or musculoskeletal diseases. Non-communicable diseases (NCDs) have both economical and ethical aspects [17, 18] (Table 13.2).

Table 13.2 What makes treatment of diseases in senior age difficult?

Somatic and psychiatric polymorbidity
Presence of non-communicable diseases
Polymorbidity – risk of side/adverse effects
Changes in pharmacokinetics
Changes in pharmacodynamics

13.3 Polypharmacy in the Elderly

The elderly are the predominant users of pharmaceuticals in the population [19].

Thus, aging of the population could be a reason for an increased use of pharmaceutical products. These patients often have multiple diseases, and so they require multiple drugs. It is well documented that polypharmacy has a greater potential to lead to drug interactions and adverse events [20].

Polypharmacy represents an administration of more medication than is in fact needed, or administration of drugs in unsuitable combination. Usually it means administration of more than four drugs at the same time. The risk of polypharmacy increases with the age of patients and polymorbidity [1, 7, 21, 22] detected high prevalence of polymorbidity, polypharmacy and inappropriate drug combination aminy seniors hospitalized due to any psychiatric condition in psychogeriatric wards (prevalence of polymorbidity: 66.1%, prevalence of polypharmacy: 51.3%, prevalence of inappropriate drug combination: 15.1%).

Pharmacological interactions contribute to the decreased in general health in the elderly, leading to disability, reduced quality of life, raising the number of hospital admissions, a longer duration of hospital stays, a greater need for ambulatory services, and increased healthcare costs [23, 24].

13.4 Changes in Pharmacokinetics and Pharmacodynamics in the Elderly

The final response (clinical effect) to a drug is influenced by pharmacokinetics (describing the fate of substances administered externally to an organism and the relationship among different types of drugs which have been administered in the same time – *drug-drug interactions*) and pharmacodynamics (studying the effects of drugs on the body and the mechanisms of drug action and the relationship between drug concentration and effect – *drug-receptor interactions*). Both pharmacokinetics and pharmacodynamics is frequently altered in senior patients, thus this may lead to changes in reactivity to the administered medication [25, 26].

Age-related changes in pharmacokinetics can be detected at different levels (changes in absorption, distribution, metabolism and excretion of drug) and they

Table 13.3 Age-related changes in pharmacokinetics [7]

Changes in	Pathophysiology	Clinical consequences
Absorption	Decreased gastrointestinal blood flow	Delayed onset of drug action
	Gastrointestinal hypomotility	Delayed onset of drug action
	Absorption surface decrease	Decreased onset of drug action
	pH increase in stomach	Delayed/changed drug action
Distribution	Decrease of total water mass	Increased plasma level of hydrosolubile drugs
	Increase of total fat mass	Risk of cummulation of liposolubile drugs
	Hypoalbuminemia	Plasma free fraction of drug increase
Metabolism	Decreased weight of liver	Decreased/slowered drug degradation
	Decreased liver blood flow	Decreased/slowered drug degradation
	Decreased liver CYP enzymes activity	Decreased/slowered drug degradation
	Decreased glucuronidization process	Decreased/slowered drug degradation
Excretion	Decreased renal blood flow	Risk of drug accumulation/toxicity
	Decreased glomerular filtration	Risk of drug accumulation/toxicity
	Decreased tubular secretion	Risk of drug accumulation/toxicity

Table 13.4 Age-related changes in pharmacodynamics

Changes in	Pathophysiology	Clinical consequences
Amount of receptors	Up-regulation	Increased clinical effect of drug
	Down-regulation/number decrease	Decreased clinical effect of drug
Sensitivity of receptors	Desenzitization	Decreased clinical effect of drug
	Hypersenzitization	Increased clinical effect of drug

may lead to different clinical consequences (Table 13.3). Decreased liver CYP enzyme activity can play an important role in altered biodegradation of psychotropic drugs. Cytochrome enzymes, such as cytochrome CYP450 and more specifically, CYP3A4,CYP2D6, CYP1A2, CYP2C9 and CYP2C19, play an important role in the metabolism of most antipsychotics, antidepressants and anxiolytic drugs. Substantial genetic variability among individuals is characterized by these enzymes. Genetic polymorphisms consequently induce an altered enzymatic activity – low activity is likely to lead to high-level drug concentrations and the potential to adverse drug reactions, and high enzymatic activity is likely to lead to reduced plasma levels and reduced drug efficacy [27].

Age-related changes in pharmacodynamics are bounded with altered sensitivity of organism to the drug. These changes might be heterogenous and very dynamic in time and they may lead to unexpected or unintended clinical effects (Table 13.4). Besides these dynamic receptor phenomena, total involutional decrease in receptor amount is a regular finding in aging organism. This may explain some of the psychiatric conditions in the elderly (memory impairment, affective disorders etc.).

Table 13.5 The most common adverse effects of inappropriate psychiatric medication

Type of adverse effect	Psychiatric medication at high risk
Sedation	Benzodiazepines, tricyclic antidepressants, antipsychotics
Hypotension	Benzodiazepines, tricyclic antidepressants, antipsychotics
Hypertension	IMAO's in inappropriate combination with food/other drugs
Dysrrhytmias	Tricyclic antidepressants, Comventional antipsychotics, Sertindol, Lithium
Anticholinergic effects	Tricyclic antidepressants, Comventional antipsychotics, Clozapine
Extrapyramidal effects	Conventional antipsychotics
Metabolic adverse effects	Antipsychotics, Tricyclic antidepressants, Mirtazapine, Valproate
Haematotoxicity	Carbamazepine, Clozapine, Valproate, Tricyclic antidepressants, Mirtazapine
Hepatotoxicity	Valproate, Carbamazepine, Tricyclic antidepressants, Antipsychotics, Benzodiazepines
Nephrotoxicity	Lithium
SIADH	SSRI, antipsychotics
Prolactine level increase	Antipsychotics, SSRI
Thyreotropic effects	Lithium

SIADH Secretion of anappropriate antidiuretine hormone

13.5 Risk of Potential Harm to a Senior Patient due to Inappropriate Psychiatric Medication

Inappropriate psychiatric drug or inappropriate drug combination can lead to potential or actual harm to a senior patient [28, 29]. Both clinicans and scientists tried to find and to publish results of their research dealing with inappropriate psychiatric drugs or their combinations which could help the clinicians in their routine practice (Table 13.5).

For instance, the PRISCUS list was created by German researchers and it can be understood as concise list revealing the most common inappropriate psychiatric drug which should be avoided in clinical practice. The PRISCUS list was created in four steps: (a) Qualitative analysis of selected PIM lists for elderly patients from other countries. Literature search – Development of a preliminary list of potentially inappropriate medications for elderly patients, specifically adapted to the German market-Generation of the final PRISCUS list by consultation of experts [30] (Table 13.6).

13.6 Inappropriate Psychotropic Drug Combination in the Elderly

Drug to drug interactions can lead to agonism (fortification of final pharmacodynamic effect), antagonism (diminishing of final effect) or risk of developping adverse effects [31]. Both somatic and psychiatric medication should be taken into account. Some of the most common inappropriate drug combinations are listed bellow [32] (Table 13.7).

Table 13.6 Potentially inappropriate medications in the elderly [30]

Drug	Adverse action	Safer alternative
Anticholinergic drugs	Anticholinergic side effects	Non-anticholinergic antihistamines
Antihistamines (*hydroxizine, clemastine, dimetindene* etc.)	Constipation, dry mouth Xerophtalmia, ECG changes (QT) Cognitive impairment, confusions	Cetirizine, loratadine, desloratadine
Urological spasmolytics (*oxybutinine, tolterodine solifenacine* etc.)	Constipation, dry mouth Xerophtalmia, ECG changes (QT) Cognitive impairment, confusions	Trospium Non-pharmacological treatment
Antidepressants		
Tricyclic antidepressants (*amitriptyline, doxepine, imipramine, clomipramine, maprotiline* etc.)	Constipation, dry mouth Ortostatic Hypotension, falls Dysrrhytmias Cognitive impairment, delirium	SSRI (citaloprame, sertraline) Mirtazapine, psychotherapy
SSRI (*fluoxetine*)	Nausea, confusional states, insomnia, dizziness, hyponatremia	Another SSRI, psychotherapy Mirtazapine, trazodone
MAO inhibitors (*tranylcypromine*)	Hypertensive cisis, cerebrál hemorrhagie Malignant Hyperthermia	SSRI except fluoxetine Psychotherapy
Antipsychotics		
Conventional (*thioridazine, fluphenazine, levomepromazine, perphenazine haloperidol >2 mg*)	Anticholinergic effects Extrapyramidal effects Hypotension, QT prolongation Increased mortality in dementia	Melperone Atypical antipsychotics
Atypical (*olanzapine >10 mg, clozapine*)	Metabolic adverse effects Risk of strokes, agranulocytosis	Melperone, Atypical antipsychotics
Sedatives, hypnotics		
Benzodiazepines (*chlordiazepoxide, diazepam, flurazepam, clorazepate, nitrazepam, flunitrazepam* etc.).	Muscle-relaxing effect, falls Sedation/paradoxical agitation Cognitive impairment Confusional states	Sedating antidepressants Antipsychotics of low potency Valeriana officinalis extractum Psychotherapy, sleep hygiene
"Z" agents (*zolpidem >5 mg/day, zopiclone >3.75 mg/day, zaleplone >5 mg/day*)	Muscle-relaxing effect, falls Sedation/paradoxical agitation Cognitive impairment Confusional states	Sedating antidepressants Antipsychotics of low potency Valeriana officinalis extractum Psychotherapy, sleep hygiene
Anti-dementia drugs (*pentoxyphylline, nicergoline, naftidrofuryl, piracetam*)	No proof of efficacy	Acetylcholinesterase inhibitors, Memantine
Mood stabilizers (*phenobarbital*) (*lithium*)	Sedation/paradoxical excitation Dysrrhytmias, Nephropathy, Thyreopathy	Lamotrigine, valproate Gabapentin, Pregabaline

SSRI Selective Serotonine Reuptake Inhibitors; *"Z"-agents* Zolpidem, zopiclone, zaleplone

Table 13.7 Inappropriate psychotropic drug combination in the elderly [30]

	Inappropriate combination with	Adverse effect of combination
Sedatives and hypnotics		
Midazolam	Calcium channel blockers	Sedation, prolongated sedation
Nitrazepame	Antimycotics	Sedation, prolongated sedation
Benzodiazepines	Opioids	Sedation, prolongated sedation
Benzodiazepines	Sedative antidepressants	Sedation, prolongated sedation
Benzodiazepines	Antipsychotics	Sedation, prolongated sedation
"Z" agents	Opioids	Sedation, prolongated sedation
"Z" agents	Sedative antidepressants	Sedation, prolongated sedation
"Z" agents	Antipsychotics	Sedation, prolongated sedation
Antidepressants		
Tricyclic	Opioids	Depression of respiration
Tricyclic	MAO inhibitors	Serotonine syndrome, hypertensive crisis
Tricyclic	SSRI	Toxic levels of TCAs, serotonine syndrome
SSRI	Anticoagulant agents	Risk of hemorrhagie
SSRI	NSAIDs	Risk of hemorrhage
SSRI	MAO inhibitors	Serotonine syndrome, hypertensive crisis
SSRI	Tricyclic antidepressants	Toxic levels of TCAs, serotonine syndrome
MAO inhibitors	Buspirone	Hypertensive cisis
MAO inhibitors	Opioids	Serotonine syndrome, hyperthermia, death
MAO inhibitors	Stimulants/dopaminergic drugs	Hypertensive cisis, death
SARI (trazodone)	Benzodiazepines	Sedation
NASSA (mirtazapine)	MAO inhibitors	Serotonine syndrome
NASSA (mirtazapine)	BZD, antipsychotics	Sedation
SNRI ((venlafaxine)	MAO inhibitors	Serotonine syndrome
NDRI (bupropione)	MAO inhibitors	Serotonine syndrom
MASSA (agomelatine)	Ofloxacine	Hepatotoxicity
Antipsychotics		
Conventional	Anticholinergic agents	Ileus states, confusional states, delirium
Conventional	Antihypertensives	Hypotension
Conventional	Benzodiazepines	Sedation, prolongated sedation
Conventional	Sedative antidepressants	Sedation, prolongated sedation
Atypical	Antihypertensives	Hypotension
Atypical	Benzodiazepines	Sedation, prolongated sedation
Atypical	Sedative antidepressants	Sedation, prolongated sedation
Mood stabilizers		
Carbamazepine	Clozapine	Agranulocytosis
Carbamazepine	TCAs, bupropione	Decreased plasma levels of TCAs, bupropione
Carbamazepine	Lithium	Sedation, prolongated sedation
Valproate	Digoxine	Increased plasma levels of digoxine free-fraction

continued

Table 13.7 continued

	Inappropriate combination with	Adverse effect of combination
Valproate	SSRI	Increased plasma levels of valproate
Valproate	Carbamazepine	Increased plasma levels of carbamazepine
Valproate	Lamotrigine	Increased plasma levels of lamotrigine
Valproate	Diazepame	Increased plasma levels of diazepame, sedation
Lamotrigine	Valproate	Increased plasma levels of lamotrigine
Anti-dementia drugs		
ACHE inhibitors	Atropine, Myorelaxatives	Complication during anesthesia
ACHE inhibitors	Digoxine, beta-blockers Antiarrhytmics	Bradycardia
ACHE inhibitors	NSAIDs	Nausea, diarrhoe, gastric ulcer
ACHE inhibitors	Nonselective beta-blockers	Bronchoconstriction
Memantine	Chinidine, chinine	Hepatotoxicity

SSRI Selective Serotonine Reuptake Inhibitors, *BZD* Benzodiazepines; *"Z"-agents* zolpidem, zopiclone, zaleplone, *MAO inhibitors* Monoaminooxidase inhibitors, *TCA's* Tricyclic antidepressants, *NSAID's* Nonsteroid anti-inflammatory drugs

13.7 Principles for Safe Psychopharmacotherapy in the Elderly

General rules for psychopharmacotherapy in elderly can be summarized into a several points [9, 33]:

A. **choice for drug with low risk potential**
(non-benzodiazepine sedativs and hypnotics,, antidepressants of higher generation – SSRI, dualistic antidepressants, MASSA, atypical antipsychotics)

B. **choice for as low dosage of drug as possible**
(lower dosage strategy compared to adult age respects changes in pharmacokinetics and pharmacodynamics in the elderly)

C. **monotherapy is prefered to combined therapy**
(this strategy prevents from drug-drug interactions)

D. **Starting dosage should be low**
(initial dosage should be just about 1/4 of final dosage is recommended to avoid initial averse effects, then we rise the dosage gradually up. This strategy is recommended both for initializing treatment and for finishing the treatment. When finishing the treatment, gradual dicrease in dosage prevents from discontinuation syndrome)

E. **when changing treatment strategy, we should stop administering the drug gradually and we should gradually switch to another medication**
(administration of all the medication should not be finished at once-risk of discontunuation syndrome and risk of abrupt changes in neurotransmiter balance in synapses)

F. **anticholinergic agent sof any kind should be strictly avoided**
(tricyclic antidepressants, conventional antipsychotics, spasmolytic agents with anticholinergic properties)

G. **benzodiazepines should be avoided whenever possible**
(especiallybenzodiazepineswithlonghalftimesuchasdiazepame,chlordiazepoxide, flunitrazepame. As for benzodiazepines, there is a high risk of addiction to them, as well as risk of withdrawal states, confusional states, iatrogenic amnesia, risk of sedation and falls with traumatic injuries).

H. **Adverse effects of treatment should be detected as soon as possible**
(hypotension, salivation, weight gain, sedation, dysrrhytmias, extrapyramidal side effects, anticholinergic side effects etc.).

I. **all the patiens mediaction should be checked, including somatic medication**
(we are aware of risk of polypharmacy, drug to drug interactions, iatropathogenic disturbances – anticholinergics followed by confusional states, adrenergic stimulans followed by sleep disturbances, corticoids followed by depression and confusional states, dopamine-acting antiparkinsonicsz followed by psychotic disorders etc.).

J. **awarenes of benefit to risk ratio and awarenes of evidence-based medicine guidelines**
(benefit for a patient, knowledge of guidelines for efficient and safe therapy)

K. **financial burden of treatment should be taken into account**
(patient can be adherent to treatment only if the medication is financially accessible to patient)

L. **patient adherence should be taken into account**
(nonadherence could be result of severe cognitive impairment and amnesia. Risk of overdosing as well as risk of underdosing the medication is not rare)

M. **good knowledge of prescribed drug profile is necessary to all the physicians**
(indications, contraindications, drug to drug interactions, averse effects, dosage, dosage corrections in nephropathy or hepatopathy, epilepsy, extrapyramidal disorders, available galenic forms of medication)

N. **patient-centered treatment strategy as well as individualized treatment strategy is a general rule**

13.8 Conclusion and Future Directions

Good knowledge both in psychiatry and in pharmacology is vitally needed for psychogeriatrists. Senior patients are at hight risk of polymorbidity which may correspond with hight risk of polypharmacy. All the clinicians treating senior patients must be aware of principles of safe and efficient pharmacotherapy, including the critical approach to polypharmacy. Benefit of pharmacotherapy on one hand and risk of pharmacotherapy on the other hand are two different scales of one balance we have to measure on.

Acknowledgement The paper was not supported by any grant or other financial support. Ethical hazard is therefore excluded.

References

1. Luzny J, Bellova J, Donek E (2010) Does gerontopsychiatry belong to medicine? cross-sectional study monitoring polymorbidity in hospitalized gerontopsychiatric patiens. Biomed Pap Med Fac Univ Palacky Czech Repub 154(1):89–92
2. Shi S, Morike K, Klotz U (2008) The clinical implications of ageing for rational drug therapy. Eur J Clin Pharmacol 64:183–199
3. Turnheim K (2000) Pharmacokinetic dosage guidelines for elderly subjects. Expert Opin Drug Metab Toxicol 1:33–48
4. Gurwitz JH, Avorn J (1991) The ambiguous relation between aging and adverse drug reactions. Ann Intern Med 114:956–966
5. Balducci L, Extermann M (2000) Management of cancer in the older person: a practical approach. Oncologist 5:224–237
6. Fried LP, Tangen CM, Walston J, Newman AB, Hirsch C, Gottdiener J, Seeman T, Tracy R, Kop WJ, Burke G, McBurnie MA (2001) Cardiovascular health study collaborative research group [6]: frailty in older adults: evidence for a phenotype. J Gerontol A Biol Sci Med Sci 56:M146–M156
7. Topinkova E (2005) Geriatrie pro praxi [Geriatrics for practice], 1st edn. Galen, Praha, pp 13–17
8. Kalvach Z, Onderková A (2006) Stáří. Pojetí geriatrického pacienta a jeho problémů v ošetřovatelské praxi. [Ageing. Concept of geriatric patient and his problems in nursing practice], 1st edn. Galen, Praha, pp 10–18
9. Spar JE, La Rue A (2002) Concise guide to geriatric psychiatry, 3rd edn. American Psychiatric Publishing, Washington, DC/London, pp 364–366
10. Sadock BJ, Kaplan HI, Sadock VA (2007) Kaplan and Sadock's synopsis of psychiatry, 10th edn. Lippincot Williams and Wilkins, Wolters Kluwer Business, Philadelphia, pp 1003–1007
11. Semple D, Smyth R, Burns J et al (2005) Oxford handbook of psychiatry, 1st edn. Oxford University Press, New York, pp 333–339
12. Luzny J, Ivanova K (2009) Quality of life in hospitalized seniors with psychiatric disorders (a cross-sectional study from the Kromeriz District, Czech Republic). Biomed Pap Med Fac Univ Palacky Czech Repub 153(4):315–318
13. Tyrer P, Silk KR (2011) Effective treatments in psychiatry, 1st edn. Cambridge University Press, Cambridge, pp 25–26
14. Cohen GD (1993) African American Issues in geriatric psychiatry: a perspective on research opportunities. J Geriatr Psychiatry Neurol 6(4):195–199
15. Engedal K et al (1991) Psychiatry for the elderly – a speciality field in progress. Tidsskr Nor Laegeforen 111(18):2258–2260
16. Nieuwenhuijzen K, Mulder WJ, Pijpers E (2007) Ageing and polymorbidity: is there a mismatch between the training of internists and the need? Neth J Med 65(10):363–365
17. Ivanova K, Spirudova L, Kutnohorska J (2005) Multikulturní ošetřovatelství. [Multicultural nursing], 1st edn. Grada, Praha, pp 12–15 (In Czech)
18. Ivanova K, Klos R (2004) Kapitoly z lékařské etiky. [Chapters from medical ethics], 1st edn. Palacky University, Olomouc, pp 99–103 (In Czech)
19. Rosenfeld S (2003) Prevalence, associated factors, and misuse of medication in the elderly: a review. Cad Saude Publica 19:717–724
20. Frankfurt SV, Tulner LR, van Campen JP, Koks CH, Beijnen JH (2006) Evaluation of pharmacotherapy in geriatric patients after performing complete geriatric assessment at a diagnostic day clinic. Clin Drug Investig 26:169–174

21. Stahl MS (2002) Essential psychopharmacology. Neuroscientific basis and practical applications, 2nd edn. Cambridge University Press, Cambridge, pp 588–591
22. Henn F, Sartorius N, Helmchen H, Lauter H (2001) Contemporary psychiatry, 1st edn. Springer, Berlin, pp 1982–1987
23. Vonbach P, Dubied A, Krahenbuhl S, Beer JH (2008) Prevalence of drug-drug interactions at hospital entry and during hospital stay of patients in internal medicine. Eur J Intern Med 19:413–420
24. Zlámal J, Ulrich M (2008) Základy ekonomie pro management zdravotnictví. [Basic economy for management of health care], 1st edn. Palacky University, Olomouc, pp 15–16 (In Czech)
25. Janicak PG (1999) Handbook of psychopharmacotherapy, 1st edn. Lippincott Williams and Wilkins, London, pp 122–125
26. Aronson JK, Grahame S, Grahame D (2004) Oxford textbook of clinical pharmacology and drug therapy, 3rd edn. Oxford University Press, Oxford, pp 17–19
27. Mackenzie B, Souza RP, Likhodi O et al (2010) Pharmacogenetics of antipsychotic treatment response and side effects. Therapy 7(2):191–198
28. Schatzberg AF, Cole JO, DeBattista C (2003) Manual of clinical psychopharmacology, 1st edn. American Psychiatric Publishing, Inc, Washington, DC, pp 688–690
29. Gelder MG, Lopez-Ibor JJ, Andreasen NC (2003) New Oxford textbook of psychiatry, 1st edn. Oxford University Press, New York, pp 2111–2117
30. Holt S, Schmiedl S, Thurmann PA (2010) Potentially inappropriate medications in the elderly: the PRISCUS list. Dtsch Arztebl Int 107(31–32):543–551
31. Shiloh R, Nutt D, Wiezman A (2003) Essentials in clinical psychiatric pharmacotherapy, 1st edn. Martin Dunitz, London, pp 104–108
32. Zieglmeier M, Hein T (2003) Interaktionen. Wirkstoffbezogene, beratungsemplepfehlungen fur die Praxis, 1st edn. Wissenschaftliche Verlagsgesellschaft mbH, Stuttgart, pp 120–132
33. Luzny J (2012) Psychogeriatry, 1st edn. Triton, Praha, pp 15–17

Chapter 14
The Role of Polypharmacy in Bipolar Disorder Treatment Guidelines

Heinz Grunze

Abstract Polypharmacy is rather the rule than the exception in the real world treatment of bipolar disorder. Guidelines do support combination treatments, but with a solitary focus of efficacy. This leads to an apparent discrepancy between the recommendations of combination treatment in guidelines and the treatment plan in clinical patient samples where factors influencing choices are more complex and not resembled by randomised controlled studies (RCTs). This article highlights the treatment recommendations of three major, up- to date guidelines and the positioning of combination treatments in acute mania, bipolar depression and maintenance treatment.

Abbreviations

AAP	Atypical antipsychotic
AD	Antidepressant
AM	Antimanic agent
AMSP	Arzneimittelsicherheit in der Psychiatrie (Surveillance study of drug safety in Psychiatry)
BAP	British Association of Psychopharmacology
BD	Bipolar Disorder
CANMAT	Canadian Network for Mood and Anxiety Treatments
ISBD	International Society for Bipolar Disorders

H. Grunze (✉)
Institute of Neuroscience, Academic Psychiatry, Campus of Aging and Vitality, Wolfson Research Centre, Newcastle University, Newcastle upon Tyne, UK
e-mail: Heinz.Grunze@ncl.ac.uk

M.S. Ritsner (ed.), *Polypharmacy in Psychiatry Practice, Volume II: Use of Polypharmacy in the "Real World"*, DOI 10.1007/978-94-007-5799-8_14,

Li	Lithium
RCT	Randomised Controlled Studies
STEP-BD	Systematic Treatment Enhancement Program for Bipolar Disorder
TEAE	Treatment emergent affective episodes
VPA	Valproate
WFSBP	World Federation of Societies of Biological Psychiatry

14.1 Real World Treatment of Bipolar Disorder

In routine practice, combination treatments in Bipolar Disorder (BD) are regularly employed to enhance efficacy of treatment directed against an acute manic, mixed or depressive episode. However, the treatment of bipolar patients may also change frequently in response to side effects, emerging comorbidities including physical health issues, and other needs to be specifically tailored for each patient. Furthermore, attention needs to be paid to the risk of manic/hypomanic/mixed switches during treatment of bipolar depression as well as to the potential risk of switch to depression while treating mania. Thus, we often find pharmacological treatment constellations where the medication effective for the respective episode is combined with a drug preventive for the opposite polarity. Consequently, many different strategies are employed by clinicians in their decision-making process and patients often receive several treatments over the course of their illness, even if not supported by controlled clinical trials. In addition, with the broadening of our concept of BD towards a Bipolar spectrum, treatment may become more challenging, and, as a matter of fact, the rate of polypharmacy is continuously rising [1–5]. Other variables influencing the choice of a given treatment strategy that have been previously identified include information resources (professional journals or reference texts), the nature and presentation of symptoms, available alternative treatment interventions and their cost-benefit analysis, physician prescriber characteristics (age, type of practice and treatment orientation) and physician-patient relationship [6].

In contrast to clinical practice, treatment guidelines elaborate on polypharmacy either only from the perspective of additional efficacy (compared to monotherapy) or, when it comes to prescribing antidepressants, in preventing treatment emergent affective episodes (TEAE). This different approach explains to a large degree why polypharmacy is much more widespread in clinical practice than someone would assume from guideline recommendations. For example, prospective data of the Stanley Foundation Bipolar Network confirmed the highly complex medication regimens in 429 naturalistically-treated bipolar patients, with lithium (51%) and valproate (42%) being the most frequently prescribed medications at the time of clinical improvement: 96.5% of the patients who responded at 6 months were on one to five medications, with over 55% of patients being on two or three medications, 31.8% requiring four or more drugs and 13.8% requiring five or more medications, and it took a mean time of 1.5years to achieve such sustained remission [7]. This is paralleled by the findings of Goldberg and collaborators [8] who examined prescribing strategies for 4,035 subjects immediately prior to enter in the STEP-BD study and observed that about 20% of patients were taking four or more drugs; complex medication strategies were most often correlated to antidepressants and atypical antipsychotics use and it was especially common in patients with substantial depressive illness burden and suicidality.

14.2 Usefulness and Limitations of Guidelines

The application of well-designed guidelines may be helpful to clinicians in reducing the variability of clinical practice and may carry substantial benefits to bipolar patients [9, 10]. Existing guidelines are quite heterogeneous as far as their methodology and degree of detail are concerned. They can be based on expert opinion, surveys among professionals, consensus panels or a just a systematic literature appraisal. They may elaborate only on general treatment principles, or may supply specific recommendations up to detailed, sequential algorithms. Guidelines may claim to be internationally applicable or resemble mainly a national approach to BD and reflect also factors independent from the illness, but of local relevance when it comes to treatment, as availability of drugs, access to health care, physician's familiarity with medication, financial constraints etc. For example, in a recent survey French psychiatrists quoted as main reason for the lack of use of guidelines that they refer mostly to an Anglo-Saxon medical practice, which they consider different from the French practice [11]. Thus, different practice and tradition of diagnosing together with the rapid growth of scientific evidence – leading to guidelines being quickly outdated – may also explain subtle differences between existing treatment recommendations.

What most guidelines, despite being considered as evidence based, share, however, are some important limitations. The rigor of the evidence – base differs across treatment phases in BD; whereas numerous randomized controlled studies (RCT) have been conducted in acute mania, remarkably less emphasis has been but on bipolar depression. In addition, the available published information can be considered as incomplete due to publication bias favouring positive trials over failed or negative studies [12, 13], and sponsor bias may not only influence publication strategies, but already outcomes of studies [14]. Finally, the developmental process of guidelines can be influenced by financial interests and bias of those compiling them. Cosgrove et al. reported that 90% of the authors of three major American clinical practice guidelines in psychiatry had financial ties to companies that manufacture drugs which were explicitly or implicitly identified in the guidelines as recommended therapies for the respective mental illnesses. However, none of the financial associations of the authors were disclosed in the guidelines [15]. As a result of the public discussion , the update of the APA guidelines, originally planned for 2007/2008 has been considerably delayed and has not been published yet at the time this chapter was written (July 2012).

BD guidelines face additional challenges. The fast majority of methodologically well designed studies are sponsored by pharmaceutical companies and serve to answer a hypothesis relevant for licensing purposes, but not necessarily of clinical interest for everyday practice. Detailed analyses on response patterns to various treatments are not available: response may be delayed for some medication that need titration or are used in lower dosages [16] but this will not be captured especially in short term studies. The nature of these RCTs also implies that they look into a population as homogenous as possible; most RCTs are therefore conducted solely in Bipolar I patients. Even within this restricted group, only a small minority will be accepted and randomized in RCTs. For example, Licht [17] reported that only about 10% of screened manic patients enter an RCT, with the fast majority failing exclusion criteria as comorbidities, episode frequency or ability to consent. Moderately or severely ill manic patients, with impaired insight and lack of cooperativeness may not be selected to participate in the RCT and, consequently, the discrepancies between highly selected patients and patients seen in clinical practice are particularly broad in mania. All these factors lead to a poor generalisability of the results. The fact that these RCTs are conducted for licensing purposes also prioritizes monotherapy studies; combination treatment studies are considered as secondary.

To overcome limits in generalisability of study results, the implementation of large, well-designed, randomized, open studies on naturalistic populations with adequate duration, using broader inclusion criteria and improving evaluation of the outcome, has been suggested by numerous experts in BD [16, 18]. These naturalistic trials should also account for combination treatments as, for example, EMBLEM, a large multinational mania and maintenance study, recently did [19].

Clinician's attitude towards guidelines appears to differ across cultures. In a recent survey, 64.1% of US psychiatrists stated that they make regularly use of guidelines for treatment decisions. Of those who did not use bipolar guidelines, the most frequently cited reason given by respondents (20.1%) was that such guidelines do not address particular features of their clinical populations [10]. A UK study published by Streeruwitz in 2007 (the year after the updated NICE guidelines for BD had been published) found that prescribing was generally in accord with published guidelines. Within the first 24 h of treatment of acute mania, monotherapy with a second generation antipsychotic was the favoured treatment; whereas at discharge, combination treatment (a mood stabilizer and a second generation antipsychotic) predominated [20]. Contrasting the use of guidelines by Anglo-American psychiatrists, one recent survey of bipolar treatment practice conducted in France found that only 1/3 of younger psychiatrists stated that they follow guidelines; however, 41% of all psychiatrists cited 'personal experience' as the key driver of medication choice, and this was especially prominent in the group of older clinicians [11].

14.3 BD Guidelines Under Review

For this review of the role of polypharmacy in BD guidelines, we selected three guidelines which have been updated more recently and appear to have some international acceptance: The World Federation of Societies of Biological Psychiatry (WFSBP) guideline (for mania: [16], for bipolar depression: [21], for maintenance: [22]), the Canadian Network for Mood and Anxiety Treatments (CANMAT) and the

International Society for Bipolar Disorders (ISBD) guideline [23], and the British Association for Psychopharmacology (BAP) guidance [24] .

All these guidelines have been developed by expert teams; whereas the WFSBP and CANMAT/ISBD guidelines are mainly compiled by psychiatrists, the BAP guideline also included input from psychologist, health care decision makers, and service users. All guidelines were created without any financial support from pharmaceutical companies and experts of the task force were selected according to their expertise. All guidelines were based on an extensive literature search and data were extracted from standard mental health related bibliographic databases. Inclusion criteria of literature data vary across the different guidelines depending also on their date of publication: the CANMAT/ISBD guideline includes data published up to 2007, the WFSBP guidelines are based on evidence published up to approximately 6 months before the publication of the respective issue. The BAP guideline does not specify the inclusion date of literature: they are based on an initial expert meeting held on 18th May 2007 followed by a literature search. Whereas the WFSBP guideline structures their recommendations according to medication, the BAP and CANMAT guideline follow different clinical scenarios for the different treatment phases, developing stepwise treatment algorithms.

14.4 Combination Treatment of Acute Mania

Although the structure of the guidelines is heterogeneous they all agree that the treatment of manic/hypomanic and mixed episodes should generally be initiated with a medication such as lithium (Li), valproate (VPA) or atypical antipsychotics (AAP), including aripiprazole, olanzapine, quetiapine, risperidone, ziprasidone and asenapine (only in WFSBP) as monotherapy (see Table 14.1). All guidelines agree on stopping ongoing antidepressant medication during mania.

The evidence for the different combination treatments is extensively discussed in Chapter nine of this book. For safety and practicability issues, monotherapy is favoured as first line approach in the WFSBP and BAP guideline. Combination therapy including Li or VPA with an AAP is suggested usually as second-line choice in the WFSBP and BAP guideline, but can be considered for severe mania as first line choice in the BAP guideline. In the WFSBP guidance, combination treatment is recommended as a subsequent step when another first line medication (second option) failed. Different from the other two guidelines, the CANMAT guideline lists some combination treatments alongside with monotherapies as first choice anti-manic treatment, specifically Li or VPA combined with different AAP. They do not link the choice of combination treatment explicitly to the severity or a special subtype of mania. Table 14.2 summarizes the positioning of combination treatments within the three guidelines.

These guideline recommendations are, as expected, quite in contrast with clinical practice, where most patients are treated with combinations of two or more antimanic agents due to illness complexity, comorbidity, lack of adherence, side effects or clinician's choice [3, 25, 26].

Table 14.1 Guideline recommendations for the treatment of acute mania

	WFSBP	CANMAT/ISBD	BAP
First line	*Monotherapy*: Li, VPA , AAPs (ARP, RISP, ZIP)	*Monotherapy*: Li, VPA, AAPs (ARP, OLZ, QTP, QTP xr, RSP, ZIP) *Combination*: Li/VPA + HAL/ RISP/QTP/OLZ/ARP *If severly agitated* im ARP, im OLZ.	*Not on AM*: If severe Mania: AAPs, VPA. If mild–mod Mania: Li, CBZ *On AM*: AM + AAPs Optimization of doses
Second line	***Best evidence***: AAPs: OLZ, QTP, ASN, CBZ, HAL *Combination*: Li/VPA + AAPs ***Less evidence***: CLZ, AMS, PLP, ZOT; OXC, PHT, Li + VPA, ECT Levetiracetam. zosinamide, retigabine	CBZ, ASN, PLP, ECT, Li + VPA, LI/VPA + ASN; Others: HAL, CLP, Li/VPA + HAL, Li + CBZ, CLZ, OXC, tamoxifen	Li/VPA + AAP, CLZ, ECT

AD antidepressant, *AM* antimanic agent, *AMS* amisulpiride, *AP* antipsychotic, *AAP* atypical antipsychotic, *ARP* aripiprazole, *ASN* asenapine, *CBZ* carbamazepine, *CLZ* clozapine, *ECT* electroconvulsive therapy, *HAL* haloperidol, *im* intramuscular, *Li* lithium, *MAO-I* monoaminooxidase inhibitor, *MDF* Modafinil, *N-Acys* N-acetyl cysteine, *OFC* olanzapine–fluoxetine combination, *OLZ* olanzapine, *Om-3FA* + omega 3 fatty acids, *OXC* oxcarbamazepine; *PHT* phenytoin, *PLP* paliperidone, *PRX* pramipexole, *QTP* quetiapine, *QTP* ^{XR} quetiapine extended release formulation, *RISP* risperidone, *RISP LAI* risperidone long-acting injectible, *SSRI* selective serotonin reuptake inhibitor, *TCA* tricyclic antidepressant, *TPR* topiramate, *VPA* valproate (the generic term of "valproate", which includes sodium valproate, valproic acid and valproate semisodium), *VLX* venlafaxine, *ZOT* zotepine, *ZIP* ziprasidone, *On AM* patient on treatment with antimanic medication, *Not on AM* patient not on treatment with antimanic medication

14.5 Combination Treatment of Bipolar Depression

A recent study by Haeberle et al. [4] describes prescription habits for bipolar depression in routine inpatient settings between 1994 and 2009. These data were generated from a large European multicenter study (AMSP). Within the period from 1994 to 2009, 85% of all hospitalized patients treated for bipolar depression received more than one class of psychotropic substances. Of the different substances, 74% of all patients received antidepressants, 55% antipsychotics, 48% anticonvulsants and 33% Li in combination therapy, i.e. in combination with other drugs of these four drug classes. Monotherapy had a low prevalence (about 15% of the patients) and showed a decreasing trend. Interestingly, quetiapine and lamotrigine which are recommended in guidelines as monotherapy were mostly administered as combination therapy, but very rarely as monotherapy (0.6 and 0.3%, respectively).

Table 14.2 Summary of positioning of combination treatments for mania in the WFSBP, BAP and CANMAT guideline

	WFSBP	CANMAT/ISBD	BAP
Initial therapy	Choose monotherapy with a recommended grade 1A agent – ARP, RISP, ZIP, VPA or LI	Either monotherapy **or combination therapy with Li/Val plus ARP, OLZ, QTP or RISP recommended as first-line treatment**	For severe mania or for mixed: oral AP or VPA For less severe patients, consider lithium or carbamazepine
If partial response to initial therapy	Optimise dosage and, if no improvement, add a second grade 1A agent	Optimise dose and check compliance	Optimise dose of first-line agent
		Add or switch to AP + or MS If insufficient response to AP + MS, replace one or both with other recommended first-line agents	**If symptoms are inadequately controlled and/or mania is severe, consider combination of lithium or valproate with an antipsychotic**
Recommendations in case of ineffective initial therapy	After 2 weeks, switch to an alternative grade 1A agent. **If still no response, add a second grade one agent**		

AP antipsychotic, *ARP* aripiprazole, *Li* lithium, *OLZ* olanzapine, *QTP* quetiapine, *RISP* risperidone, *VPA* valproate (the generic term of "valproate", which includes sodium valproate, valproic acid and valproate semisodium), *ZIP* ziprasidone

More recently, there has also been a growing interest in RCTs examining the treatment of bipolar depression which constitute the scientific base of evidence based medicine guidelines. Besides the WFSBP, CANMAT and BAP guidance, other consensus guidelines focusing specifically on bipolar depression have been developed, namely, the ECNP Consensus Meeting on Bipolar depression [27] and the International Consensus Group on the Evidence-Based Pharmacologic Treatment of Bipolar I and II Depression [28].

All of the recent guidelines acknowledge the role of quetiapine as the only medication which has shown efficacy both in monotherapy and combination with lithium or valproate in several RCTs in bipolar depression. The role of lamotrigine, however, differs slightly between guidelines: it is recommended on an equal level to quetiapine in the BAP and CANMAT; however, although recommended, the weak evidence is explicitly mentioned only in the WFSBP guidelines. In addition, CANMAT and WFSBP mention also Li or Valproate (VPA) monotherapy as another first line option. Different to mania, however, all three guidelines argue in favour of different combination treatments. In severe depression, the use of an antidepressant (preferably an SSRI or Bupropion) together with an antimanic agent (AM) is endorsed. In addition, CANMAT recommends to combine LI with VPA, whereas the WFSBP guideline favour the combination of lamotrigine and Li based on a study which was published after the CANMAT and BAP guidelines came out [29]. Other combination strategies backed up by either of these guidelines include Modafinil + AM, pramipexole + AM, Omega three fatty acids + AM, N-acetyl cysteine + AM, topiramate + AM, riluzole + AM, and different antidepressants (MAO-I, Venlafaxine , tricyclics) + AM. In part, this cornucopia of different combinations may resemble the relative absence of well established evidence for specific treatments; however, it may also hint towards the greater challenge of successfully treating bipolar depression compared to mania [30]. Table 14.3 summarizes recommendations of the three guidelines.

14.6 Maintenance Combination Treatment

A general principle of most guidelines is to continue any successful acute treatment for maintenance, and this may include various combinations effective during the acute episode. This practice differs from what has been recommended not too long ago when acute treatment and prophylaxis were strictly divided, and establishing patients on monotherapies (mostly lithium) for prophylactic purposes was considered best clinical practice. Since then, a persistent pattern in RCT has merged demonstrating that “what gets you well, keeps you well”. Thus, complex medication regimens are nowadays well accepted for long-term treatment, as long as tolerability or safety issues do not limit their extended use. And as matter of fact, monotherapy is not any more the rule, but the exception in BD maintenance treatment [25, 31, 32].

Table 14.3 Guideline recommendations for the treatment of bipolar depression

	WFSP	CANMAT/ISBD	BAP
1st line	QTP, adj QTP, OFC, OLZ, LTG, LTG + Li, VPA	Li, LTG, QTP, QTP ^{XR}, Li/VPA + SSRI, OLZ + SSRI, Li + VPA, Li/VPA + bupropion	QTP, LTG, Li, VPA, SSRIs + AM (Li, DVP, AP) less severe: Li, LTG, VPA. If no history of mania: ADs
2nd line	Optimization of 1st line treatment. Augmentation with Li ot throid hormiones. MDF + Li/VPA/ADs Other: AM together with Inositol, zonisamide, Om-3FA or N-Acys, ECT	Optimization of 1st line treatment VPA/QTP + SSRI, Li/VPA + LTG, others: CBZ, OLZ, Li + CBZ, Li + PRX, Li/DVP + VLX, Li + MAOI, ECT, Li/VPA/ AAP + TCA, Li/VPA/ CBZ + SSRI + LTG, Adjunctive Om-3FA, adjunctive riluzole, adjunctive TPR	Augmentation strategies, TCAs, ECT

AD antidepressant, *AM* antimanic agent, *AP* antipsychotic, *AAP* atypical antipsychotic, *CBZ* carbamazepine, *ECT* electroconvulsive therapy, *Li* lithium, *MAO-I* monoaminooxidase inhibitor, *N-Acys* N-acetyl cysteine, *OLZ* olanzapine, *Om-3FA* omega 3 fatty acids, *PRX* pramipexole, *QTP* quetiapine, *SSRI* selective serotonin reuptake inhibitor, *TCA* tricyclic antidepressant, *TPR* topiramate, *VPA* valproate (the generic term of "valproate", which includes sodium valproate, valproic acid and valproate semisodium), *VLX* venlafaxine

The acceptance of combination treatments as a primary choice appears to be more recognised in the WFSB and CANMAT guidelines, where several combinations are mentioned as first and second choice treatments alongside with monotherapies. These evidence-based combinations consist of an AAP and Li or VPA. The long-term use of ADs together with an AM is backed up by the WFSBP guidelines, but with less support (recommendation grade 4). Different from WFSBP and CANMAT/ISBD, the BAP guidelines follow a more traditional approach and consider long-term combination treatments only when first and second choice monotherapies have failed. Table 14.4 summarizes the treatment recommendations of WFSBP, CANMAT/ISBD and BAP for BD maintenance treatment.

In conclusion, there appears to be some uncertainty about the optimal long-term treatment. No RCTs and only few naturalistic trials beyond 2 years duration exist, and the impact of complex medication regimens on long-term physical health issues is poorly researched. In addition, not only efficacy and tolerability, but other factors such as the impact on suicide risk, cognition and quality of life become of additional importance when tailoring long-term treatment.

14.7 Conclusions and Future Directions

Combinations treatments of BD are part of recommendations in the consulted guideline (WFSP, CANMAT, BAP), more frequent in bipolar depression than in mania or maintenance. The positioning of polypharmacy in mania differs among guidelines and, in part, depends on the severity of mania. For long-term treatment, WFSBP and CANMAT appear to be more liberal with the use of polypharmacy than the BAP guideline. But given the intrinsic limitations of guidelines, especially their sole scope on efficacy and their low representativeness of clinical samples, it is not surprising that the use of polypharmacy in clinical settings has little in common with what guidelines recommend. Clinical reality is unlikely to change, so in order to bridge this gap guidelines need to adapt. A first step could be the acceptance of pragmatic and representative real world studies, such as EMBLEM [33] or the BALANCE study [34] as equally valid evidence as RCTs. Of note, the BALANCE study demonstrated that, contrary to the outcome of most RCT where combination treatment was more efficacious than monotherapy, Li + VPA combination is not better than just Li monotherapy. It would be an innovative approach to identify in a first step what combination treatments are favored by clinicians in (sub) group of BD patients, and then test their efficacy in a pragmatic study against evidence based comparators.

Table 14.4 Guideline recommendations for the maintenace treatment of bipolar disorder

	WFSP	CANMAT/ISBD	BAP
1st line	Li, LTG, QTP, ARP, ARP + Li or VPA, QTP + Li or VPA	Li, LTG,VPA, OLZ, QTP, QTP + Li or VPA, RISP LAI, RISP LAI + Li or VPA, ZIP + Li or VPA	For manic polarity: Li, ARP, QTP, VPA, OLZ For depresssive polarity: QTP, LTG
2nd line	CBZ, VPA, OLZ, RISP, OLZ + Li or VPA, RIS + Li or VPA, ZIP + Li or VPA	CBZ, Li + VPA, Li + CBZ, OLZ + Li or VPA, Li + RISP, Li + LTG, OFC	For manic polarity: CBZ For depressive polarity : Li *Combination treatments only when monotherapy has failed* (*3rd line option*)

ARP aripiprazole, *CBZ* carbamazepine, *Li* lithium, *OFC* olanzapine–fluoxetine combination, *OLZ* olanzapine, *QTP* quetiapine, *RISP* risperidone, *RISP LAI* risperidone long-acting injectible, *VPA* valproate (the generic term of "valproate", which includes sodium valproate, valproic acid and valproate semisodium), *ZIP* ziprasidone

References

1. Frye MA, Ketter TA, Leverich GS et al (2000) The increasing use of polypharmacotherapy for refractory mood disorders: 22 years of study. J Clin Psychiatry 61:9–15
2. Mojtabai R, Olfson M (2010) National trends in psychotropic medication polypharmacy in office-based psychiatry. Arch Gen Psychiatry 67:26–36
3. Wolfsperger M, Greil W, Rossler W, Grohmann R (2007) Pharmacological treatment of acute mania in psychiatric in-patients between 1994 and 2004. J Affect Disord 99:9–17
4. Haeberle A, Greil W, Russmann S, Grohmann R (in press) Mono- and combination drug therapies in hospitalized patients with bipolardepression. Data from the European drug surveillance program AMSP. BMC Psychiatry
5. Walpoth-Niederwanger M, Kemmler G, Grunze H, Weiss U, Hoertnagl C, Strauss R et al (in press) Treatment patterns in inpatients with bipolar disorder at a psychiatric university hospital over a 9-year period: focus on mood stabilizers. Int Clin Psychopharmacol
6. Poulsen RL (1992) Some current factors influencing the prescribing and use of psychiatric drugs. Public Health Rep 107:47–53
7. Post RM, Altshuler LL, Frye MA, Suppes T, Keck PE Jr, McElroy SL et al (2010) Complexity of pharmacologic treatment required for sustained improvement in outpatients with bipolar disorder. J Clin Psychiatry 71:1176–1186
8. Goldberg JF, Brooks JO III, Kurita K et al (2009) Depressive illness burden associated with complex polypharmacy in patients with bipolar disorder: findings from the STEP-BD. J Clin Psychiatry 70:155–162
9. Dennehy EB, Suppes T, Rush AJ et al (2005) Does provider adherence to a treatment guideline change clinical outcomes for patients with bipolar disorder? Results from the Texas medication algorithm project. Psychol Med 35:1695–1706
10. Perlis RH (2007) Use of treatment guidelines in clinical decision making in bipolar disorder: a pilot survey of clinicians. Curr Med Res Opin 23:467–475
11. Samalin L, Guillaume S, Auclair C, Llorca PM (2011) Adherence to guidelines by French psychiatrists in their real world of clinical practice. J Nerv Ment Dis 199:239–243
12. Turner EH, Matthews AM, Linardatos E et al (2008) Selective publication of antidepressant trials and its influence on apparent efficacy. N Engl J Med 358:252–260
13. Ghaemi NS, Shirzadi AA, Filkowski M (2008) Publication bias and the pharmaceutical industry: the case of lamotrigine in bipolar disorder. Medscape J Med 10:211
14. Heres S, Davis J, Maino K, Jetzinger E, Kissling W, Leucht S (2006) Why olanzapine beats risperidone, risperidone beats quetiapine, and quetiapine beats olanzapine: an exploratory analysis of head-to-head comparison studies of second-generation antipsychotics. Am J Psychiatry 163:185–194
15. Cosgrove L, Bursztajn HJ, Krimsky S, Anaya M, Walker J (2009) Conflicts of interest and disclosure in the American Psychiatric Association's Clinical Practice Guidelines. Psychother Psychosom 78:228–232
16. Grunze H, Vieta E, Goodwin GM et al (2009) The World Federation of Societies of Biological Psychiatry (WFSBP) guidelines for the biological treatment of bipolar disorders: update 2009 on the treatment of acute mania. World J Biol Psychiatry 10:85–116
17. Licht RW (2002) Limits of the applicability and generalizability of drug trials in mania. Bipolar Disord 4(Suppl 1):66–68
18. Nivoli AM, Murru A, Goikolea JM et al (2012) New treatment guidelines for acute bipolar mania: a critical review. J Affect Disord 140:125–141
19. Vieta E, Panicali F, Goetz I, Reed C, Comes M, Tohen M (2008) Olanzapine monotherapy and olanzapine combination therapy in the treatment of mania: 12-week results from he European Mania in Bipolar Longitudinal Evaluation of Medication (EMBLEM) observational study. J Affect Disord 106:63–72
20. Streeruwitz A, Barnes TR, Fehler J, Ohlsen R, Curtis VA (2007) Pharmacological management of acute mania: does current prescribing practice reflect treatment guidelines? J Psychopharmacol 21:206–209

21. Grunze H, Vieta E, Goodwin GM et al (2010) The World Federation of Societies of Biological Psychiatry (WFSBP) guidelines for the biological treatment of bipolar disorders: update 2010 on the treatment of acute bipolar depression. World J Biol Psychiatry 11:81–109
22. Grunze H, Vieta E, Goodwin GM, et al (in press) The World Federation of Societies of Biological Psychiatry (WFSBP) guidelines for the biological treatment of bipolar disorders: update 2012 on the Long-term Treatment of Bipolar Disorder. World J Biol Psychiatry
23. Yatham LN, Kennedy SH, Schaffer A et al (2009) Canadian Network for Mood and Anxiety Treatments (CANMAT) and International Society for Bipolar Disorders (ISBD) collaborative update of CANMAT guidelines for the management of patients with bipolar disorder: update 2009. Bipolar Disord 11:225–255
24. Goodwin GM (2009) Evidence-based guidelines for treating bipolar disorder: revised second edition –recommendations from the British Association for Psychopharmacology. J Psychopharmacol 23:346–388
25. Grunze H, Forsthoff A, Born C (2005) Polypharmazie in der behandlung bipolarer störungen. In: Messer T, Schmauss M (eds) Polypharmazie in der behandlung psychischer erkrankungen. Springer, Wien/New York, pp 81–102
26. Ghaemi SN, Hsu DJ, Thase ME et al (2006) Pharmacological treatment patterns at study entry for the first 500 STEP-BD participants. Psychiatr Serv 57:660–665
27. Goodwin GM, Anderson I, Arango C et al (2008) ECNP consensus meeting. Bipolar depression. Nice, March 2007. Eur Neuropsychopharmacol 18:535–549
28. Kasper S, Calabrese JR, Johnson G, Tajima O, Vieta E, Viguera AC et al (2008) International consensus group on the evidence-based pharmacologic treatment of bipolar I and II depression. J Clin Psychiatry 69:1632–1646
29. van der Loos ML, Mulder PG, Hartong EG, Blom MB, Vergouwen AC, de Keyzer HJ et al (2009) Efficacy and safety of lamotrigine as add-on treatment to lithium in bipolar depression: a multicenter, double-blind, placebo-controlled trial. J Clin Psychiatry 70:223–231
30. Kupfer DJ, Frank E, Grochocinski VJ et al (2000) Stabilization in the treatment of mania, depression and mixed states. Acta Neuropsychiatrica 12:3–114
31. Rybakowski J (2007) Long-term pharmacological treatment of bipolar disorders. Neuro Endocrinol Lett 28(Suppl 1):71–93
32. Goodwin G, Vieta E (2005) Effective maintenance treatment – breaking the cycle of bipolar disorder. Eur Psychiatry 20:365–371
33. Goetz I, Tohen M, Reed C, Lorenzo M, Vieta E (2007) Functional impairment in patients with mania: baseline results of the EMBLEM study. Bipolar Disord 9:45–52
34. Geddes JR, Goodwin GM, Rendell J et al (2010) Lithium plus valproate combination therapy versus monotherapy for relapse prevention in bipolar I disorder (BALANCE): a randomised open-label trial. Lancet 375:385–395

Appendix 1. Annotated Bibliography on Polypharmacy

Rena Kurs

Abstract Treatment resistance in schizophrenia and other mental disorders often challenges guideline-recommended monotherapy. Antipsychotic polypharmacy is thus increasingly encountered in clinical practice, and surveys of prescribing in psychiatric services internationally have identified the relatively frequent and consistent use of combined psychotropic medications, usually for people with established psychotic disorders. To date there are no clear cut acknowledged evidenced based clinical practice guidelines for the use of psychotropic polypharmacy. The following annotated bibliography is a collection of representative publications on this controversial subject. The articles presented were chosen based on timeliness, and generalizability. They will be of interest to clinicians, multidisciplinary care-givers, and families of patients treated with psychotropic medications. There are links to the full text of open access publications, and to abstracts of articles available for purchase or to subscribers of the specific journals. For convenience sake, the publications have been divided into the following sections: General polypharmacy reviews and guidelines, Pediatric polypharmacy, and Disease specific polypharmacy. The last section includes links to various clinical practice guidelines for psychiatric disorders.

Publications appear in descending order of year of publication

R. Kurs, B.A. (✉)
Medical Library, Sha'ar Menashe Mental Health Center, Hadera, Israel
e-mail: rena@sm.health.gov.il

M.S. Ritsner (ed.), *Polypharmacy in Psychiatry Practice, Volume II: Use of Polypharmacy in the "Real World"*, DOI 10.1007/978-94-007-5799-8,

General Polypharmacy Reviews and Guidelines

Antipsychotic Polypharmacy: Update and Guidelines for Practice
Rajiv Tandon

An evaluation of the appropriateness of the many rationales for antipsychotic combinations with a brief outline of recommendations for the role of polypharmacy in antipsychotic therapy.

http://medicaidmentalhealth.org/files/Guidelines/Antipsychotic%20 Polypharmacy%20Update%20and%20Guidelines%20for%20 Practice201201170826337 6.pdf (Full text).

Polypharmacy with antipsychotics, antidepressants, or benzodiazepines and mortality in schizophrenia.
Tiihonen J, Suokas JT, Suvisaari JM, Haukka J, Korhonen P. *Archives of General Psychiatry. 2012 May;69(5):476–83.*

The authors investigated whether the use of benzodiazepines, antidepressants, or multiple concomitant antipsychotics is associated with increased mortality among patients with schizophrenia

http://www.ncbi.nlm.nih.gov/pubmed/22566579 (Abstract)

Antipsychotic polypharmacy: review of mechanisms, mortality and management
Julie LanganPolash Shajahan *The Psychiatrist (2010) 34: 58–62*

In this review the authors consider the reasons behind antipsychotic polypharmacy and the patterns of its use. They consider the evidence of effectiveness of combined therapy *v.* monotherapy and the rationale behind the potentially beneficial combinations that are used. The potential dangers of antipsychotic polypharmacy are also discussed and the limited research regarding switching from polypharmacy to monotherapy is reviewed. Some provisional recommendations regarding antipsychotic polypharmacy are proposed.http://pb.rcpsych.org/content/34/2/58.full (Full text).

Polypharmacy or medication washout: an old tool revisited
Hoffman DA, Schiller M, Greenblatt JM Iosifescu D

The authors discuss the role of washout, and whether it can help physicians select appropriate polypharmacy more effectively and safely, if necessary.

Neuropsychiatric Disease and Treatment 2011:7 639–648

http://www.ncbi.nlm.nih.gov/pmc/articles/PMC3215520/pdf/ndt-7-639.pdf (Full text)

Psychiatric Polypharmacy: Identifying Risks and Seeking Solutions
The Joint Commission Perspectives on Patient Safety, November 2008, Volume 8, Issue 11

Copyright 2008 Joint Commission on Accreditation of Healthcare Organization

Discusses four types of polypharmacy: same-class polypharmacy, multiclass polypharmacy, adjunctive polypharmacy, augmentation.

http://ebookbrowse.com/polypharmacy-pdf-d98995356 (Full text)

Quality Concerns in Psychotropic Prescribing: Reducing Psychotropic Polypharmacy

Reference Guide

New York State Office of Mental Health

In 2007, the NYS Office of Mental Health convened a Scientific Advisory Committee of national experts in psychopharmacology. Six workgroups (schizophrenia, depression, bipolar disorder, older adults, youth, and women) identified approximately 80 quality concerns in psychotropic prescribing that are common, costly, and measurable. This clinical module provides information on the quality domain of polypharmacy, including an overview of the evidence base and definitions of each indicator.

http://www.omh.ny.gov/omhweb/psyckes_medicaid/quality_concerns/reference_guide/polypharmacy.pdf (Full text)

A Critical Review of Atypical Antipsychotic Utilization: Comparing Monotherapy with Polypharmacy and Augmentation

S.M. Stahl, M.M. Grady *Current Medicinal Chemistry, 2004, 11, 313–327*

This article reviews evidence for the increasingly common means of treating schizophrenia and psychosis, with particular emphasis on polypharmacy and augmentation.

http://www.nascos.org/library_files/Atypicals%20Review.pdf (Full text).

Polypharmacy in Psychiatry

S. Nassir Ghaemi *New York, NY: Dekker; 2002, 346 pages.*

This practical reference book examines the advantages and disadvantages of polypharmacy in psychiatry, and provides up-to-date clinical guidelines on the appropriate use of combinations of pharmacological therapy in major psychiatric disorders-including multidisciplinary approaches to treatment. The book consolidates available and current material on polypharmacy and psychiatry into one comprehensive volume. Polypharmacy in Psychiatry also discusses the use of alternative and herbal medications psychosocial aspects of polypharmacy the psychology of polypharmacy cultural components of polypharmacy historical background

http://books.google.co.il/books?id=TthcnM15c0sC&printsec=frontcover&hl=iw&source=gbs_ge_summary_r&cad=0#v=onepage&q&f=false (Excerpts from google books)

Decision Making in Psychopharmacology: Pocketbook

Siegfried Kasper, Joseph Zohar, Dan J. Stein

Martin Dunitz, Oct 10, 2002–112 pages

Rather than providing treatment guidelines this book highlights the different available avenues of treatment for mental disorders. Decision Making in Psychopharmacology is intended to stimulate discussion and clear thinking about the evaluative process.

http://books.google.co.il/books/about/Decision_Making_in_Psychopharmacology_Po.html?id=cvq5lNZCI_QC&redir_esc=y

NASMHPD Medical Directors' Technical Report on Psychiatric Polypharmacy
Approved by the NASMHPD Medical Directors Council October 9, 2001, for distribution to the NASMHPD Membership

This report is the seventh in a continuing series of reports initiated by the Medical Directors Council of the National Association of State Mental Health Program Directors (NASMHPD) (Alexandria, Virginia, USA).

The purpose of this report is to review information on the use of polypharmacy, to outline guidelines for the use of polypharmacy, and to make recommendations that decrease the inappropriate use of multiple psychiatric medications in patients with psychiatric illness.

http://www.nasmhpd.org/docs/publications/archiveDocs/2001/Polypharmacy.PDF (Full text).

Polypharmacy: When is it rational?
Sheldon H. Preskorn *Journal of Practical Psychiatry and Behavioral Health, July 1995, 92–98*

Though published in 1995, this is a landmark paper in which the author discusses when it makes sense to consider using more than one medication to treat a single condition. He gives a brief history of the use of polypharmacy in psychiatry and discusses how new discoveries in psychotropic drug development are making polypharmacy an increasingly important topic. The author then presents a list of ten criteria to guide the rational use of psychotropic polypharmacy and explains each in detail with examples drawn from clinical practice.

http://www.preskorn.com/columns/9507.html (Full text).

Pediatric Polypharmacy

The definition and prevalence of pediatric psychotropic polypharmacy
Chen H, Patel A, Sherer J, Aparasu R

Psychiatric Services. 2011 Dec;62(12):1450–5.

Using increasingly stringent criteria, this study evaluated the prevalence of psychotropic polypharmacy among children on the basis of duration of overlap between two or more psychotropic medications.

http://www.ncbi.nlm.nih.gov/pubmed/22193792 (Abstract)

Antipsychotic polypharmacy in the treatment of children and adolescents in the fee-for-service component of a large state Medicaid program.
Constantine RJ, Boaz T, Tandon R.

Clinical Therapeutics 2010;32(5):949–59.

The aims of this study were to quantify and describe antipsychotic polypharmacy use among patients aged 6–12 years (children) and 13–17 years (adolescents) and to identify the characteristics of polypharmacy recipients.

http://www.ncbi.nlm.nih.gov/pubmed/20685503

Predictors of polypharmacy and off-label prescribing of psychotropic medications: A national survey of child psychiatrists
Marcia Kearns

Thesis – Master of Arts 2011, University of Missouri

Anational survey of child psychiatrists to examine typical prescribing practices for children with anxiety, depression, and disruptive behavior disorders from a social judgment theory perspective. The author examined the extent to which polypharmacy and off-label prescribing occur in routine practice and the degree to which child characteristics, child psychiatrist characteristics, and medication availability may influence these prescribing practices.

https://mospace.umsystem.edu/xmlui/bitstream/handle/10355/11178/research.pdf.pdf?sequence=3 (Full text)

National trends in child and adolescent psychotropic polypharmacy in office-based practice, 1996–2007.
Comer JS, Olfson M, Mojtabai R.

Journal of the American Academy of Child & Adolescent Psychiatry. 2010;49(10):1001–10.

Analysis of the annual data from the 1996–2007 National Ambulatory Medical Care Surveys that examined patterns and trends in multi-class psychotropic treatment within a nationally representative sample of 3466 child and adolescent visits to office-based physicians in which a psychotropic medication was prescribed. http://www.ncbi.nlm.nih.gov/pmc/articles/PMC2952543/ (Abstract)

Pediatric Psychotropic Polypharmacy
Zonfrillo MR, Penn JV, Leonard HL. *Psychiatry (Edgmont (Pa.: Township) 2005 Aug;2(8):14-9.*

A literature review of relevant articles pertaining to polypharmacy using the Pub Med database from 1994 through April 2004 for pediatric populations under 18 years old.

http://www.ncbi.nlm.nih.gov/pmc/articles/PMC3000211/ (Abstract)

Disease Specific Polypharmacy

Depression

Medication Augmentation after the Failure of SSRIs for Depression
Madhukar H. Trivedi, Maurizio Fava, Stephen R. Wisniewski, Michael E. Thase, Frederick Quitkin, Diane Warden, Louise Ritz, Andrew A. Nierenberg, Barry D. Lebowitz, Melanie M. Biggs, James F. Luther, Kathy Shores-Wilson,

A. John Rush, for the STAR*D Study Team *New England Journal of Medicine 2006;354:1243–52.*

This study might be considered a "real-world" trial of the augmentation of an SSRI—citalopram—with sustained-release bupropion or buspirone after a consistent, well-implemented trial of citalopram was performed. Remission rates in this trial were similar to thosefound in most previous uncontrolled trials of augmentation of SSRIs, which have typically been conducted in research clinics and have involved symptomatic volunteers with nonchronic depression and few general medical and psychiatric coexisting illnesses. Remission rates in this trial should be generalizable to most outpatients with nonpsychotic major depressive disorder who are seen in both primary and psychiatric settings and who have not had adequate benefit with the use of an SSRI alone.

http://www.nejm.org/doi/pdf/10.1056/NEJMoa052964 (Full text).

Schizophrenia

Polypharmacy with antipsychotics, antidepressants, or benzodiazepines and mortality in schizophrenia.

Tiihonen J, Suokas JT, Suvisaari JM, Haukka J, Korhonen P.

Archives of General Psychiatry. 2012;69(5):476–83.

In a registry based linkage study, the authors investigated if the use of benzodiazepines, antidepressants, or multiple concomitant antipsychotics is associated with increased mortality among patients with schizophrenia.

They linked national databases of mortality and medication prescriptions among a complete nationwide cohort of 2588 patients hospitalized in Finland for the first time with a diagnosis of schizophrenia between January 1, 2000, and December 31, 2007. Hazard ratios (HRs) were computed for all-cause mortality during the use of antipsychotics, antidepressants, or benzodiazepines in outpatient care,

http://archpsyc.jamanetwork.com/article.aspx?articleid=1151489 (Abstract)

Treatment-resistant Schizophrenia: Evidence-based Strategies.

Englisch S., Zink M. *Mens Sana Monographs 2012;10:20–32.*

The authors report on findings of frequent use of polypharmacy in treatment-refractory cases, addressing psychotic positive, negative and cognitive symptoms, treatment-emergent side effects caused by antipsychotics and comorbid depressive or obsessive-compulsive symptoms.

http://www.msmonographs.org/article.asp?issn=0973-1229;year=2012;volume=10;issue=1;spage=20;epage=32;aulast=Englisch (Full text).

Effects of polypharmacy on outcome in patients with schizophrenia in routine psychiatric treatment.

Längle G, Steinert T, Weiser P, Schepp W, Jaeger S, Pfiffner C, Frasch K, Eschweiler GW, Messer T, Croissant D, Becker T, Kilian R.

Acta Psychiatrica Scandinavica. 2012;125(5):372–81.

The authors evaluated the effects of different types of psychotropic polypharmacy on clinical outcomes and quality of life (QOL) in patients with schizophrenia and schizoaffective disorder in routine care.

http://www.ncbi.nlm.nih.gov/pubmed/22321029 (Abstract)

Antipsychotic Polypharmacy in Schizophrenia: Benefits and Risks
Barnes, Thomas R.E.; Paton, Carol *CNS Drugs: 2011; 25(5) 383–399*

This review addresses the clinical trial data and other evidence for the following pharmacological approaches: the addition of a second antipsychotic to boost therapeutic response, the use of as-required antipsychotic medication (mainly to treat disturbed behaviour), gradual cross-titration while switching from one antipsychotic to another, and augmentation of clozapine with a second antipsychotic where the illness has failed to respond adequately to an optimized trial of clozapine. Also reviewed are examples of systematic, practice-based interventions designed to reduce the prevalence of antipsychotic polypharmacy, most of which have met with only modest success.

http://adisonline.com/cnsdrugs/Abstract/2011/25050/Antipsychotic_Polypharmacy_in_Schizophrenia_.3.aspx (Abstract)

Antipsychotic polypharmacy in the treatment of schizophrenia—a health technology assessment
Baandrup L, Lublin H, Nordentoft M, Peacock L, Srensen J, Andersen SE, Glenthj B

Copenhagen: National Board of Health, Danish Centre of Health Technology Assessment (DACEHTA), 2011.

Health Technology Assessment—funded projects 2011; 11(1)

Language: English summary of the full report in Danish

Version date: January 25 2011

This health technology assessment explored how antipsychotic polypharmacy may be reduced by intervention methods and organisational changes. The report is directed at decision-makers at the level of the management board of regions and mental health centres. This report only discusses antipsychotic polypharmacy in the context of schizophrenia spectrum disorders, because the principles of treatment regarding other psychiatric disorders, e.g. bipolar affective disorder, differ substantially.

http://www.sst.dk/publ/Publ2011/MTV/Polyfarmaci/polyfarmaciMTVsummary.pdf (Full text)

Combination and augmentation strategies in treatment-resistant schizophrenia
Susanne Englisch, Mathias Zink

Drug Discovery Today: Therapeutic Strategies Vol.8 (1–2) 2011, 17–23

This review discusses risks, benefits and levels of evidence of combination strategies involving multiple psychotropic substances, with a focus on their clinical relevance.

http://www.sciencedirect.com/science/article/pii/S1740677311000313 (Abstract)

Polypharmacy in schizophrenia
Zink M, Englisch S, Meyer-Lindenberg A.

Current Opinion in Psychiatry. 2010;23(2):103–11.

This review summarizes the current state of evidence of combined antipsychotic treatment strategies and the augmentation of antipsychotics with mood stabilizers, antidepressants and experimental substances. http://www.ncbi.nlm.nih.gov/pubmed?term=Curr%20Opin%20Psychiatry%20AND%20Polypharmacy%20in%20schizophrenia.%20AND%20Zink%20M (Abstract)

Antipsychotic combinations vs monotherapy in schizophrenia: a meta-analysis of randomized controlled trials.

Correll CU, Rummel-Kluge C, Corves C, Kane JM, Leucht S.

Schizophrenia Bulletin 2009 Mar;35(2):443–57.

This paper reports on the evaluation of therapeutic and adverse effects of antipsychotic cotreatment vs monotherapy in schizophrenia, based on Cochrane Schizophrenia Group register and hand searches of relevant journals/conference proceedings. Study Selection included randomized controlled trials comparing antipsychotic monotherapy to cotreatment with a second antipsychotic. The authors concluded that in certain clinical situations, antipsychotic cotreatment may be superior to monotherapy. However, the database is subject to possible publication bias and was too heterogeneous to derive firm clinical recommendations, underscoring the need for future research.

http://www.ncbi.nlm.nih.gov/pmc/articles/PMC2659301/pdf/sbn018.pdf (Full text)

Antipsychotic monotherapy and polypharmacy in the naturalistic treatment of schizophrenia with atypical antipsychotics

Douglas Faries, Haya Ascher-Svanum, Baojin Zhu, Christoph Correll, John Kane

BMC Psychiatry 2005, 5:26 doi:10.1186/1471-244X-5-26

This study assessed the annual rate and duration of antipsychotic monotherapy and its inverse, antipsychotic polypharmacy, among schizophrenia patients initiated on commonly used atypical antipsychotic medications. The authors concluded that despite guidelines recommending the use of polypharmacy only as a last resort, the use of antipsychotic polypharmacy for prolonged periods is very common during the treatment of schizophrenia patients in usual care settings. Reasons for and the impact of the predominant use of polypharmacy will require further study.

http://www.biomedcentral.com/1471-244X/5/26 (Full text).

Validation of Polypharmacy Process Measures in Inpatient Schizophrenia Care

Birgit Janssen, Stefan Weinmann, Mathias Berger, Wolfgang Qaebel *Schizo-phrenia Bulletin,* Vol. 30, No. 4, 2004 1023–1033

As part of a comprehensive quality management program, the authors prospectively evaluated two schizophrenia polypharmacy performance measures in a cohort of 1,075 consecutively recruited individuals with schizophrenia in seven psychiatric hospitals. The results show the strengths and limits of polypharmacy performance measures to compare clinical practice in inpatient schizophrenia care and to detect possible treatment problems.

http://schizophreniabulletin.oxfordjournals.org/content/30/4/1023.full.pdf (Full text)

Polypharmacy in patients with schizophrenia.

McCue RE, Waheed R, Urcuyo L. *Journal of Clinical Psychiatry. 2003 Sep;64(9):984–9.*

The objective of this report was to describe the changes in prescription practices with psychotropic medications for patients diagnosed with schizophrenia in 1995 and 2000. No patients were discharged on treatment with more than 1 antipsychotic in 1995, whereas in 2000, 15.9% of patients were. Results of increased used of polypharmacy are discussed.

http://www.ncbi.nlm.nih.gov/pubmed/14628972 (Abstract)

General Practice Guidelines

Handbook of Schizophrenia Spectrum Disorders, Volume III:

Therapeutic Approaches, Comorbidity, and Outcomes
Michael S. Ritsner (Editor), Springer, 2011, 462 p.

This collection of monographs by eminent investigators reviews recent research regarding the origins, onset, course, and outcome of schizophrenia spectrum disorders. The book provides an up-to-date overview of the rapid advances made in the clinical and basic science studies supporting our understanding of the relationship between cerebral processes and clinical, cognitive and other presentations of the schizophrenia spectrum disorders. In addition, this book aims to monitor important research developments, relevant to the treatment and rehabilitation of patients.

http://www.springer.com/biomed/neuroscience/book/978-94-007-0833-4

Royal Australian and New Zealand College of Psychiatrists Clinical Practice Guidelines

The Australian and New Zealand versions of RANZCP's Consumer and Carer Clinical Practice Guidelines are free of charge to download, using the links on the webpage. These booklets are a valuable resource to support consumers, their carers, families and friends in learning more about mental illness and the treatments that are available.

The RANZCP has developed Clinical Practice Guidelines (CPGs) to provide mental health practitioners, consumers, and carers with evidence-based information about particular mental illnesses and appropriate treatment options.Available guidelines: anorexia nervosa, bipolar disorder, deliberate self harm, depression, panic disorder and agoraphobia, schizophrena.

http://www.ranzcp.org/Publications/Clinical-Practice-Guidelines.aspx

National Institute for Health and Clinical Excellence (NICE)

Guidelines—National Institute for Health and Clinical Excellence—Links to guidelines in psychiatry

http://www.nice.org.uk/Search.do?searchText=psychiatry&newsearch=true&x=17&y=12&page=2#/search/?reload

Borderline personality disorder Borderline personality disorder: treatment and management

NICE clinical guideline 78 Developed by the National Collaborating Centre for Mental Health

Issue date: January 2009

http://www.nice.org.uk/nicemedia/live/12125/42900/42900.pdf

Generalised anxiety disorder and panic disorder (with or without agoraphobia) in adults

Management in primary, secondary and community care

Issue date: January 2011

http://www.nice.org.uk/nicemedia/live/13314/52599/52599.pdf

Schizophrenia

Core interventions in the treatment and management of schizophrenia in adults in primary and secondary care

NICE clinical guideline 82

Developed by the National Collaborating Centre for Mental Health, National Institute for Health and Clinical Excellence

http://www.nice.org.uk/nicemedia/live/11786/43608/43608.pdf

APA Practice Guidelines

http://www.psych.org/practice/clinical-practice-guidelines

American Psychiatric Association Clinical Practice Guidelines provide evidenced—based recommendations for the assessment and treatment of psychiatric disorders. The guidelines are published on PsychiatryOnline. Below are direct links to guidelines for some of the major psychiatric disorders.

Schizophrenia

Guideline Watch (September 2009): Practice guideline for the treatment of patients with schizophrenia

Dixon L, Perkins D, Calmes C.

The original guideline was published in February 2004. The November 2009 Guideline Watch associated with this guideline provides additional information that has become available since publication of the guideline, but it is not a formal update of the guideline.

http://psychiatryonline.org/data/Books/prac/Schizophrenia_Guideline%20 Watch.pdf

Major Depressive Disorder

Practice guideline for the treatment of patients with major depressive disorder, Third Edition

Gelenberg AJ, Freeman MP, Markowitz JC, Rosenbaum JF, Thase ME, Trivedi MH, Van Rhoads, RX

American Psychiatric Association (APA). Practice guideline for the treatment of patients with major depressive disorder. 3rd ed. Arlington (VA): American Psychiatric Association (APA); 2010 Oct. 152 p. (1170 references)

http://psychiatryonline.org/content.aspx?bookid=28&sectionid=1667485

Guideline Watch: Practice Guideline for the Treatment of Patients With Bipolar Disorder, 2nd Edition

Robert M. A. Hirschfeld

APA's *Practice Guideline for the Treatment of Patients With Bipolar Disorder,* 2nd Edition, was published in April 2002 (1). Since that time, a number of controlled treatment studies on aspects of bipolar disorder have been completed and published. This guideline watch briefly reviews the most important of the studies. The majority of the studies were industry supported.

http://psychiatryonline.org/data/Books/prac/Bipolar.watch.pdf

Practice guideline for theTreatment of Patients With Obsessive-Compulsive Disorder

Koran, LM, Hanna GL, Hollander E, Nestadt G, Simpson HB.

This practice guideline was approved in October 2006 and published in July 2007

http://psychiatryonline.org/data/Books/prac/OCDPracticeGuidelineFinal 05-04-07.pdf

U.S. Department of Health & Human Services, Agency for Healthcare Research and Quality

National Guideline Clearinghouse—Guidelines for Mental Disorders

Includes 292 links to clinical practice guidelines from around the globe, for various mental disorders

http://guideline.gov/browse/by-topic-detail.aspx?id=1180&ct=1

Appendix 2. List of Psychotropic Medications

Rena Kurs

Abstract The following is a list of psychotropic medications arranged in alphabetical order, by generic names. The list is divided into the following subsections: Antipsychotic agents, Antidepressant Medications (also used for anxiety disorders), Mood Stabilizing and Anticonvulsant Medications, Anti-anxiety Medications, Sleep Agents.

This list was compiled for the convenience of the reader. It is not intended or implied to be a substitute for professional medical or pharmacological advice. The information on psychotropic medications in this list is provided as an information resource only, and is not to be used or relied on for any diagnostic or treatment purposes. This information is not intended to be patient education, and should not be used as a substitute for professional diagnosis and treatment. Following the psychotropic drug list, there is an annotated list of internet links to sites with current psychotropic drug lists that include additional information such as dosage facts, recommended dosages/blood levels, half life, anticholinergic effects, sedation, orthostatic hypotension, sexual dysfunction, gastrointestinal effects, activation/insomnia, detailed side effects, medication management and black box warnings.

Abbreviations

FGA	1st generation antipsychotic agent
MAOI	Monoamine oxidase inhibitor
MAOI-B	Monoamine oxidase -B inhibitor
SGA	2nd generation antipsychotic agent
SNRI	Serotonin norepinephrine reuptake inhibitor

R. Kurs, B.A. (✉)
Medical Library, Sha'ar Menashe Mental Health Center, Hadera, Israel
e-mail: rena@sm.health.gov.il

M.S. Ritsner (ed.), *Polypharmacy in Psychiatry Practice, Volume II: Use of Polypharmacy in the "Real World"*, DOI 10.1007/978-94-007-5799-8,

SPARI	Selective partial agonist and reuptake inhibitor
SSRI	Selective serotonin reuptake inhibitor
TCA	Tricyclic antidepressant

Antipsychotic agents			
Generic name	Trade/Brand names	Therapeutic class	Chemical class
Aripiprazole	Abilify, Abilitat, Abilify Discmeltv	SGA	Benzisoxazole derivatives
Asenapine	Saphris	SGA	Dibenzo-oxepino pyrroles
Chlorpromazine	Largactil, Contomin, Thorazine, Propaphenin, Megaphen, Chlorderazin, Chloropromazine, Aminazine, Fenactil, Clozine	FGA	Phenothiazine
Clozapine	Clozaril, Leponex, FazaClo, Clopine	SGA	Dibenzodiazepine
Fluphenazine	Anatensol, Fludecasin, Dapotum D, Fludecate	FGA	Phenothiazine antipsychotics
Haloperidol	Aloperidol, Eukystol, Aloperidin, Aloperidolo, Brotopon, Galoperidol, Halopoidol, Serenace	FGA	Phenyl-piperidinyl-butyrophenone
Iloperidone	Zomaril, Fanapt, Fanapta, Fiapta	SGA	Piperidinyl-benzisoxazole derivatives
Loxapine	Cloxazepine, Dibenzoazepine, Oxilapine, Dibenzacepin, Loxapin, Loxapac	Tricyclic antipsychotic agents has been classed as FGA and SGA	Dibenzoxazepine
Lurasidone	Latuda	SGA	Benzisothiazol derivatives.
Molindone*	Moban, Molindone, Molindone Hydrochloride Tablets	Has been classed as both FGA and SGA	Dihydroindolone compound
Olanzapine	Zyprexa, Zyprexa Zydis, Olansek, Symbyax, Zalasta, Lanzac, Zyprexa Velotab	SGA	Thienobenzodiazepine class
Paliperidone	Invega, Paliperidone	SGA	Benzisoxazole derivatives
Perphenazine	Trilafon, Perfenazine, Etaperazine, Etaperazin, Ethaperazine, Fentazin, Perphenazin, Chlorpiprazine, Thilatazin	FGA	Piperazinyl phenothiazine

(continued)

(continued)

Antipsychotic agents			
Generic name	Trade/Brand names	Therapeutic class	Chemical class
Pimozide (for Tourette's syndrome)	Orap, Opiran, Neoperidole, Halomonth, Pimozidum	FGA	Diphenylbutylpiperidine
Quetiapine	Seroquel, Quetiapine fumarate	SGA	Dibenzothiazepine derivatives
Risperidone	Risperdal, Risperidal, Rispolept, Risperin, Rispolin, Sequinan, Risperdal Consta, Risperidonum, Risperdal M-Tab	SGA	Benzisoxazole derivatives
Thioridazine	Mellaril, Melleril, Meleril, Mallorol, Malloryl, Mellerets, Mellerette, Melleretten, Thioridazin, Novoridazine, Thiori	FGA	Phenothiazine
Thiothixene	Tiotixene, cis-Thiothixene, Navane, (E)-Thiothixene, Thiothixine, Navan, trans-Thiothixene	FGA	Thioxanthene derivative
Trifluoperazine	Trifluperazine, Trifluoroperazine, Triperazine, Triflurin, Trifluoperazin, Trifluoperazina, Flurazine, Stelazine, Eskazine, Jatroneuroal, Modalina Trifluoromethylperazine	FGA	Phenothiazine
Ziprasidone	Geodon, Zeldox, Zipfasidone Hydrochloride	SGA	Benzisoxazole derivatives
Antidepressant medications (also used for anxiety disorders)			
Amitriptyline	Damilen, Elavil, Triptanol, Flavyl, Lantron, Seroten, Damitriptyline, Proheptadiene, Tryptanol, Tryptomer, Tryptizol, Laroxyl, Sarotex, Lentizol, Endep, Vanatrip	TCA	Dibenzocycloheptadiene derivative

(continued)

(continued)

Antipsychotic agents			
Generic name	Trade/Brand names	Therapeutic class	Chemical class
Amoxapine	Asendin, Demolox, Amoxepine, Moxadil, Desmethylloxapin, Amoxapina, Amoxapinum, Asendis, Defanyl, Amoksian, Demolox, Asendin	TCA	Dibenzoxazepine class
Bupropion	Bupropion hydrochloride, Wellbutrin, Zyban, Wellbutrin SR, Wellbutrin XL, Amfebutamone hydrochloride	Unicyclic antidepressant	Aminoketones
Citalopram	Nitalapram, Cipram, Celexa, Citalopramum, Cytalopram, Celapram, Ciprapine, Citabax	SSRI	Racemic bicyclic phthalane derivative
Clomipramine	Clomipramine hydrochloride, Anafranil, Clomipramine HCL, Anaphranil, Chlorimipramine hydrochloride	TCA	Dibenzazepine
Desipramine	Desipramine hydrochloride, Norpramin, Pertofran, Pertofrane, Norpolake, Nortimil, DMI hydrochloride, Pertofrin, Petylyl	TCA	Dibenzazepine
Desvenlafaxine	Pristiq extended release,	SNRI	
Doxepin	Doxepine, Zonalon, Quitaxon, Doxepinum	TCA	Dibenzoxepin
Duloxetine	Cymbalta, Yentreve, Xeristar Ariclaim, Duzela	SNRI	Naphthalenes
Escitalopram	Escitalopram, Cipralex, Seroplex, Nexito, anxiset-E, Lexapro, Lexamil, Lexam, Entact, Losita, Animaxen	SSRI	Furancarbonitrile
F`luoxetine	Prozac, Fluctin, Flunirin, Fluoxeren, Sarafem, Adofen, Lovan, Equilibrane, Rowexetina, Fontex, Fluval	SSRI	Phenylpropylamines

(continued)

(continued)

Antipsychotic agents			
Generic name	Trade/Brand names	Therapeutic class	Chemical class
Fluvoxamine	Luvox, Faverin, Dumyrox, Dumirox, Favoxil, Floxyfral, Maveral	SSRI	2-aminoethyl oxime ethers of aralkylketones
Imipramine	Imidobenzyle, Antideprin, Melipramine, Berkomine, Dimipressin, Melipramin, Intalpram, Nelipramin, Dynaprin	TCA	Dibenzazepines and derivatives
Imipramine pamoate	Tofranil-PM	TCA	Dibenzazepines and derivatives
Isocarboxazid	Isocarbonazid, Isocarboxazide, Benazide, Enerzer, Marplan, Isocarbossazide, Isocarboxyzid, Maraplan, Marplon	MOAI	Hydrazine
maprotiline	Dibencycladine, Deprilept, Maprotilin, Maprotylina, Ludiomil	TCA	anthracenes
Mirtazapine	Remergil, Remeron, Zispin, Remergon, Rexer, Remeron SolTab, Mepirzepine, Promyrtil, Norset	TCA	Piperazino-azepine
Nefazodone*	Dutonin, Serzone	Synthetically derived phenylpiperazine antidepressant	Phenols and derivatives
Nortriptyline	Sensaval, Avantyl, Noritren, Pamelor, Ateben, Desitriptilina, Nortryptiline, Nortrilen, Demethylamitriptyline, Aventyl, Lumbeck	TCA	Dibenzocycloheptenes
Paroxetine	Paxil, Seroxat, Aropax, Paxil CR, Paroxetinum, Frosinor, Motivan, Paroxetina, Paxetil	SSRI	Phenylpiperidine
Paroxetine mesylate	Pexeva	SSRI	Mesylate salt of a phenylpiperidine compound
Phenelzine	Phenelzine sulfate, Estinerval, Nardelzine, Kalgan, Nardil, Alacine, Alazine, Alazin	MAOI	Hydrazine

(continued)

(continued)

Antipsychotic agents			
Generic name	Trade/Brand names	Therapeutic class	Chemical class
Protriptyline	Amimetilina, Vivactil, Protryptyline, Triptil, Novopramine, Protriptilina, Protriptylinum, Rhotrimine	TCA	Dibenzocycloheptene
Selegiline	Eldepryl, Emsam, Jumex, L-Deprenalin, Carbex, Zelapar, Selegilinum, Selegilina, Selegyline, Anipryl,	MAOI-B	Levorotatory acetylenic derivative of phenethylamine
Sertraline	Sertraline hydrochloride, Zoloft, Gladem, Serad, Lustral, Atruline, Tresleen, Tatig	SSRI	Tametralines
tranylcypromine	Parnate, Transamine, Jatrosom, Tranylcypromine	MAOI	phenethylamine and amphetamine class
Trazodone	Desyrel, Oleptro, Beneficat, Deprax, Desirel, Molipaxin, Thombran, Trazorel, Trialodine, Trittico, and Mesyrel	SARI	Triazolopyridine
Trimipramine	Surmontil, Rhotrimine, Stangil, Trimeprimine, Sapilent, Surmontil, Surmontyl, bcta-Methylimipramine, Trimeproprimin, Stangyl,	TCA	Dibenzazepines and Derivatives
Venlafaxine	Elafax, Venlafaxina, Venlafaxinum, Effexor, Efectin, VenlafaxineXR	SNRI	Phenols and derivatives
Vilazodone	Vibryd	SPARI	Carboxamide derivative
Mood stabilizing and anticonvulsant medications			
Carbamazepine	Tegretol, Carbamazepen, Finlepsin, Carbazepine, Tegretal, Neurotol, Biston, Epitol	Anticonvulsant	Dibenzazepines and Derivatives
Divalproex sodium (valproic acid)	Depakote, Epival, Valproate semisodium, Depakote ER, Sodium divalproate, Divalproate, Delepsine, Sprinkle, Valcote, Zalkote	Anticonvulsant	

(continued)

(continued)

Antipsychotic agents			
Generic name	Trade/Brand names	Therapeutic class	Chemical class
Gabapentin	Neurontin, Gabapentine, Aclonium, Fanatrix, Horizant, Gabarone, Gralise, Nupentin	Anticonvulsant.	GABA analogue
Lamotrigine	Lamictal, Lamotrigine	Anticonvulsant.	Phenyltriazine
Lithium carbonate	Eskalith, Lithobid, Dilithium carbonate, Lithonate, Liskonum, Lithane, Lithotabs, Micalith, Priadel, Limas	Mood-stabilizing agent	Inorganic ions and gases
Lithium citrate (generic only)	Lithium citrate, Trilithium citrate Demalit, Litarex, Eskalith	Mood-stabilizing agent	
Oxcarbazepine	Trileptal, Oxcarbamazepine, Timox, Epilexter	Anticonvulsant and mood stabilizer	Structural derivative of carbamazepine
Topiramate	Topamax, Epitomax, Topimax, Topomax, Topina, Tipiramate	Anticonvulsant.	Sulfamate-substituted monosaccharide
Anti-anxiety medications			
Alprazolam	Xanax, Trankimazin, Cassadan, Esparon, Tafil, Xanax XR, Alpronax, Intensol, Tranquinal	Antianxiety and sedative-hypnotic	Triazolobenzodiazepine compound
Buspirone	BuSpar, Ansial, Buspirona, Buspironum, Bespar, Ansiced, Anxiron, Buspisal	Anxiolytic agent	Azaspirodecanedione
Chlordiazepoxide	Librium, Chlozepid, Elenium, Helogaphen, Ifibrium, Kalmocaps, Librelease, Librinin	Anxiolytic agent	Benzodiazepine
Clonazepam	Klonopin, Rivotril, Clonex, Paxam, Kriadex, Antelepsin, Cloazepam, Iktorivil, Klonopin, Landsen	Anxiolytic, anticonvulsant, muscle-relaxant	Benzodiazepine
Clorazepate	Tranxene, Novo-Clopate	Anxiolytic, anticonvulsant, muscle-relaxant	Benzodiazepine
Diazepam	Valium, Ansiolisina, Assival, Diazemuls, Relanium, Stesolid, Apaurin, Faustan, Seduxen, Sibazon	Anticonvulsant, anxiolytic, sedative, muscle relaxant	Benzodiazepine

(continued)

(continued)

Antipsychotic agents			
Generic name	Trade/Brand names	Therapeutic class	Chemical class
Lorazepam	Ativan, Temesta, Idalprem, Tavor, Bonatranquan, Delormetazepam, Almazine	Anti-anxiety agent hypnotic, anticonvulsant, sedative	Benzodiazepine
Oxazepam	Adumbran, Tazepam, Serax, Vaben, Ansioxacepam, Droxacepam, Anxiolit, Aplakil, Astress, Drimuel	Anti- anxiety, alcohol withdrawal, and insomnia	Benzodiazepine
ADHD medications			
Amphetamine	Mydrial, Adderall, dexedrine, Dextrostat, Desoxyn, Didrex, ProCentra. Fenopromin, Vivanxe, Benzedrine, Psychedrine	CNS stimulant	Phenethylamine
Atomoxetine	Strattera, Tomoxetine, Attentin	Non stimulant SNRI	Phenylpropylamines
Dexmethyl-phenidate	Focalin	CNS stimulant	
Dextroam-phetamine	Dexedrine, Dextrostat, Dexamphetamine	CNS stimulant	Phenethylamines Amphetamines
Guanfacine	Intuniv, Estulic, Tenex, Guanfacinum, Guanfacina	Centrally acting antihypertensive agent	Phenethylamines
Lisdexamfetamine dimesylate	Vyvanse, Lisdexamfe-tamine mesilate	CNS stimulant	Phenethylamines amphetamines
Methamphe-tamine	Desoxyn, Desyphed, Metamfetamine, Norodin, Stimulex	CNS stimulant	Phenethylamines amphetamines
Methylphenidate	Ritalin, Concerta, Daytrana, Metadate, Methylin, Riphenidate, Ritaline, Meridil,	CNS stimulant	Adrenergic agent, dopamine uptake inhibitors, adrenergic uptake inhibitors,
Sleep agents			
Eszopiclone	Estorra, Lunesta	Hypnotic	Lactams, cyclopyrrolones
Ramelteon	Roserem	Hypnotic	Benzofurans, indanes, phenylpropylamines
Zaleplon	Sonata, Zalaplon	Hypnotic	Acetanilides, pyrazolopyrimidines
Zolpidem	Ambien CR, Lorex, Stilnoct, Stilnox, Sanval	Hypnotic	Phynylporpenes, imidazopyridines

*Medications discontinued in some countries

Bibliography

1. Mental Health Medications. National Institute of mental Health
http://www.nimh.nih.gov/health/publications/mental-health-medications/complete-index.shtml#pub11
2. PubChem Compound
The PubChem Compound Database contains validated chemical depiction information provided to describe substances in PubChem Substance. Structures stored within PubChem Compounds are pre-clustered and cross-referenced by identity and similarity groups.
http://www.ncbi.nlm.nih.gov/pccompound
3. Daily Med: Current Medication Information
DailyMed provides high quality information about marketed drugs. Drug labeling on this Web site is the most recent submitted to the Food and Drug Administration (FDA) and currently in use.
http://dailymed.nlm.nih.gov/dailymed/
4. DrugBank: Open Data Drug and Drug Target Database
http://www.drugbank.ca/
5. BehaveNet. BehaveNet is the Web's most comprehensive encyclopedic taxonomy of psychiatric drugs (including drugs of abuse), diagnoses (including diagnostic criteria), terminology and notable people with references to associated media and other resources
http://behavenet.com/
Links to Psychotropic Drug Lists

1. **Review of Psychotropic Drugs 2012**
Includes Medication categories, brand name, generic name, dosage facts, half life, anticholinergic effect, sedation, orthostatic hypotension, sexual dysfunction, GI effects, activation/insomnia, detailed side effects Authors' disclaimer: These Medication tables are NOT exhaustive for drug categories, dosage facts, side effects, adverse effects, indications or any special instructions (comments) and should only be used to guide learning. Use a pharmacologic text, drug guide such as the Physician's Desk Reference (PDR), or package insert for more complete medication information.
http://www.dhs.state.il.us/OneNetLibrary/27896/documents/By_Division/Division%20of%20DD/HumanRights/PsychotropicDrugsList.pdf

2. **Contemporary Psychotropic Medications listed alphabetically.**
Metro Crisis Services
In this table, both the generic or chemical names and the U.S. brand names are listed alphabetically. Brand names used in the United States, these medications may be sold outside the U.S. under different brand names. Includes links to Medline Plus for additional information for each drug.
http://www.metrocrisisservices.org/7-learn-more/medications/medications-listed-alphabetically

3. **National Alliance on Mental Illness, NAMI, Policy Research Institute**
   Commonly Prescribed Psychotropic Medications
   Brand names are followed by the generic in parenthesis. A second chart below provides cross-referencing by generic name.
   *Although this medication has been approved by the FDA for the treatment of other disorders, it has not been approved for this particular use. Some evidence of this medication's efficacy for such use does exist however. This type of medication use is referred to as "off label."
   Remember, always consult your doctor or pharmacist with any specific medication questions http://www.nami.org/Template.cfm?Section=Policymakers_Toolkit&Template=/ContentManagement/HTMLDisplay.cfm&ContentID=18971

4. **University of Illinois at Chicago, Department of Children and Family Services (DCFS) Psychotropic Medication List**
   Includes Generic name, trade name, recommended doses/blood levels, medication management, black box warning, FDA indication for children
   http://www.psych.uic.edu/csp/DCFS_Psychotropic_Medication.pdf

5. **National Institute of Mental Health**
   This guide describes the types of medications used to treat mental disorders, side effects of medications, directions for taking medications, and includes any FDA warnings. http://www.nimh.nih.gov/health/publications/mental-health-medications/complete-index.shtml

6. **International Narcotics Control Board. Green List (24th edition, May 2010)**
   Annex to the annual statistical report on psychotropic substances (form P). List of Psychotropic Substances under International Control
   http://www.incb.org/pdf/e/list/Green_list_ENG_2010_53991.pdf

7. **Medication Safety team, Department of Health, Australia. Psychotropic Drug List**
   Current at January 2011.
   This is a list of pyschotropic medications available in Australia.
   This table has been developed in collaboration with the Medication Safety team, Department of Health. For ease of uses, the medications are listed alphabetically, whether by generic name, or by brand name.
   http://www.fallssa.com.au/documents/hp/Drug_list_in_SA_Health_Template_V2.pdf

Contents to Volume I

M.S. Ritsner (ed.), *Polypharmacy in Psychiatry Practice, Volume II: Use of Polypharmacy in the "Real World"*, DOI 10.1007/978-94-007-5799-8,

Contributors to Volume I

Rebecca Ahlbrand, B.S. Cincinnati Veterans Affairs Medical Center, Psychiatry Service (V116A), Cincinnati, OH, USA

Department of Psychiatry and Behavioral Neuroscience, University of Cincinnati College of Medicine, Cincinnati, OH, USA

Petr Bob, Ph.D. Department of Psychiatry, 1st Faculty of Medicine, Center for Neuropsychiatric Research of Traumatic Stress, Charles University, Prague, Czech Republic

Jessica L. Gören, PharmD, BCPP University of Rhode Island, Kingston, RI, USA

Harvard Medical School, Boston, MA, USA

Cambridge Health Alliance, Cambridge, MA, USA

Maureen M. Grainger, B.S. Cincinnati Veterans Affairs Medical Center, Psychiatry Service (V116A), Cincinnati, OH, USA

Paul S. Horn, Ph.D. Division of Neurology, Cincinnati Children's Hospital Medical Center, Cincinnati, OH, USA

Department of Mathematical Sciences, University of Cincinnati, Cincinnati, OH, USA

Grigori Joffe, M.D., Ph.D. Department of Psychiatry, Helsinki University Central Hospital (HUCH), Hospital District of Helsinki and Uusimaa, Helsinki, Finland

Ahsan Y. Khan, M.D. Department of Psychiatry and Behavioral Sciences, College of Medicine, University of Oklahoma Health Sciences Center, Oklahoma City, OK, USA

Dimitrios Kontis, M.D., Ph.D. 1st Psychiatric Department, Psychiatric Hospital of Attica, Athens, Greece

M.S. Ritsner (ed.), *Polypharmacy in Psychiatry Practice, Volume II: Use of Polypharmacy in the "Real World"*, DOI 10.1007/978-94-007-5799-8,

Daniela Krause, M.D. Department of Psychiatry and Psychotherapy, Faculty of Medicine, Ludwig-Maximilians-University of Munich, Munich, Germany

Rena Kurs, B.A. Medical Library, Sha'ar Menashe Mental Health Center, Hadera, Israel

Hans-Jürgen Möller, M.D. Department of Psychiatry and Psychotherapy, Faculty of Medicine, Ludwig-Maximilians-University of Munich, Munich, Germany

Debbi A. Morrissette, Ph.D. California State University, San Marcos, San Marcos, CA, USA

Neuroscience Education Institute, Carlsbad, CA, USA

Adrian P. Mundt, M.D., Ph.D. Departamento de Psiquiatría y Salud Pública, Universidad de Chile, Clínica Psiquiátrica Universitaria, Santiago de Chile, Chile

Unit for Social & Community Psychiatry, Barts & The London School of Medicine & Dentistry, Queen Mary University of London, London, UK

Richard Musil, M.D. Department of Psychiatry and Psychotherapy, Faculty of Medicine, Ludwig-Maximilians-University of Munich, Munich, Germany

Michael Obermeier Department of Psychiatry and Psychotherapy, Faculty of Medicine, Ludwig-Maximilians-University of Munich, Munich, Germany

Sheldon H. Preskorn, M.D. Department of Psychiatry & Behavioral Sciences, University of Kansas School of Medicine-Wichita, Wichita, KS, USA

Neil M. Richtand, M.D., Ph.D. Cincinnati Veterans Affairs Medical Center, Psychiatry Service (V116A), Cincinnati, OH, USA

Department of Psychiatry and Behavioral Neuroscience, University of Cincinnati College of Medicine, Cincinnati, OH, USA

Neuroscience Graduate Program, University of Cincinnati, Cincinnati, OH, USA

Michael Riedel, M.D. Department of Psychiatry and Psychotherapy, Faculty of Medicine, Ludwig-Maximilians-University of Munich, Germany

Vincent-von-Paul-Hospital, Rottweil, Germany

Michael S. Ritsner, M.D., Ph.D. Rappaport Faculty of Medicine, Technion – Israel Institute of Technology, Haifa and Chair, Acute Department, Sha'ar Menashe Mental Health Center, Hadera, Israel

Rebecca Schennach, M.D. Department of Psychiatry and Psychotherapy, Faculty of Medicine, Ludwig-Maximilians-University of Munich, Munich, Germany

Florian Seemüller, M.D. Department of Psychiatry and Psychotherapy, Faculty of Medicine, Ludwig-Maximilians-University of Munich, Munich, Germany

Ilja Spellmann, M.D. Department of Psychiatry and Psychotherapy, Faculty of Medicine, Ludwig-Maximilians-University of Munich, Munich, Germany

Stephen M. Stahl, M.D., Ph.D. Neuroscience Education Institute, Carlsbad, CA, USA

Department of Psychiatry, University of California, San Diego, CA, USA

Viacheslav Terevnikov, M.D. Hospital District of Helsinki and Uusimaa, Kellokoski Hospital, Tuusula, Finland

Ashley Tewksbury, PharmD Community Health Network, Indianapolis, IN, USA

Eirini Theochari, M.D. 1st Psychiatric Department, Psychiatric Hospital of Attica, Athens, Greece

Joachim G. Witzel, M.D. Central State Forensic Psychiatric Hospital of Saxony-Anhalt, Stendal, Germany

Index

M.S. Ritsner (ed.), *Polypharmacy in Psychiatry Practice, Volume II: Use of Polypharmacy in the "Real World"*, DOI 10.1007/978-94-007-5799-8,

MIX
Papier aus verantwortungsvollen Quellen
Paper from responsible sources
FSC® C105338

If you have any concerns about our products,
you can contact us on
ProductSafety@springernature.com

In case Publisher is established outside the EU,
the EU authorized representative is:
Springer Nature Customer Service Center GmbH
Europaplatz 3, 69115 Heidelberg, Germany

Printed by Libri Plureos GmbH
in Hamburg, Germany